HUMAN GENETIC DISEASES

Edited by **Dijana Plaseska-Karanfilska**

Human Genetic Diseases
Edited by Dijana Plaseska-Karanfilska

Published by InTech
Janeza Trdine 9, 51000 Rijeka, Croatia

Publishing Process Manager Davor Vidic

Technical Editor Teodora Smiljanic

Cover Designer InTech Design Team

Additional hard copies can be obtained from orders@intechopen.com

Human Genetic Diseases, Edited by Dijana Plaseska-Karanfilska
p. cm.
ISBN 978-953-307-936-3

For EU product safety concerns:
IN TECH d.o.o., Prolaz Marije Krucifikse Kozulić 3, 51000 Rijeka, Croatia,
info@intechopen.com or visit our website at intechopen.com.

Meet the editor

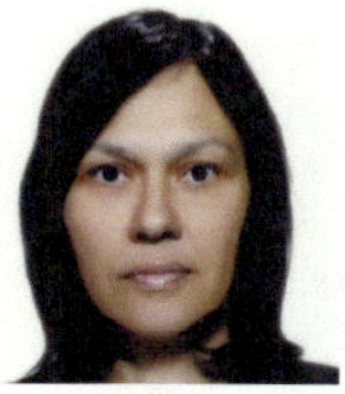

Dr. Dijana Plaseska-Karanfilska graduated from the Faculty of Medicine, University "St. Cyril and Methodius" in Skopje, Republic of Macedonia in 1987. She defended the PhD thesis "Micromethodology for the characterization of haemoglobin variants" in 1994 at the Limburg University, in Maastricht, the Netherlands. Since 1988 Dr. Plaseska-Karanfilska has been employed at the Research Centre for Genetic Engineering and Biotechnology (RCGEB), Macedonian Academy of Sciences and Arts (MASA) where at present she holds a position of a senior scientist, group leader and head of laboratory. In 2010 she has been elected for Associate Professor of molecular biology and pharmacogenetics at the Faculty of Pharmacy, University "St. Cyril and Methodius", Skopje, R. Macedonia. During her professional career Dr. Plaseska-Karanfilska made a contribution to the molecular characterization of different monogenic diseases in Macedonia, such as hemoglobinopathies, cystic fibrosis, cystinuria, Fragile X syndrome, etc. She has been also involved in the research of different infectious diseases, such as HPV, HBV, HCV infections and molecular basis of several malignant diseases as well as forensic DNA identification. Dr. Plaseska-Karanfilska's recent special research interest is in the field of reproductive genetics, such as male infertility, spontaneous abortion, rapid and non-invasive prenatal diagnosis and breast cancer.

Contents

Preface

The genetics science is less than 150 years old, but its accomplishments have been astonishing. Genetics has become an indispensable component of almost all research in modern biology and medicine. Human genetic variation is associated with many, if not all, human diseases and disabilities. Nowadays, studies investigating any biological process, from the molecular level to the population level, use the "genetic approach" to gain understanding of that process.

This book contains many diverse chapters, dealing with human genetic diseases, methods to diagnose them, novel approaches to treat them and molecular approaches and concepts to understand them. The chapters have been written by contributors from thirteen different countries from four continents. Thus, population specific genetic variation and genetics practices in relation to the religion are part of the book chapters as well.

The book is composed of 16 chapters. The first two chapters are devoted to signaling pathways. Chapter 1 describes the general structure of signalling pathways, the relevance of signalling for normal development and for the appearance of multitude of human diseases, and underlines several strategies that Drosophila genetics offers in biomedical research. Chapter 2_provides a review of the fibroblast growth factor (FGF) family in humans, mice, and zebrafish and their developmental physiological and pathophysiological roles.

Chapter 3 deals with osteoclast biology and provides examples of genetic osteoclast diseases, including osteopetrosis, pycnodysostosis and Paget's disease of bone. Chapter 4 gives an overview of the rare Ataxia telangiectasia like disorder (ATLD) caused by MRE11A gene mutations and describes the study initiated to assess the frequency of the c.630G>C mutation in the population of Saudi Arabia.

The next three chapters deal with different aspects of three common monogenic diseases. Chapter 5 gives an overview of Gaucher disease and describes the glucocerebrosidase gene mutations associated with neurological forms of this genetic disease. Chapter 6 gives an overview of the different forms of thalassemias, methods used for their diagnosis and describes the spectrum of β-thalassemia mutations found in Iran. Chapter 7 describes a study that investigates the role of chemokines in the pathogenesis of ocular changes in patients with cystic fibrosis (CF).

Chapter 8 presents the genetic make-up of Azoreans in comparison with mainland Portugal population and emphasizes how this genetic research has allowed the implementation of molecular diagnosis in the hospital of the Azores archipelago.

Chapters 9 and 10 are devoted to preimplantation genetic diagnosis. Chapter 9 evaluates the effect of Double-Factor Preimplantation Genetic Diagnosis (DF-PGD) on implantation in couples with monogenic diseases. Chapter 10 presents one of the world's largest experiences on preimplantation HLA typing in families with genetic and acquired disorders.

Chapters 11 and 12 describe molecular methods for diagnosis of the most common chromosomal abnormalities. Chapter 11 describes the usefulness of two rapid molecular techniques, Multiplex Ligation-dependent Probe Amplification (MLPA) and Quantitative Fluorescent-Polymerase Chain Reaction (QF-PCR) for prenatal diagnosis and post mortem fetuses with multiple malformations. Chapter 12 describes a multiplex QF-PCR method that allows simultaneous detection of the most common genetic causes of male infertility, i.e. sex chromosomal aneuploidies and azoospermia factor (AZF) deletions, and some potential risk factors such as partial AZFc deletions/duplications and androgen receptor CAG repeats.

Chapters 13 and 14 deal with the treatment of genetic diseases. Chapter 13 describes a Spliceosome Mediated RNA *Trans*-splicing (SMaRT) as a promising tool for gene therapy of epidermolysis bullosa simplex. Chapter 14 discusses some of the technological advances regarding the application of nanomedicine in the treatment of genetic conditions.

Chapters 15 and 16 are related to genetics in relation to Islamic religion. Chapter 15 examines the effect of consanguinity on selected multi-factorial diseases and congenital disorders in a target population of the Arab community in Israel. Chapter 16 presents the medical genetic practices in Islamic community of Iran in relation to the Islamic Teaching.

Although this book does not give a comprehensive overview of human genetic diseases, I believe that the sixteen book chapters will be a valuable resource for researchers and students in different life and medical sciences.

Dijana Plaseska-Karanfilska, MD, PhD
Macedonian Academy of Sciences and Arts,
Research Center for Genetic Engineering
and Biotechnology "Georgi D. Efremov", Skopje,
Republic of Macedonia

1

Signalling Pathways in Development and Human Disease: A Drosophila Wing Perspective

Cristina Molnar, Martín Resnik-Docampo, María F. Organista, Mercedes Martín, Covadonga F. Hevia and Jose F. de Celis
Centro de Biología Molecular "Severo Ochoa", CSIC and UAM
C/Nicolás Cabrera 1, Universidad Autónoma de Madrid, Madrid
Spain

1. Introduction

The proteins involved in signalling are organised in several signalling pathways, and both these proteins and their molecular interactions are conserved during evolution. In this chapter we describe the genetic structure of the main conserved signalling pathways identified in multicellular organisms, focusing in those signalling pathways in which the activation of cell receptors by proteins with ligand activity is linked to transcriptional responses. These pathways play key roles during normal development, and their de-regulation has been implicated in a variety of human diseases. We will emphasize the conservation of the proteins and mechanisms involved in each of these pathways, and describe the Drosophila wing imaginal disc as an experimental system to dissect cell signalling in vivo. Finally, we will discuss some of the strategies that are been used to identify additional components of signalling pathways in Drosophila. Our main aim is to underline the general structure of signalling pathways, the relevance of signalling for normal development and for the appearance of multitude of human diseases, and describe several strategies that Drosophila genetics offers in biomedical research.

2. General structure of signalling pathways in multi-cellular organisms: Ligands, receptors, transducers and transcriptional outputs of the Notch, EGFR, InR, Wnt, TGFβ, BMP, Hippo and JNK pathways

Signalling pathways are molecular modules used to convey information among cells. Each pathway is formed by several components connected by molecular recognition and organised in a hierarchical manner, starting with a ligand and ending with a transcription factor. The temporal and spatial expression of the ligands determines the domain of activation of each signalling pathway. The expression of ligands is subject to transcriptional regulation defined by the combination of transcription factors present in the ligand-producing cell (see for example Bachmann and Knust, 1998; Haenlin et al., 1990; Haenlin et al., 1994; Parks et al., 1995; Vargesson et al., 1998). The outcome of each pathway is the activation of a specific transcription factor, and consequently, in many respects a signalling pathway is a molecular device used to coordinate gene expression programs in cell populations. In these roles they are instrumental during multicellular development and

adult tissue homeostasis, regulating a variety of cell behaviours including cell division, apoptosis, migration and differentiation.
The components of each signalling pathway can be operationally grouped into ligands, receptors, transducers and transcription factors (Table 1).

	Ligands		Receptors		Transducers		Transcription Factors	
Pathway/Organism	Fly	Human	Fly	Human	Fly	Human	Fly	Human
	Argos	Argos	EGFR	EGFR	Sos	Sos1	Yan	ETV
		EGF	Sevenless	ROS1	Grb	Grb2	Pointed 1-2	ETS (ELK1)
		HB-EGF	Torso		Ras	K-Ras /H-Ras/N-RAS		AP1
		TGF-a		HER 2-4	Raf	SHC		SRF
		NRG1-4			dMEK	MEK 1/2		
EGFR	Spitz					MEKK 1/3		
	Vein				rolled	ERK 1/2		
	Gurken				dPI3K	PI3K		
	Keren				dPTEN	PTEN		
		EPR			dPDK1	PDK1		
					AKT	AKT		
	dachsous	DCHS 1		Fat 1-3	Hippo	MST1,2	Yorkie	YAP,TAZ
		DCHS 2	Fat	Fat 4	Salvador	hWW45/SAV1		
			CRB		Kibra	Kibra		
					Expanded	Willin/FRMD6/Ex2		
SWH					Merlin	MER/NF2		
					Mats	MOBK1B		
					Warts	LAT 1-2		
					dRassf1	RASSF1		
					Dachs			
	Delta	Delta-4/A-D	Notch	Notch1			Su(H)	CSL
	Serrate	Serrate		Notch2-4			Notch-i	NICD
NOTCH		Jagged1-2						
		Dll3-4						
	Ilp1-7	Insulin	InR	IGF1R	dPI3K	PI3K	dFOXO	FOXO
		IGF1-3			dPTEN	PTEN		
InR					dPDK1	PDK1		
					AKT	AKT		
					dRheb	Rheb		
					dTSC1/2	TSC1/2		
	Leucine	Leucine	Slimfast		dRagA/C	RRAG B/C		UBF
	Glutamine	Glutamine	pathetic		dMAP4K3	hMAP4K3	Tif-IA	TIF-1A
				SLC7AS/SLC3A2	dTOR	TOR		SL1
TOR					draptor	Raptor		Pol I
					drictor	Rictor		
					dS6K	S6K		
					d4EBP1	4EBP1		
	Eiger	TNF	Wengen	TNFR1	dTRAF1-2	TRAF1-2	Jra	Jun
	PVF	PDGF		TNFR2	dRac1	Rac1	Kayak	Fos
			PVR	PDGFR	Msn			
					Dsh			
					MAP4K3	MAP4K3		
JNK					dTAK1	TAK1		
					dASK1	ASK1		
					Slpr			
					dMekk1	MEKK1/4		
					Hep	MKK4/7		
					BSK	JNK1/2/3		
	Spaetzle		Toll	TLR1,2,4,5,6,11	Pelle	IRAK1,3	Dif/Dorsal	NFKB1
					Cactus kinase		Deaf1	DEAF1
					Tube			
					Pellino			
					Myd88	MYD88		
					Gprk2			
TOLL						TIRAP		
						IRAK4		
						TRAF6		
						TAK1		
						TAB1		
						MKK3-4/6-7		
						TBK1		
						IRF3,7		
	Upd 1-3	IFN I (a/b)	Dome	Gp130	Hop	JAK1/2/3		STAT1a/ b
		IFN II (g)	Mom			TYK2		STAT2
JAK/STAT							STAT92E	STAT3a/b
								STAT4a/b
								STAT5A /B/6

Continuation	Ligands		Receptors		Transducers		Transcription Factors	
Pathway/Organism	Fly	Human	Fly	Human	Fly	Human	Fly	Human
WNT	Wingless	WNT 1	Frizzled	Frizzled	Dishevelled	Dishevelled	Pangolin	LEF/TCF
		WNT 2-16	Arrow	LRP 5	Axin	Axin		
				LRP 6	Zeste-White 3	GSK3		
				ROR2	APC	APC		
					Armadillo	b-Catenin		
						DVL		
TGF-β	Dpp	BMP2,4	Tkv	BMPR IA,IB	Mad	Smad1,5,8	Mad	Smad1,5,8
		BMP5-8		ALK-1,2,6	dSmad2	Smad2,3	dSmad2	Smad2,3
	Gbb		Sax		Medea	Smad4,4b	Medea	Smad4,4b
	Activinb	Activin A,B	Wit		Dad	Smad6,7		
		TGFb1,2,3	Babo	ActRIB/AcvR-i/ALK4/TbRI				
		Nodal		BMPR-II/ TGbR-II/				
		GDF 5	Put					
		MIS		AMHR				
	Scw			ActR-II, IIB				
	Daw							
	Mav							
	Myo							
Hh	hh	Shh	Ptc	Ptc1	Smo	SMO	Cubitus-i	Gli-1
		Ihh		Ptc2	Costal2	KIF7		Gli-2,3
		Dhh				KIF3A		
						IFT88/IFT172		
					Fused	Fused		
					Su(Fu)	SUFU		
						MIM		
						Iguana		
						FKBP8		
						SIL		
						Rab23		
					PKA	PKA		
					CKI	CKI		
					GSK3	GSK3		
					Kurtz	b-arrestin-2		
					Slimb	{beta}TrCP		
					Gprk2	GRK2		

Table 1. Main components of the principal signalling pathways in *Drosophila melanogaster* and *Homo sapiens*.
For references see: EGFR: Kataoka, 2009/Shilo, 2003; SWH:Gruscne et al., 2010/Kango-Singh and Singh, 2009/Matallanas et al., 2008; Notcn:Bray 2006/Scnwanbeck et al., 2010; InR: Ma and Blenis, 2009; TOR: Hietakangas and Cohen, 2009/Rosner et al., 2008/Zoncu et al 2011; JNK: Igaki 2009- Toll' So and Oucni 2010/ Valanne et al., 2011; JAK/STAT: Rane and Reddy, 2000/Hou et al., 2002/Wright et al., 2011; Wnt: Seto and Bellen, 2004/Chien et al., 2009; TGF-B: Raftery and Sutherland, 1999/Massague and Wotton, 2000/Waite and Eng, 2003 and Hh: Ruiz-Gomez et al., 2007/Jacob and Lum, 2007.

In the simplest example, that of steroid hormones, a single protein can recognise a ligand molecule and also acts as a transcription factor (Stanisic et al., 2010), but, in general, different proteins can be unequivocally assigned to each category in different pathways. Ligands are mostly proteins that can be secreted from the cell or directly presented in the cell membrane to neighbouring cells (Figure 1). In general, ligands are subject to considerable post-transcriptional modifications, including ubiquitination (Delta/Serrate in the Notch pathway; Le Bras et al., 2011), lipid modifications (Hedgehog family of proteins; Steinhauer and Treisman, 2009), proteolytic processing from a larger precursor to form the active peptide (TGFß superfamily members and EGF/FGF ligands; Zhu and Burgess, 2001; Urban et al., 2002), palmitoylation and glycosylation (Wnt and EGFR ligands; Miura et al., 2006; Steinhauer and Treisman, 2009) and glycosylation (JAK/STAT ligands) (Figure 1). These modifications are required for the secretion of the ligand and its spreading through the tissue, and they also determine their ability to bind and activate their receptors. In addition,

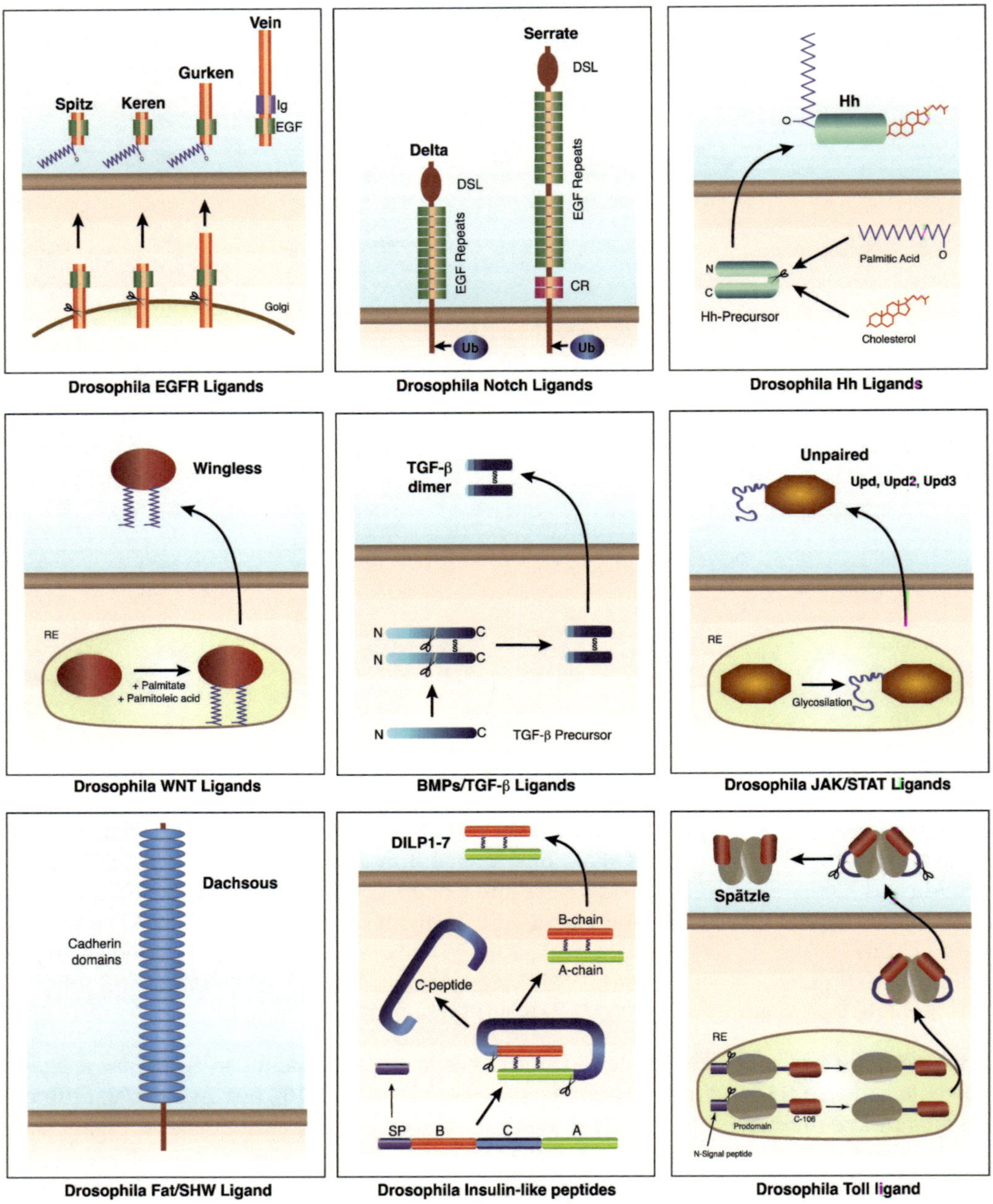

Fig. 1. Schematic representation of the ligands and their post-transcriptional modifications. Upper panels: EGFR, Notch and Hh ligands, middle panels: Wnt, BMP/TGFβ and JAK/STAT ligands and bottom panels (SWH, Insulin and Toll ligands.

most secreted ligands display strong interactions with several components of the extracellular matrix, which help to establish their diffusion range and to shape the concentration of active ligand at a distance from the ligand-producing cells (Jackson et al., 1997; Baeg et al., 2001; Araujo et al., 2003; Bartscherer and Boutros, 2008). The distribution of the ligands is also affected by interactions with their receptors, as ligand-receptor interactions remove the ligand from the extra-cellular milieu and regulate the concentration of the ligand through endocytosis and subsequent lysosomal degradation or recycling of ligand-receptor complexes (Lecuit and Cohen, 1998; Chen and Struhl, 1996; Funakoshi et al., 2001; Pfeiffer and Vincent, 1999).

Receptors are in general transmembrane proteins with two well-differentiated activities. Thus, they interact with the ligand through their extra-cellular domain, and recruit different components of the transduction machinery in their intra-cellular domain (Figure 2). The cell biology of receptors is complex and diverse, but in general includes mechanisms to ensure the correct trafficking of the receptor through the Endoplasmic reticulum-Golgi network, post-transcriptional modifications during trafficking to synthesize the active form of the protein, localization of the receptor to apical domains in the cell membrane, interaction of the receptor with different co-receptor molecules, and turn-over mechanisms that regulate the number of activated-receptors in the cell membrane and other intracellular compartments (Piddini and Vincent, 2003; Hoeller et al., 2005; Mills, 2007; Sorkin and von Zastrow, 2009; Bethani et al., 2010). Similarly, the activation of the receptor by binding to appropriate ligands uses different mechanisms that rely in the clustering of receptor complexes, phosphorylation of receptor molecules after complex formation (EGFR and TGFß), or conformational changes that allow the proteolytic processing of the receptor (Notch) or its interaction with specific transduction components (Wnt; Figure 2).

The receptors act on their downstream transducers through a variety of mechanisms that include phosphorylation (EGFR/InR and JAK; Arbouzova and Zeidler, 2006; Pfeifer et al., 2008; Hombria and Sotillos, 2008 Avraham and Yarden, 2011) and TGFß receptor complexes; Miyazono et al., 2010), the recruitment of intracellular transducers after conformation changes (Wnt receptors; Angers and Moon, 2009), or the indirect modification of the phosphorylation state and subcellular localization of its transducer (Hedgehog receptors; Ruiz-Gomez et al., 2007). In a particular case (Notch; Bray, 2006), the receptor itself directly contributes to modify the composition and activity of transcription complexes (Figure 2).

The components of the transduction machinery downstream of the receptor are also heterogeneous, ranging from the simplest cases in which the receptor itself becomes part of a transcription complex (Notch) or directly modifies by phosphorylation a transcription factor, triggering a change in its subcellular localization from the cytoplasm to the nucleus (Smad and Stat proteins in TGFβ and JAK pathways, respectively; Miyazono et al., 2010; Hou et al., 2002). In other cases the receptor (Wnt receptors; Angers and Moon, 2009) or a transducer regulated by the receptor (Smoothened in the Hh pathway; Ruiz-Gomez et al., 2007) acts as a scaffold to recruit and sequester different components that prevent the accumulation of a transcription factor in the nucleus (ß-catenin and Gli, respectively). Finally, in the cases of Sav/Warts/Hippo (SWH; Harvey and Tapon, 2007; Halder and Johnson, 2011), Toll (Valanne et al., 2011), and receptors with tyrosin-kinase activity such as EGFR (Shilo, 2003) and InR (Brogiolo et al., 2001), the activation of the receptor is communicated to the responding transcription factor through a linear cascade of phosphorylation (EGFR, InR and SWH) or proteolytic events (Toll) that end in the generation of active forms of the transcription factor localised in the nucleus (ETS proteins for EGFR and Rel/Dorsal for Toll), or in the exclusion from the nucleus of the transcriptional co-activator Yorki/YAP (SWH) (Table 2).

By using these mechanisms, the state of the pathway changes the nuclear localization of a transcription factor that binds to the DNA with sequence-specificity. In the simplest cases

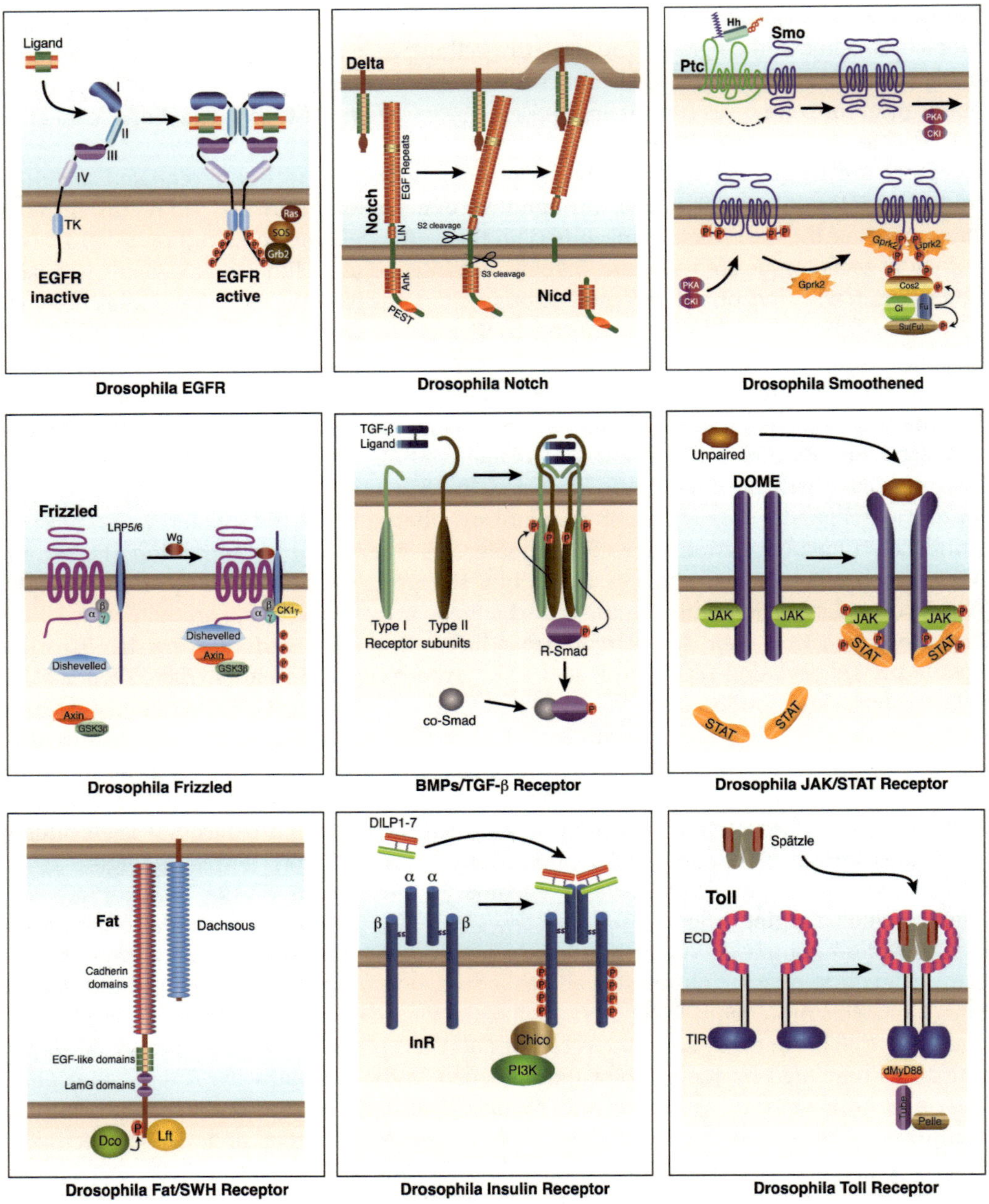

Fig. 2. Schematic representation of the receptors and their mechanisms of activation

this is accomplished directly by the receptor itself, which re-localise to the nucleus upon ligand binding (Notch). In the case of Yorki/YAP (SWH; Harvey and Tapon, 2007) and Foxo (InR; Van Der Heide et al., 2004; Greer and Brunet, 2008), pathway activity prevents or promote, respectively, their entrance into the nucleus, and in the case of Dorsal/Rel (Gerondakis et al., 2006) the pathway triggers the proteolytic processing of a protein that sequesters this transcription factor in the cytoplasm (Table 2). In other pathways the transcription factor resides in the nucleus, where it acts as a member of a transcriptional repressor complex. In these cases, the transcriptional output of signalling is determined by the induction of a transition, regulated by the pathway, from a transcriptional repressor to a transcriptional activator (Table 2). This transition is accomplished using different mechanisms such as the generation of an intracellular fragment of the receptor (Notch; Bray, 2006), the phosphorylation of the transcription factors (ETS in EGFR; Baonza et al., 2002 and Smads in TGFß; Miyazono et al., 2005) or the inhibition of the proteolytic processing of the transcription factor (Gli in Hh and ß-Catenin in Wnt: Nusse, 1999).

	TF		Activation of TF		Localization/State of TF		Co-TF	
Pathway / Organism	Fly	Human	Fly	Human	Fly	Human	Fly	Human
EGFR	Pnt/Yan	ETS/ETV	Phosphorylation		C/N; R/A		Gro MAE	TLE -
Hh	Ci	Gli-1, Gli-2, Gli-3	Proteolisis		C/N; R/A		dCBP	CBP
InR/TOR	dFOXO	FOXO	Phosphorylation		N/C; R/A		-	
JAK/STAT	Stat92E	STAT1-2-3-4-5-6	Phosphorylation		C/N; A		Ept	TSG101
JNK	Jra/Kay	Jun/Fos	Phosphorylation		C/N; A		-	
NOTCH	Su(H)-NICD	CSL-NICD	Proteolisis		C/N; R/A		Mam -	MANL1-3 SKIP
SWH	Yki	Yap, Taz	Phosphorylation		N/C; A		Sd Hth	TEAD1-4 Meis1-3
TGFβ	DSmad2-Med/Mad-Med	Smad2-Smad4/Smad3,Smad5-Smad4	Phosphorylation		C/N; R/A		Shn dCBP dSki/dSno	HIVEP3 CBP SKIL
TOLL	Dif/Dorsal	NFκβ	Proteolisis		C/N; A		dCBP Gro $TAF_{II}60/TAF_{II}110$ Twi	CBP TLE TAF6 TWIST1
WNT	Arm-Pan	β-catenin-TCF	Proteolisis		C/N; R/A		Gro dCBP Lgs Brm	TLE CBP BCL9L BRG1

Table 2. Transcription factors and their mechanism of activation. Abbreviations: Transcription Factor (TF), Pointed (Pnt), Cubitus interruptus (Ci), Signal-transducer and activator of transcription protein at 92E (Stat92E), Jun-related antigen (Jra), Kayak (Kay), Suppressor Hairless (Su(H)), Notch intracellular domain (NICD), Yorki (Ykl), Mothers against dpp (Mad), Medea (Med), Dorsal-related inmmunity factor (Dif), Armadillo (Arm), Pangolin (Pan), Groucho (Gro), CREB-bincing protein (CBP), Erupted (Ept), Tumor Susceptibility Gene-101 (TSG101), Mastermind (Mam), Skl-interacting Protein (SKIP), Scalloped (Sd), Homothorax (Hth), Schnurri (Shn), Human immunodeficiency virus type I enhancer binding protein 3 (HIVEP3), Sno oncogene (Sno), SKI-like oncogene (SKIL), TBP-associated factor "60/110 (TAF"60/110), Twist (Twi), Legless (Lgs), Brahma (Brm). Localization/State of TF: Citosolic (C) and nuclear (N) subcellular localization. Function as a transcriptional activator (A) or repression (R). TF that traslocate to the nucleus upon activation (C/N) or from the nucleus to the cytoplasm (N/C). For references see: EGFR: Vivekanand et al., 2004/Hassen and Paroush, 2007; Hn: Akimarti et al., 1997a/Chen et al., 2000; InR/Tor: Ma and Blenis, 2009/Hietakangas and Cohen, 2009/Resnik-Docampo and de Celis, 2011; JAK/STAT: Gilbert et al., 2009 ; JNK: Igaki, 2009; NOTCH: Zhou et al., 2000/Petcherski and Kimble, 2000/Bray, 2006; SWH: Halder and Johnson, 2011; TGFb: Feng et al., 1998/Janknecht et al., 1998/Pouponnot et al., 1998/Waltzer and Bienz, 1999/Luo et al., 1999/Strochein et al., 1999/Sun et al., 1999a/Sun et al., 1999b/Dai et al., 2000/Barrio et al., 2007; Toll: Dubnicoff et al., 1997/Aklkmaru et al., 1997b/Pham et al., 1999 and Wnt: Waltzer and Bienz, 1998/Roose et al., 1998/Nusse, 1999/Barker et al., 2001/Hoffmans and Basler, 2004.

In all cases, the presence in the nucleus of a transcriptional activator in response to signalling modifies the expression of a battery of target genes, leading to changes in cell behaviour that are conditioned by the state of the responding cell. In this manner, some aspects of the transcriptional landscape of the ligand expressing cells are communicated to the receiving cells, where a novel pattern of transcription can be established. Thus, the transcription factors regulated by each signalling pathway contribute to the combinatory of regulators present in a given cell, and this, combined with the structure of gene regulatory sequences, makes the transcriptional responses to a pathway cell type specific (Bonn and Furlong, 2008; Chopra and Levine, 2009). At this time, little is known about the number and identity of target genes whose expression are directly regulated by signalling and whose function contributes significantly to the cellular response to signalling. This is an area of intensive research, and the use of chromatin immunoprecipitation techniques coupled with microarrays or deep-sequencing, the development of reporter systems for cell culture assays and the functional analysis of the identified target genes promise a much better understanding of the transcriptional responses to signalling in the near future (Yang et al., 2004; Miyazono et al., 2005; Friedman and Perrimon, 2006; Mummery-Widmer et al., 2009; Bernard et al., 2010; Kim and Marques, 2010).

3. General aspects of the biological roles play by signalling pathways during development

The development of multicellular organisms relies to a large extent in the spatial and temporal generation of gene expression domains (Arnone and Davidson, 1997). In this manner, and under the perspective that signalling pathways are mostly elaborate devices to regulate transcription, it is no wonder that these pathways play prominent roles during the development of all organisms. Their key contribution is mostly based in their ability to communicate transcriptional stages between cell populations and generate spatial domains of gene expression. Other characteristics that make signalling a powerful system to regulate cell behaviour are the quantitative response to signalling, the operation of elaborate feed-back mechanisms, positive and negative, that modulate the intensity and duration of signalling (Perrimon and McMahon, 1999), and the existence of cross-interactions between pathways (McNeill and Woodgett, 2010). These cross-interactions occur both at the level of transcription, in which one pathway regulates the expression of others pathway ligands, or by interactions in which one pathway affects the activity of components belonging to a different pathway (Hasson and Paroush, 2007; McNeill and Woodgett, 2010). All these characteristics confer a great versatility to the function of signalling during development, and also contribute to the disastrous consequences that signalling miss-regulation has in different genetic disorders (Harper et al., 2003; Logan and Nusse, 2004; Inoki et al., 2005; Bentires-Alj et al., 2006; Jacob and Lum, 2007; Gordon and Blobe, 2008; Rosner et al., 2008; Gordon and Blobe, 2008; Table 3). To summarize, we have divided the biological roles played by signalling into the following categories:

1. Cellular responses that directly modify the metabolic state of the cell. This is best exemplified by the action of the InR/TOR pathway, which activity is used as a way to adjust the growth of the cell to the availability of nutrients (Brogiolo et al., 2001). In addition, this pathway is also used to coordinate the growth of different organs during development and adult tissue homeostasis (Zoncu et al., 2011).

2. Cellular responses that make cells to progress through the cell cycle, acquire migratory behaviour, enter into the apoptotic pathway or in general to make a transition between cell states. All pathways contribute in different cellular settings to modify a pre-existing cellular state (Thompson, 2010). For example, inputs from the BMP and FGF pathways regulate the entrance in apoptosis of inter-digital epidermal cells during vertebrate limb development (Pajni-Underwood et al., 2007); and TGFß/BMPs also participate in regulating epithelial-mesenchymal transitions (Zavadil and Böttinger, 2005). BMP together with JNK also promote changes in the cytoskeleton that influence the movement of layers of cells during morphogenesis (Fernandez et al., 2007). On the other hand, several pathways have direct links with the cell cycle, either promoting the transitions between different phases of the cycle or triggering the entrance of cells in senescence (Campisi and d'Adda, 2007; Jones and Kazlauskas, 2001).
3. Regulation of alternative cell fates within populations of competent cells. Many pathways are engaged in the allocation of cell fates during development. The Notch and EGFR pathways fall in this class, regulating neural fates within proneural clusters in a process that employs Notch signalling to prevent neural fate and EGFR to promote this fate (Lage et al., 1997; Bray, 2006; Axelrod, 2010).
4. Regulation of spatial domains of gene expression within growing epithelia. The patterning of epithelial tissues is generally organised with respect to signalling centres. These centres operate as the source of ligands belonging to the EGFR, TGFß/BMP, Wnt and Hh signalling pathways. Because these ligands act in a concentration-dependent manner at a distance from the cells expressing them, they can set adjacent domains of gene expression that partition the epithelium into different territories with specific gene expression patterns. This process is used reiteratively during the development of all multicellular organisms, and some examples are the patterning of segments in the embryonic epidermis and the subdivision of the imaginal discs into different territories in flies (Moussian and Roth, 2005), the generation of cell diversity in the vertebrate neural tube (Lupo et al., 2006), the establishment of the antero-posterior patterning in the vertebrate limbs and many others (Kumar, 2001; Duboc and Logan, 2009; Towers and Tickle, 2009; Arnold and Robertson, 2009).
5. Interactions between independent layers of cells. The development of tridimensional structures implies the coordination of cellular fates between cell layers of independent origin. This type of information transfer is at the base of the chains of inductive processes that pervade vertebrate development, and also contribute to set temporal and spatial patterns of cell migration during neurogenesis and myogenesis (Carmena et al., 1998; Kimelman, 2006; Lupo et al., 2006; Wackerhage and Ratkevicius, 2008; Steventon et al., 2009; Mok and Sweetman, 2011).

The correct regulation of cell proliferation, differentiation and survival is essential for the proper development and homeostasis of all organisms. The key roles that signalling plays in these processes are likely behind the multitude of human diseases caused by genetic alterations in the components of most signalling pathways. We outlined in Table 3 some examples illustrating human pathologies associated to defects in signalling, showing that changes in the activity of almost any component of different pathways, from the ligands to the transcription factors, lead to specific pathologies. In this manner, both loss and gain of function mutations in different pathways have been described as potential causes of developmental disorders and disease. For example, the loss of TGFß and SWH function, as well as increase in JAK/STAT and EGFR, Wnt and Hh signalling are linked to tumour formation and progression in a variety of cell types (Massague et al., 2000; Waite and Eng, 2003; Harvey and Tapon, 2007), the miss-regulation of Toll signalling is related with defects in the immune response (O'Neill, 2003), and is associated to the increase in the susceptibility of immune diseases such as Lupus and arthritis (Constantinescu et al., 2008; Schindler, 2002). Mutations in Hh, TGFß and Notch pathways have also been related with blood and circulatory system diseases such as hypertension or CADASIL, and defects in JNK pathway to neurodegenerative diseases including Parkinson and Alzheimer. Similarly, the mTOR pathway is implicated in metabolic diseases including diabetes and obesity as well as in ageing (Inoki et al., 2005). Finally, many developmental disorders, including Noonan syndrome, Cleft palate, Pallister Hall syndrome, Polydactyli or Tetra-Amelia, have been found associated to EGFR, TGFß, Hh, and Wnt de-regulation (Tartaglia and Gelb, 2005).

Pathway	Component		Disease	References
EGFR	Receptors	EGFR	Most carcinomas (including Breast, Ovarian and Stomatch)	Downward, 2003; Mendelsohn and Baselga, 2000; Kuan et al., 2001
		HER2	Breast cancer	Downward, 2003
	Transducer	B-Raf	Cardio-fascio-cutaneus syndrome, Colorectal cancer, Melanoma	Downward, 2003; Schubbert et al., 2007; Bentires-Alj et al., 2006
		Sos1	Noonan syndrome, JMML	Schubbert et al., 2007
		K-Ras	AML, JMML, Noonan, Myelodysplastic, Cardio-fascio-cutaneus and Leopard syndromes, Lung adenocarcinoma, Bladder, Colorectal, Kydney, Liver, Pancreas, and Thyroid tumors, Seminoma, Melanoma	Schubbert et al., 2007; Tartaglia and Gelb, 2005; Bentires-Alj et al., 2006; Downward, 2003; Bos, 1989
		H-Ras	AML, Costello and Myelodysplastic syndromes, Rhabdomyosarcoma, Neuro and Ganglioneuroblastoma, Adenocarcinoma, Bladder, Colorectal, Kydney, Liver, Lung, Pancreas and Thyroid cancers, Seminoma, Melanoma	Schubbert et al., 2007; Aoki et al., 2005; Bentires-Alj et al., 2006; Downward, 2003
		MEK 1/2	Cardio-fascio-cutaneus syndrome	Schubbert et al., 2007; Bentires-Alj et al., 2006
		C-Raf	AML	Zebisch et al., 2006; Kim and Choi, 2010

Pathway	Component		Disease	References
Hh	Ligand	Shh	Basal cell carcinoma	Beachy et al., 2004
	Receptor	Ptc1	Basal cell carcinoma, Medulloblastoma, Rhabdo and Fibrosarcoma	Taipale and Beachy, 2001; Peacock et al., 2007; Wechsler-Reya and Scott, 2001; Jacob and Lum, 2007
	Transducer	SUFU	Basal cell carcinoma, Medullobastoma	Beachy et al., 2004
		Smo	Basal cell carcinoma, Sporadic tumours, Medulloblastoma	Taipale and Beachy, 2001; Beachy et al., 2004; Peacock et al., 2007
	TF	Gli	Glioma, GCPS, PHS, PAP-A	Ruiz i Altaba et al., 2002; Beachy et al., 2004; Ruiz-Gomez et al., 2007; Zhu and Lo, 2010
InR	Ligand	IGF1	Colorectal neoplasia	Jacobs, 2008
		IGF2	Colonic adenocarcinoma	Jacobs, 2008
	Receptor	IGF2R	Breast and Hepatocellular carcinomas	Jacobs, 2008
	Transducer	PKD1	Polycystic kidney disease	Rosner et al., 2008
		PTEN	Bannayan-Riley-Ruvalcaba and Proteus syndromes, Cowden and Lhermitte-Duclos diseases	Inoki et al., 2005
		TSC 1/2	Tuberous sclerosis and Lymphangiomatosis	van Slegtenhorst et al., 1997; Rosner et al., 2008
		STK11	Peutz-Jeghers syndrome	Hernan et al., 2004
		AMPK	Cardiac hypertrophy	Blair et al., 2001
		VHL	Angiomas, Hemangioblastomas, Renal carcinoma	Rosner et al., 2008
TOR	Transducer	MAP4K3	Pancreas cancer	Zoncu et al., 2011
		mTORC1	Obesity	Zoncu et al., 2011
		S6K1-IRS1	Diabetes type 2	Zoncu et al., 2011
		NF1	Neurofibromatosis	Zoncu et al., 2011
		p14	Growth defects, Inmunodeficiency	Zoncu et al., 2011

Pathway	Component		Disease	References
JAK/ STAT	Receptor	IL-2Rgc	X-linked SCID	O'Sullivan et al., 2007
		IL-7Ra	SCID	O'Sullivan et al., 2007
		IFNgRI	Susceptibility to Mycobacterial infection	O'Sullivan et al., 2007
	Transducer	JAK2	ALL, AML, MPDs, PV,	Constantinescu et al., 2008
		JAK3	SCID	Schindler, 2002; O'Sullivan et al., 2007
	TF	STAT1	ALL, AML, CLL, Brain, Breast, Lung, Head and Neck tumours, Erytroleukemia, Susceptibility to Mycobacterial infection	Bromberg, 2002; O'Sullivan et al., 2007
		STAT3	AML, CLL, LGL, Crohn's disease, Brain, Breast, Head, Lung, Neck, Ovarian, Pancreas, Prostate and Renal tumours, Mycosis fungoides, Burkitt's, Hodgkins and Anaplastic large cell lymphomas, Myeloma, Melanoma	Bromberg, 2002; O'Sullivan et al., 2007
		STAT4	Chronic obstructive pulmonary disease	O'Sullivan et al., 2007
		STAT5	ALL, AML, CML, Crohn's disease, Erytroleukemia	Bromberg, 2002; O'Sullivan et al., 2007
JNK	Transducer	JNK1	Diabetes type 2	Waeber et al., 2000
		JNK2	Atherosclerosis	Ricci et al., 2004; Sumara et al., 2005
		JNK3	Parkinson Disease	Resnick and Fennell, 2004
		p38	Alzheimer Disease	Smith et al., 2006
		MKK4	Breast, Biliary and Pancreatic carcinomas	Su et al., 1998
Notch	Ligand	Dll-3	Spondylocosta dysotosis	Harper et al., 2003
		Jagged-1	Alagille Syndrome	Harper et al., 2003
	Receptor	Notch-1	ALL	Ellisen et al., 1991; Harper et al., 2003
		Notch-3	CADASIL	Harper et al., 2003
		Notch-4	Lung Cancer, Esquizophrenia and Aloppecia aerata	Dang et al., 2000; Wei and Hemmings, 2000; Ujike et al., 2001; Tazi-Ahnini et al., 2003

Pathway	Component		Disease	References
TGFβ	Ligand	TGFβ	Mammary, Prostate and Renal cancers	Rooke and Crosier, 2001
		TGF1	Camurati-Englemann disease	Gordon and Blobe, 2008
		GDF-5	Hunter-Thompson and Grebe-type chondrodysplasias, Brachydactyly type C, Symphalangism, Hereditary chondrodysplasia	Massague et al., 2000; Gordon and Blobe, 2008
		BMP-15	Premature ovarian failure	Gordon and Blobe, 2008
		MIS	Persistent Müllerian duct syndrome	Massague et al., 2000; Gordon and Blobe, 2008
		NODAL	Situs Ambiguus	Gordon and Blobe, 2008
		TGFβ-2,3	Cleft palate	Gordon and Blobe, 2008
	Receptor	TGFBRI	Breast cancer, Loeys-dietz, Marfan and Furlong syndromes, Familial thoracic aortic aneurysm	Rooke and Crosier, 2001; ten Dijke and Arthur, 2007; Gordon and Blobe, 2008
		BMPRII	PAH, TADD	Massague et al., 2000; Waite and Eng, 2003; ten Dijke and Arthur, 2007; Gordon and Blobe, 2008
		TGFBRII	CML, Colorectal, Gastric, Head and Neck tumours, Small cell lung cancer and Hereditary non-polyposis colorectal cancers, Loeys-dietz, Marfan and Sphrintzen-Goldberg syndromes, B and T-cell lymphoma, Retinoblastoma, Glioma, TADD	Rooke and Crosier, 2001; Gordon and Blobe, 2008
		BMPRI	Brachydactyly type A2, JPS, Bannayan-Riley-Ruvalcaba and Cowden syndrome, TADD	Waite and Eng, 2003 ; Gordon and Blobe, 2008
		ALK1	HTT2	Massague et al., 2000; Waite and Eng, 2003; ten Dijke and Arthur, 2007; Gordon and Blobe, 2008
		AMHR2	Persistent Müllerian duct syndrome	Massague et al., 2000 ; Gordon and Blobe, 2008
	Transducer/TF	Smad4	Pancreatic, Colorectal and Ovarian cancers, JPS, HHT	Massague et al., 2000; Waite and Eng, 2003; ten Dijke and Arthur, 2007; Gordon and Blobe, 2008
		Smad2	Colorectal cancer	Rooke and Crosier, 2001
		Smad3	CML	Rooke and Crosier, 2001

Pathway	Component		Disease	References
SWH	Receptor	Fat4	Breast cancer	Qi et al., 2009; Pan, 2010
	Transducer	MST 1/2	Soft tissue sarcoma	Seidel et al., 2007; Pan, 2010
		RASSF1	Lung and Kidney cancers	Kango-Singh and Singh, 2009
		NF2	NF2, Schwanomas	Evans et al., 2000; Jiang et al., 2006; Pan, 2010; Bao et al., 2011
		Lat 1/2	Breast tumours	Turenchalk et al., 1999; Zeng and Hong, 2008
	TF	YAP TAZ	Breast, Colorectal, Hepatocellular, Lung, Ovarian, Pancreatic and Prostate carcinomas	Overholtzer et al., 2006; Zender et al., 2006; Dong et al., 2007; Steinhardt et al., 2008
Toll	Receptor	TLR1	Colon cancer Gram-positive sepsis	So and Ouchi, 2010
		TLR2	Colon, Gastric and Hepatocellular carcinomas	So and Ouchi, 2010
		TLR3	Breast, Colon and Hepatocellular cancinomas, Melanoma	So and Ouchi, 2010
		TLR4	Atheroesclerosis, Arthritis, Breast, Colon, Gastric, Hepatocellular, Lung and Ovarian cancers, Carcinoma, Melanoma, Chronic inflamation	So and Ouchi, 2010; Zhu and Mohan, 2010
		TLR5	Gastric and Cervical squamous cell carcinomas	So and Ouchi, 2010
		TLR6	Hepatocellular carcinoma	So and Ouchi, 2010
		TLR7	CLL, Lupus	So and Ouchi, 2010; Zhu and Mohan, 2010
		TLR9	Breast, Cervical, Gastric, Hepatocelular and Prostate and Aquamus cell carcinomas, Glioma Diabetes type 1	So and Ouchi, 2010 ; Meyers et al. 2010
	TF	NF-KB	Diabetes type 2	Baker et al. 2011

Pathway	Component		Disease	References
Wnt	Ligand	WNT 3	Tetra-amelia	Logan and Nusse, 2004
	Receptor	LRP 5	Bone density defects, OPPG, FEVR	Logan and Nusse, 2004
		FZD 4	FEVR	Logan and Nusse, 2004
	Transducer	APC	Colon, Adeno and Basal cell carcinoma, Turcot's syndrome, FAP	Peifer and Polakis, 2000; Wechsler-Reya and Scott, 2001; Beachy et al., 2004; Logan and Nusse, 2004
		Axin	Adenocarcinoma	Beachy et al., 2004
		Axin-2	Tooth agenesis, Predisposition to Colon cancer	Logan and Nusse, 2004
		b-catenin	Adenocarcinoma	Beachy et al., 2004
	TF	TCF	Susceptibility to Diabetes type 2	Jin, 2008

Table 3. Genetic diseases associated to signalling pathways. Abbreviations: Acute lymphoblastic leukemia (ALL), Acute myeloid leukemia (AML), Chronic lymphocytic leukemia (CLL), Chronic myeloid leukemia (CML), Familial adenomatous polyposis (FAP), Familial exudative vitreoretinopathy (FEVR), Familial thoracic aortic aneurysm syndrome (TADD), Greig cephalopolysyndactyly syndrome (GCPS), Hereditary hemorrhagic telangiectasia (HHT) or Rendu-Osler-Weber syndrome, Juvenile myelomonocytic leukaemia (JMML), Juvenile polyposis syndrome (JPS), Large granular lymphocyte leukemia (LGL), Myeloproliferative diseases (MPDs), Osteoperosis-pseudoglioma syndrome (OPPG), Primary pulmonary arterial hypertension (PAH), Postaxial polydactyly type A (PAP-A), Pallister–Hall syndrome (PHS), Polycythemia vera (PV), Severed combined immunodeficiency (SCID).

4. Drosophila as a model organism to analyse the genetic and cellular biology of signalling

Because of the prominent roles that signalling plays during development, and its relevance in maintaining adult homeostasis and normal physiology (see Table 3), the analysis and experimental manipulation of signalling pathways has a central role in biomedical research. In this context, a key aspect in the analysis of signalling is the use of experimental systems allowing the identification of novel components of the different pathways, the manipulation of their activity by genetic and pharmacological approaches and the understanding of the mechanisms by which they regulate cell behaviour. Not surprisingly, the organisms that most have contributed to the analysis of signalling are those allowing a robust and efficient genetic approach to unravel gene function, in particular *Caenorhabditis elegans* and *Drosophila melanogaster*. In fact, many known components of all signalling pathway were identified in these organisms through genetic screens. The rationale of these experiments is straightforward: mutations affecting the same signalling pathway result in a similar phenotype and in general display genetic interactions. Thus, exhaustive genetic screens aimed to identify

genes regulating embryonic segmentation in flies were instrumental to identify many components of the Notch, BMP, Hh and Wnt pathways (Nusslein-Volhard and Wieschaus, 1980), and genetic screens carried out in sensitized genetic backgrounds resulted in the identification of additional components of these pathways and also of the EGFR and InR pathways (Greaves et al., 1999; Rebay et al., 2000; Huang and Rubin, 2000; Guichard et al., 2002; Mahoney et al., 2006). More recently, mosaic screens in adult structures of the fly uncovered the SWH pathway, because of its contribution to the regulation of cell proliferation, competition and apoptosis (Cho et al., 2006; Harvey and Tapon, 2007 Tyler et al., 2007).
Signalling in *C. elegans* and *D. melanogaster* has been analysed in many different developmental settings, including the formation of the gonads (Horvitz and Sternberg, 1991), the development of the imaginal discs (Sotillos and de Celis, 2005; de Celis, 2003) and the patterning of the embryonic segments (Irish and Gelbart, 1987; Wesley, 1999), among many others. In general these studies rely in a good cellular description of the tissue and its development, the possibility of directly monitoring the domains of signalling using specific reporter assays, and the availability of sophisticated techniques to manipulate the activity of any pathway component and analyse its phenotypic consequences. We will describe in what follows and from the perspective of signalling some relevant aspects of the development of the Drosophila wing imaginal disc, one experimental system that has been instrumental in the analysis of cell signalling during the development of epithelial tissues.

5. The wing imaginal disc of Drosophila as a developmental model to analyse the structure, interactions and biological outcomes of signalling pathways

Imaginal discs are epithelial structures that give rise to most of the adult external structures of the fly. The wing imaginal disc starts its development as a group of about 20 embryonic ectodermal cells (Cohen et al., 1993). These cells proliferate during larval development to form the mature third instar disc, composed by approximately 50000 cells primed to differentiate during metamorphosis the fly wing and part of the thorax (Figure 3) (de Celis, 2003). Cell signalling pervades the development of the wing imaginal disc; from the initial step of primordium specification to the last stages of cellular differentiation. In this manner, the cells that constitute the wing disc primordium are determined by the combined actions of the BMP, EGFR and Wnt signalling pathways, which regulate the expression of the transcription factors specifying the group of wing disc precursor cells (Cohen et al., 1993; Goto and Hayashi, 1997). From this point onwards, the primordium enters a developmental program that involves cell division and different stages of territorial organization by which all cells acquire their individual genetic specification (Zecca and Struhl, 2002).
Territorial subdivisions in the wing disc are regulated by coordinate signalling events involving the EGFR, BMP, Notch, Hh and Wnt pathways (Figure 3). First, the wing primordium is subdivided into anterior and posterior compartments, which correspond to independent cell lineages of polyclonal origin. The posterior compartment is the source of the ligand Hh, which signalling contributes to the maintenance of the anterior-posterior compartment boundary and sets specific domains of gene expression in anterior cells from this early stage onwards (Tabata and Kornberg, 1994) (Figure 3). The subdivision into anterior-posterior compartments is followed later in development by patterning along the proximo-distal axes of the disc, a process that relies in the establishment of complementary domains of signalling by the EGFR pathway in proximal cells and by the Wnt pathway in distal cells (Zecca and Struhl, 2002). These two complementary signalling centers determine the expression of transcription factors such as Apterous, the Iroquois gene complex and Spalt in proximal cells, defining what will become the thorax of the mature wing disc (Cavodeassi et

al., 2002). The establishment of the domain of *apterous* expression also triggers the initiation of the wing region, which will appear centred along the boundary between *apterous* expressing cells, the future dorsal compartment, and *apterous* non-expressing cells, corresponding to the ventral compartment. This boundary corresponds to the future dorso-ventral compartment boundary of the wing, and is the place where Notch signalling is activated to regulate the expression of the co-factor Vestigial, which labels the primordium of the wing blade (Figure 3). The establishment of the wing blade territory as a domain of cells expressing vestigial along the dorso-ventral boundary also requires *wingless* function, which expression in distal cells is also regulated by the transcription factors defining the proximo-distal axes of the wing disc (Wu and Cohen, 2002; Whitworth and Russell, 2003; Zirin and Mann, 2007). At this stage, which corresponds to the second instar larvae, the wing disc already contains the future thorax and wing territories, and the wing is already subdivided into anterior-posterior and dorso-ventral compartments. The subsequent development of the wing disc epithelium involves the generation of the wing hinge, originated in the proximal part of the wing blade and specified by two novel rings of *wingless* expression (Perea et al., 2009), and the establishment of smaller domains of expression in both the thorax and wing regions (Figure 3).

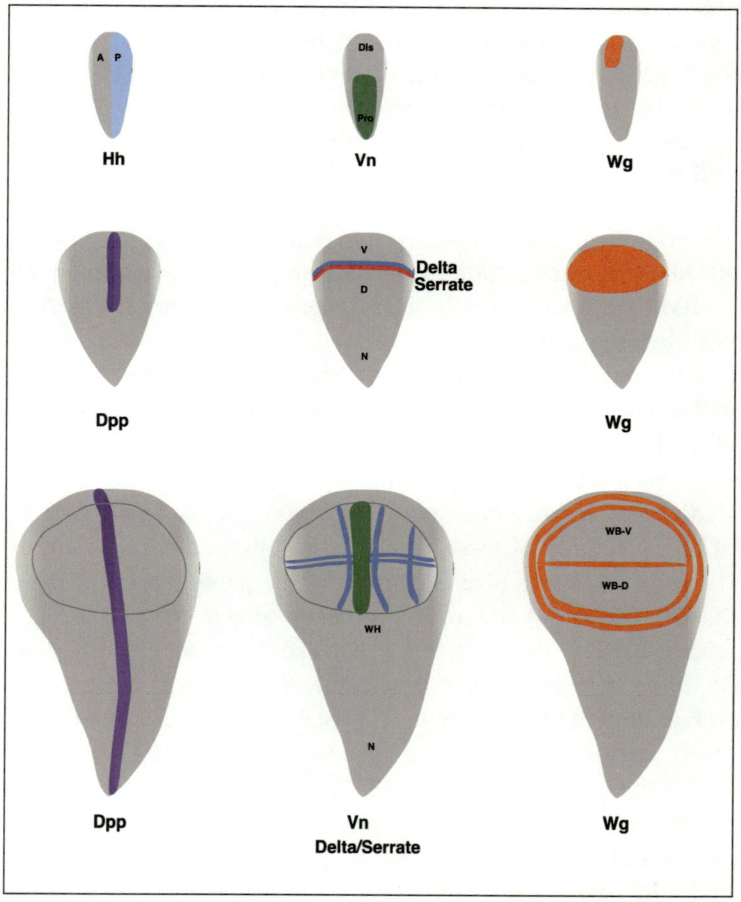

Fig. 3. Schematic representation of the wing disc during the second (upper panels), mid-third (middle panel) and late-third (bottom panel) larval instard, showing the expression of ligands in coloured stripes.

The global subdivision of the wing disc into large territories described above is followed by the regional specification of the pattern elements characteristic of the wing and thorax. These elements, the sensory organs decorating the thorax and wing margin and the longitudinal veins running along the proximo-distal length of the wing blade and hinge, differentiate from fields of competent cells, the proneural clusters and the provein territories, respectively. As it happened with the earlier territorial subdivisions, the positioning of each proneural cluster and provein territory also relies on the function of different signalling pathways, mainly the Wnt, Hh and BMP pathways for the proneural clusters and the BMP and Hh pathways for the proveins (Tomoyasu et al., 1998; Sato et al., 1999; de Celis et al., 1999; Cavodeassi et al., 2001; de Celis, 2003). These pathways now regulate the expression of several transcription factors that control the expression of the proneural and provein genes, constituting a landscape of transcriptional regulators that has been named the "pre-pattern" (Stern, 1954; Cavodeassi et al., 2001). At this stage, all patterned elements are genetically specified in the form of groups of cells with a competence to differentiate individual cell types. The last stage before cell differentiation is the assignation of cell fates within proneural clusters and provein territories. This process relies in a complex set of cell interactions mediated by the Notch and EGFR pathways and generally named "lateral inhibition". During lateral inhibition, the EGFR pathway promotes the acquisition of the sensory organ precursor and vein fates and the Notch pathway prevents other competent cells from following these fates. In this manner, the end result is that only one cell from the proneural clusters will acquire the sensory organ precursor fate and enter a particular pattern of cell divisions (Pi and Chien, 2007). A similar process operates in the provein fields using the same two pathways, but in this case the maintenance of stripes of cells ready to differentiate as veins during pupal development also requires the activity of the BMP pathway, which ligand becomes expressed at this stage in the developing veins (de Celis, 2003).

The patterning of the disc is accompanied by a continuous increase in its size (Baker, 2007). Wing disc growth occurs mainly by cell proliferation, with cells taking about 10 hours to go through the cell cycle (González Gaitán et al., 1994; Milan et al., 1996; Neufeld et al., 1998). Several pathways such as the EGFR, Wnt, SWH, Notch and TGFβ play key roles in promoting cell division. In this manner, a reduction (EGFR, Wnt, Notch and TGFβ) or increase (SWH) in the activity of these pathways results in the formation of smaller adult structures, and this reduction in size is caused by the generation of a lower than normal number of cells (see Figure 4). Interestingly, these effects have a strong component of territorial specificity, because the reduction of each pathway activity affects each territory of the wing disc to different extents. For example, the Wnt pathway is particularly required to promote cell proliferation in the wing hinge (Dichtel-Danjoy et al., 2009), whereas the Notch pathway is mostly required in the wing blade (de Celis and Garcia-Bellido, 1994). As mutations affecting the activity of the EGFR, Wnt, BMP and Notch pathways also affect territorial specification, the defects in cell proliferation are accompanied by changes in the general organization of the disc and its patterning. Cell division is coupled with cell growth in a manner that wing disc cells maintain a similar size during their proliferative phase. From the perspective of cellular growth, the most relevant pathway operating in the wing disc is the InR/Tor signalling system (Hietakangas and Cohen, 2009). The activity of InR/Tor is mostly required as a sensor to translate nutritional and humoral signals into

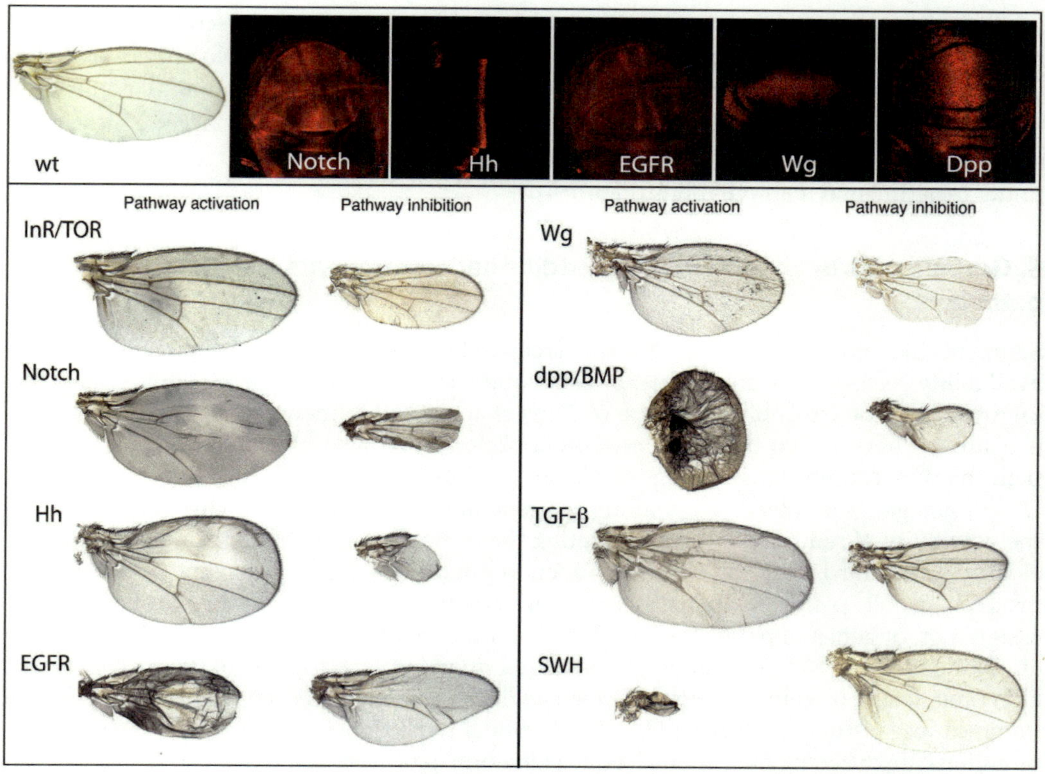

Fig. 4. Upper panel: Pictures of a wild type wing (wt, left) and third instar imaginal discs showing the domains of Notch, Hh, EGFR, Wg and Dpp signalling. Bottom panel: Pictures of mutant wings in which the activity of the InR/Tor, Notch, Hh and EGFR (left two columns), and Wg, dpp/BMP, TGF-β and SWH (right two columns) is either increased (Pathway activation columns) or decreased (Pathway inhibition columns)

adequate rates of protein synthesis, but also provides survival signals for the cell and stimulates cell division (Hietakangas and Cohen, 2009). In general, mutations reducing InR/Tor signalling result in the formation of adult structures smaller than normal, due to both a reduction in cell size and a diminution in the number of cells (see Figure 4).

Although the wing disc is probably one of the best understood biological systems, there are still many caveats regarding the molecular mechanisms that drive cell division during the growth of the disc. Similarly, it is not entirely understood how the progress through the cell cycle is coordinated with cellular growth, and what makes the disc stop its proliferative phase when it reaches a particular size. In this manner, the molecular mechanisms ensuring the formation of patterned structures of the appropriate dimensions are still elusive. Despite of this, the current knowledge about imaginal disc development is robust enough to use this system as a model to unravel the intricacies and roles played by signalling pathways during development, and to model human diseases, using the advantages of fly genetics. There are two key aspects of the analysis of signalling in the wing disc that favours this system as an experimental model. First is the facility by which mutant phenotypes can be assigned to specific failures in particular signalling pathways. This simplifies the identification of additional components of each signalling pathway by the phenotype caused by mutations in the corresponding genes (Figure 4), and also allows the design of genetic screens aimed to identify novel elements of the pathway. Secondly, the spatial and temporal domains of signalling can be precisely described by monitoring the expression of target genes in the disc, and this allows the visualization of receptor activity both in normal conditions and under experimental manipulations (Figure 4).

6. Genetic approaches to identify additional components of signalling pathways

Some of the main reasons to choose Drosophila for the study of signalling are the availability of sophisticated genetic techniques to manipulate gene activity and the knowledge of the Drosophila genome (Adams et al., 2000; Matthews et al., 2005). First, there is a strong conservation between Drosophila proteins involved in signalling pathways and their human counterparts (Reiter et al., 2001; Chien et al., 2002 see Table 1). Second, Drosophila genes involved in signalling are generally represented in single copies, reducing the possibility of redundancy and facilitating the characterization of gene functions (Adams et al., 2000). Third, loss- and gain-of-function conditions in genes coding for signalling proteins of all pathways usually result in complementary phenotypes, allowing the assignation of genes to pathways based on mutant phenotypes (Molnar et al., 2006; Cruz et al., 2009 see Figure 4). The phenotypes observed upon hyper-activation of the pathways also allow the design of gain-of-function screens, which have the potential to uncover genes not found in loss-of-function screens due to functional redundancy (Rorth et al., 1998). Finally, mutations in different elements of each signalling pathway generally display gene-dose dependent phenotypic interactions in genetic combinations, allowing the hierarchical ordering of pathway components through genetic analysis.

There are two main ways in which genetic screens have been used to identify the components of different signalling pathways. In a first approach, newly induced mutants are tested for a phenotype in a particular structure which development depends on the normal activity of specific signalling pathways. In these cases, the mutants can be induced by chemical mutagenesis or by mobilizing transposable elements, and they can be analyzed either in homozigosity in the entire animal, or in mosaics in adult tissues using a combination of the Gal4/UAS and FRT/FLP systems. A recent example of this approach is the search for novel components of the Notch signalling pathway, in which a large collection of interference RNAs is expressed in the wing disc to systematically reduce the expression of the endogenous genes, resulting in the identification of Notch pathway candidates based on the resulting mutant phenotypes (Mummery-Widmer et al., 2009). In addition, whereas chemical mutagenesis and the expression of interference RNA result in loss of gene function, the use of transposable elements with UAS sequences allows the generation of gain-of-function conditions, which can be restricted to the tissue of interest (Rorth et al., 1998). Complementary to these approaches, the search for novel components of signalling pathways has also relied in the design of "modifier" screens, in which both loss- and gain-of-function mutants are tested in particular mutant backgrounds. In these cases, the screen aims to identify genes belonging to a pre-determined set of interacting genes. Some examples of successful screens aiming to identify members of known signalling pathways are those targeting the Sevenless and EGFR (Karim et al., 1996; Huang and Rubin, 2000; Taguchi et al., 2000; Rebay et al., 2000), Notch (Verheyen et al., 1996; Go and Artavanis-

Tsakonas, 1998; Muller et al., 2005a), Dpp (Raftery et al., 1995; Chen et al., 1998; Su et al., 2001), JAK/STAT (Bach et al., 2003; Mukherjee et al., 2006), Hh (Haines and van den Heuvel, 2000; Collins and Cohen, 2005), TNF (Geuking et al., 2005) and Wnt (Greaves et al., 1999; Cox et al., 2000; Desbordes et al., 2005) pathways.

Although the use of genetic screens in vivo has many advantages, they are time-consuming and difficult to escalate genome-wide. For these reasons, and based on the knowledge of the Drosophila genome, several techniques using Drosophila cells in culture and interference RNA have been adopted in the search for novel signalling components. These screens allow the identification of genes affecting the expression of reporter constructs that reveal the activity of specific signalling pathways (Clemens et al., 2000; Flockhart et al., 2006). This approach has been used to search for novel components of the Hh (Lum et al., 2003; Nybakken et al., 2005), and of the Wnt (DasGupta et al., 2005), JAK/Stat (Muller et al., 2005b), TNF (Kleino et al., 2005), Tor (Lindquist et al., 2011) and ERK (Friedman and Perrimon, 2006) signalling pathways.

7. Drosophila models of genetic diseases

It is clear that the main advantage of the Drosophila model from a biomedical perspective is the possibility of designing genetic screens aimed to the identification of genes involved in a particular phenotypic outcome. In this context, it is worth noticing that an estimated 60% of genes related to human diseases have orthologs in Drosophila, and this category includes all genes involved in cell signalling (Chien et al., 2002; Reiter et al., 2001). The possibility of generating transgenic flies expressing modified non-Drosophila proteins is allowing the design of "humanized" fly models for a variety of human genetic diseases such as Multiple Endocrine Neoplasia Type 2 (Read et al., 2005), cardiomyopathies (Vu Manh et al., 2005) and Adenomatous Polyposis Coli (APC; Bhandari and Shashidhara, 2001) and several neurodegenerative diseases (Fernandez-Funez et al., 2000; Crowther et al., 2004; Sang and Jackson, 2005; Botas, 2007; Branco et al., 2008; Cukier et al., 2008; Miller et al., 2010). The aim of these experiments is to recreate in a fly tissue some of the cellular aspects of the pathology caused by the human protein, and to use this genetic background as a platform to search for genes affecting the phenotype caused by the miss-expression of this protein (Botas, 2007). In the long term, it is expected that the identification of additional genes involved in a particular phenotypic outcome will allow the search for chemotherapeutic agents with therapeutical value. In addition to genetic searches, Drosophila also permits to recapitulate the biology of particular diseases in vivo systems, an approach that is been applied to the study of tumorigenesis using among other tissues the imaginal discs (Janic et al., 2010). In this manner Drosophila tissues can be used not only to track down the steps leading to tumour initiation, progression and metastasis in vivo, but also to manipulate in genetic mosaics the activity of genes leading to tumoral growth and to assay therapeutic drugs (Kango-Singh and Halder, 2004; Vidal and Cagan, 2006; Jang et al., 2007; Januschke and Gonzalez, 2008; Read et al., 2009; Caldeira et al., 2009; Das and Cagan, 2010; Bina et al., 2010; Wu et al., 2010). This approach is contributing to dissect the effects of tumour-promoting and tumour-suppressing genes in the regulation of proliferation, apoptosis, cell-adhesion, trafficking and cell polarity, and revealed the importance of cellular interactions in the outcome of tumoral progression. Finally, the modelling of specific cancers, such as type 2 multiple endocrine neoplasia (MEN2, caused by hyper-activation of RET; Read et al., 2005b) has allowed the design and use of pharmacological approaches to modify the phenotype caused by oncogenic forms of dRET (Das and Cagan, 2010). In addition, a similar approach prove successful in interfering with the activation of the EGFR (Aritakula and Ramasamy, 2008), suggesting that *Drosophila* has also the potential to be a robust model system for the screening of anticancer drugs in vivo.

8. Acknowledgements

We are very grateful to Ana Ruiz-Gómez and Antonio Baonza for criticism that greatly improved the manuscript. Work in our laboratory is funded by Grants BFU2009-09403 and CSD2007-00008 and by an institutional grant from Fundación Ramón Areces to the Centro de Biología Molecular Severo Ochoa. We apologize to all scientists whose contributions were not referenced in this review because of space limitations.

9. References

Adams, M. D. Celniker, S. E. Holt, R. A. Evans, C. A. Gocayne, J. D. Amanatides, P. G. Scherer, S. E. Li, P. W. Hoskins, R. A. Galle, R. F. et al. (2000). The genome sequence of Drosophila melanogaster. *Science* 287, 2185-95.

Akimaru, H., Chen, Y., Dai, P., Hou, D. X., Nonaka, M., Smolik, S. M., Armstrong, S., Goodman, R. H. and Ishii, S. (1997a). Drosophila CBP is a co-activator of cubitus interruptus in hedgehog signalling. *Nature* 386, 735-8.

Akimaru, H., Hou, D. X. and Ishii, S. (1997b). Drosophila CBP is required for dorsal-dependent twist gene expression. *Nat Genet* 17, 211-4.

Angers, S. and Moon, R. T. (2009). Proximal events in Wnt signal transduction. *Nat Rev Mol Cell Biol* 10, 468-77.

Aoki, Y.,Nihori,T, Kawame, H., Kurosawa, K., Ohashi, H., Tanaka, Y., Filocamo, M., Kato, K., Suzuki, Y., Kure, S. et al. (2005). Germline mutations in HRAS proto-oncogene cause Costello syndrome. *Nat Genet* 37, 1038-40.

Araujo, H., Negreiros, E. and Bier, E. (2003). Integrins modulate Sog activity in the Drosophila wing. *Development* 130, 3851-64.

Arbouzova, N. I. and Zeidler, M. P. (2006). JAK/STAT signalling in Drosophila: insights into conserved regulatory and cellular functions. *Development* 133, 2605-16.

Aritakula, A. and Ramasamy, A. (2008). Drosophila-based in vivo assay for the validation of inhibitors of the epidermal growth factor receptor/Ras pathway. *J. Biosci.* 33, 731-742.

Arnold, S. J. and Robertson, E. J. (2009). Making a commitment: cell lineage allocation and axis patterning in the early mouse embryo. *Nat Rev Mol Cell Biol* 10, 91-103.

Arnone, M. I. and Davidson, E. H. (1997). The hardwiring of development: organization and function of genomic regulatory systems. *Development* 124, 1851-64.

Avraham, R. and Yarden, Y. (2011). Feedback regulation of EGFR signalling: decision making by early and delayed loops. *Nat Rev Mol Cell Biol* 12, 104-17.

Axelrod, J. D. (2010). Delivering the lateral inhibition punchline: it's all about the timing. *Sci Signal* 3, pe38.

Bach, E. A., Vincent, S., Zeidler, M. P. and Perrimon, N. (2003). A Sensitized Genetic Screen to Identify Novel Regulators and Components of the Drosophila Janus Kinase/Signal Transducer and Activator of Transcription Pathway. *Genetics* 165, 1149-1166.

Bachmann, A. and Knust, E. (1998). Dissection of cis-regulatory elements of the Drosophila gene Serrate. *Dev. Genes Evol.* 208, 346-351.

Baeg, G.-H., Lin, X., Khare, N., Baumgartner, S. and Perrimon, N. (2001). Heparan sulfate proteoglycans are critical for the organization of the extracellular distribution of Wingless. *Development* 128, 87-94.

Baker, N. E. (2007). Patterning signals and proliferation in Drosophila imaginal discs. *Curr Opin Genet Dev* 17, 287-93.

Baker, R. G., Hayden, M. S. and Ghosh, S. (2011). NF-kappaB, inflammation, and metabolic disease. *Cell Metab* 13, 11-22.

Baonza, A., Murawsky, C. M., Travers, A. A. and Freeman, M. (2002). Pointed and Tramtrack69 establish an EGFR-dependent transcriptional switch to regulate mitosis. *Nat Cell Biol* 4, 976-980.

Bartscherer, K. and Boutros, M. (2008). Regulation of Wnt protein secretion and its role in gradient formation. *EMBO Rep* 9, 977-82.

Bao, Y., Hata, Y., Ikeda, M. and Withanage, K. (2011). Mammalian Hippo pathway: from development to cancer and beyond. *J Biochem* 149, 361-79.

Barker, N., Hurlstone, A., Musisi, H., Miles, A., Bienz, M. and Clevers, H. (2001). The chromatin remodelling factor Brg-1 interacts with beta-catenin to promote target gene activation. *EMBO J* 20, 4935-43.

Barrio, R., Lopez-Varea, A., Casado, M. and de Celis, J. F. (2007). Characterization of dSnoN and its relationship to Decapentaplegic signalling in Drosophila. *Dev Biol* 306, 66-81.

Beachy, P. A., Karhadkar, S. S. and Berman, D. M. (2004). Tissue repair and stem cell renewal in carcinogenesis. *Nature* 432, 324-31.

Bentires-Alj, M., Kontaridis, M. I. and Neel, B. G. (2006). Stops along the RAS pathway in human genetic disease. *Nat Med* 12, 283-5.

Bernard, F., Krejci, A., Housden, B., Adryan, B. and Bray, S. J. (2010). Specificity of Notch pathway activation: twist controls the transcriptional output in adult muscle progenitors. *Development* 137, 2633-42.

Bethani, I., Skanland, S. S., Dikic, I. and Acker-Palmer, A. (2010). Spatial organization of transmembrane receptor signalling. *EMBO J* 29, 2677-88.

Bhandari, P. and Shashidhara, L. S. (2001). Studies on human colon cancer gene APC by targeted expression in Drosophila. *Oncogene* 20, 6871-80.

Bina, S., Wright, V. M., Fisher, K. H., Milo, M. and Zeidler, M. P. (2010). Transcriptional targets of Drosophila JAK/STAT pathway signalling as effectors of haematopoietic tumour formation. *EMBO Rep* 11, 201-7.

Blair, E., Redwood, C., Ashrafian, H., Oliveira, M., Broxholme, J., Kerr, B., Salmon, A., Ostman-Smith, I. and Watkins, H. (2001). Mutations in the gamma(2) subunit of AMP-activated protein kinase cause familial hypertrophic cardiomyopathy: evidence for the central role of energy compromise in disease pathogenesis. *Hum Mol Genet* 10, 1215-20.

Bonn, S. and Furlong, E. E. (2008). cis-Regulatory networks during development: a view of Drosophila. *Curr Opin Genet Dev* 18, 513-20.

Bos, J. L. (1989). ras oncogenes in human cancer: a review. *Cancer Res* 49, 4682-9.

Botas, J. (2007). Drosophila researchers focus on human disease. *Nat Genet* 39, 589-91.

Branco, J., Al-Ramahi, I., Ukani, L., Perez, A. M., Fernandez-Funez, P., Rincon-Limas, D. and Botas, J. (2008). Comparative analysis of genetic modifiers in Drosophila points to common and distinct mechanisms of pathogenesis among polyglutamine diseases. *Hum Mol Genet* 17, 376-90.

Bray, S. J. (2006). Notch signalling: a simple pathway becomes complex. *Nat Rev Mol Cell Biol* 7, 678-89.

Brogiolo, W., Stocker, H., Ikeya, T., Rintelen, F., Fernandez, R. and Hafen, E. (2001). An evolutionarily conserved function of the Drosophila insulin receptor and insulin-like peptides in growth control. *Curr Biol* 11, 213-21.

Bromberg, J. (2002). Stat proteins and oncogenesis. *J Clin Invest* 109, 1139-42.

Caldeira, J., Pereira, P. S., Suriano, G. and Casares, F. (2009). Using fruitflies to help understand the molecular mechanisms of human hereditary diffuse gastric cancer. *Int J Dev Biol* 53, 1557-61.

Campisi, J. and d'Adda, F. (2007). Cellular senescence: when bad things happen to good cells. *Nature Reviews Molecular Cell Biology* 8, 729-740.

Carmena, A., Gisselbrecht, S., Harrison, J., Jimenez, F. and Michelson, A. M. (1998). Combinatorial signalling codes for the progressive determination of cell fates in the Drosophila embryonic mesoderm. *Genes Dev* 12, 3910-22.

Carbone, D. P. (2000). Chromosome 19 translocation, overexpression of Notch3, and human lung cancer. *J Natl Cancer Inst* 92, 1355-7.

Cavodeassi, F., Modolell, J. and Gomez-Skarmeta, J. L. (2001). The Iroquois family of genes: from body building to neural patterning. *Development* 128, 2847-55.

Cavodeassi, F., Rodriguez, I. and Modolell, J. (2002). Dpp signalling is a key effector of the wing-body wall subdivision of the Drosophila mesothorax. *Development* 129, 3815-3823.

Chen, Y., Riese, M. J., Killinger, M. A. and Hoffmann, F. M. (1998). A genetic screen for modifiers of Drosophila decapentaplegic signalling identifies mutations in punt, Mothers against dpp and the BMP-7 homologue, 60A. *Development* 125, 1759-1768.

Chen, Y., Goodman, R. H. and Smolik, S. M. (2000). Cubitus interruptus requires Drosophila CREB-binding protein to activate wingless expression in the Drosophila embryo. *Mol Cell Biol* 20, 1616-25.

Chen, Y. and Struhl, G. (1996). Dual roles for Patched in sequestering and transducing Hedgehog. *Cell* 87, 553-563.

Chien, S., Reiter, L. T., Bier, E. and Gribskov, M. (2002). Homophila: human disease gene cognates in Drosophila. *Nucleic Acids Res* 30, 149-51.

Chien, A. J., Conrad, W. H. and Moon, R. T. (2009). A Wnt survival guide: from flies to human disease. *J Invest Dermatol* 129, 1614-27.

Cho, E., Feng, Y., Rauskolb, C., Maitra, S., Fehon, R. and Irvine, K. D. (2006). Delineation of a Fat tumor suppressor pathway. *Nat Genet* 38, 1142-50.

Chopra, V. S. and Levine, M. (2009). Combinatorial patterning mechanisms in the Drosophila embryo. *Brief Funct Genomic Proteomic* 8, 243-9.

Clemens, J. C., Worby, C. A., Simonson-Leff, N., Muda, M., Maehama, T., Hemmings, B. A. and Dixon, J. E. (2000). Use of double-stranded RNA interference in Drosophila cell lines to dissect signal transduction pathways. *P.N.A.S.* 97, 6499-6503.

Cohen, B., Simcox, A. A. and Cohen, S. M. (1993). Allocation of the thoracic imaginal primordia in the Drosophila embryo. *Development* 117, 397-608.

Collins, R. T. and Cohen, S. M. (2005). A Genetic Screen in Drosophila for Identifying Novel Components of the Hedgehog Signalling Pathway. *Genetics* 170, 173-184.
Constantinescu, S. N., Girardot, M. and Pecquet, C. (2008). Mining for JAK-STAT mutations in cancer. *Trends Biochem Sci* 33, 122-31.
Cox, R. T., McEwen, D. G., Myster, D. L., Duronio, R. J., Loureiro, J. and Peifer, M. (2000). A screen for mutations that suppress the phenotype of Drosophila armadillo, the beta-catenin homolog. *Genetics* 155, 1725-40.
Crowther, D. C., Kinghorn, K. J., Page, R. and Lomas, D. A. (2004). Therapeutic targets from a Drosophila model of Alzheimer's disease. *Curr Opin Pharmacol* 4, 513-6.
Cruz, C., Glavic, A., Casado, M. and de Celis, J. F. (2009). A gain-of-function screen identifying genes required for growth and pattern formation of the Drosophila melanogaster wing. *Genetics* 183, 1005-26.
Cukier, H. N., Perez, A. M., Collins, A. L., Zhou, Z., Zoghbi, H. Y. and Botas, J. (2008). Genetic modifiers of MeCP2 function in Drosophila. *PLoS Genet* 4, e1000179.
Dai, H., Hogan, C., Gopalakrishnan, B., Torres-Vazquez, J., Nguyen, M., Park, S., Raftery, L. A., Warrior, R. and Arora, K. (2000). The zinc finger protein schnurri acts as a Smad partner in mediating the transcriptional response to decapentaplegic. *Dev Biol* 227, 373-87.
Dang, T. P., Gazdar, A. F., Virmani, A. K., Sepetavec, T., Hande, K. R., Minna, J. D., Roberts, J. R. ,
Dong, J., Feldmann, G., Huang, J., Wu, S., Zhang, N., Comerford, S. A., Gayyed, M. F., Anders, R. A., Maitra, A. and Pan, D. (2007). Elucidation of a universal size-control mechanism in Drosophila and mammals. *Cell* 130, 1120-33.
Das, T. and Cagan, R. (2010). Drosophila as a novel therapeutic discovery tool for thyroid cancer. *Thyroid* 20, 689-95.
DasGupta, R., Kaykas, A., Moon, R. T. and Perrimon, N. (2005). Functional genomic analysis of the Wnt-wingless signalling pathway. *Science* 308, 826-33.
de Celis, J. F. (2003). Pattern formation in the Drosophila wing: the development of the veins. *BioEssays* 25, 443-451.
de Celis, J. F., Barrio, R. and Kafatos, F. C. (1999). Regulation of the spalt/spalt-related gene complex and its function during sensory organ development in the Drosophila thorax. *Development* 126, 2653-2662.
de Celis, J. F. and Garcia-Bellido, A. (1994). Roles of the Notch gene in Drosophila wing morphogenesis. *Mech. Dev.*, 109-122.
Desbordes, S. C., Chandraratna, D. and Sanson, B. (2005). A Screen for Genes Regulating the Wingless Gradient in Drosophila Embryos. *Genetics* 170, 749-766.
Dichtel-Danjoy, M. L., Caldeira, J. and Casares, F. (2009). SoxF is part of a novel negative-feedback loop in the wingless pathway that controls proliferation in the Drosophila wing disc. *Development* 136, 761-9.
Downward, J. (2003). Targeting RAS signalling pathways in cancer therapy. *Nat Rev Cancer* 3, 11-22.
Duboc, V. and Logan, M. P. (2009). Building limb morphology through integration of signalling modules. *Curr Opin Genet Dev* 19, 497-503.
Dubnicoff, T., Valentine, S. A., Chen, G., Shi, T., Lengyel, J. A., Paroush, Z. and Courey, A. J. (1997). Conversion of dorsal from an activator to a repressor by the global corepressor Groucho. *Genes Dev* 11, 2952-7.

Ellisen, L. W., Bird, J., West, D. C., Soreng, A. L., Reynolds, T. C., Smith, S. D. and Sklar, J. (1991). TAN-1, the human homolog of the Drosophila notch gene, is broken by chromosomal translocations in T lymphoblastic neoplasms. *Cell* 66, 649-61.

Evans, D. G., Sainio, M. and Baser, M. E. (2000). Neurofibromatosis type 2. *J Med Genet* 37, 897-904.

Feng, X. H., Zhang, Y., Wu, R. Y. and Derynck, R. (1998). The tumor suppressor Smad4/DPC4 and transcriptional adaptor CBP/p300 are coactivators for smad3 in TGF-beta-induced transcriptional activation. *Genes Dev* 12, 2153-63.

Fernandez, B. G., Arias, A. M. and Jacinto, A. (2007). Dpp signalling orchestrates dorsal closure by regulating cell shape changes both in the amnioserosa and in the epidermis. *Mech Dev* 124, 884-97.

Fernandez-Funez, P., Nino-Rosales, M. L., de Gouyon, B., She, W. C., Luchak, J. M., Martinez, P., Turiegano, E., Benito, J., Capovilla, M., Skinner, P. J. et al. (2000). Identification of genes that modify ataxin-1-induced neurodegeneration. *Nature* 408, 101-6.

Flockhart, I., Booker, M., Kiger, A., Boutros, M., Armknecht, S., Ramadan, N., Richardson, C., Xu, T., Perrimon, N. and Mathey-Prevot, B. (2006). FlyRNAi: the Drosophila RNAi screening center database *Nucleic Acids Research* 34, 489-494.

Friedman, A. and Perrimon, N. (2006). A functional RNAi screen for regulators of receptor tyrosine kinase and ERK signalling. *Nature* 444, 230-4.

Funakoshi, Y., Minami, M. and Tabata, T. (2001). mtv shapes the activity gradient of the Dpp morphogen through regulation of thickveins. *Development* 128, 67-74.

Gerondakis, S., Grumont, R., Gugasyan, R., Wong, L., Isomura, I., Ho, W. and Banerjee, A. (2006). Unravelling the complexities of the NF-kappaB signalling pathway using mouse knockout and transgenic models. *Oncogene* 25, 6781-99.

Geuking, P., Narasimamurthy, R. and Basler, K. (2005). A Genetic Screen Targeting the Tumor Necrosis Factor/Eiger Signalling Pathway: Identification of Drosophila TAB2 as a Functionally Conserved Component. *Genetics* 171, 1683-1694.

Gilbert, M. M., Beam, C. K., Robinson, B. S. and Moberg, K. H. (2009). Genetic interactions between the Drosophila tumor suppressor gene ept and the stat92E transcription factor. *PLoS One* 4, e7083.

Go, M. J. and Artavanis-Tsakonas, S. (1998). A genetic screen for novel components of the Notch signalling pathway during Drosophila bristle development. *Genetics* 150, 211-220.

González Gaitán, M., Capdevila, M. P. and García Bellido, A. (1994). Cell proliferation patterns in the wing imaginal disc of Drosophila. *Mech. Dev.* 46, 183-200.

Gordon, K. J. and Blobe, G. C. (2008). Role of transforming growth factor-beta superfamily signalling pathways in human disease. *Biochim Biophys Acta* 1782, 197-228.

Goto, S. and Hayashi, S. (1997). Specification of the embryonic limb primordium by graded activity of Decapentaplegic. *Development* 124, 125-132.

Greaves, S., Sanson, B., White, P. and Vincent, J. P. (1999). A screen for identifying genes interacting with armadillo, the Drosophila homolog of beta-catenin. *Genetics* 153, 1753-66.

Greer, E. L. and Brunet, A. (2008). FOXO transcription factors in ageing and cancer. *Acta Physiol (Oxf)* 192, 19-28.

Grusche, F. A., Richardson, H. E. and Harvey, K. F. (2010). Upstream regulation of the hippo size control pathway. *Curr Biol* 20, R574-82.

Guichard, A., Srinivasan, S., Zimm, G. and Bier, E. (2002). A screen for dominant mutations applied to components in the Drosophila EGF-R pathway. *Proc Natl Acad Sci U S A* 99, 3752-7.

Haber, D. A. (2006). Transforming properties of YAP, a candidate oncogene on the chromosome 11q22 amplicon. *Proc Natl Acad Sci U S A* 103, 12405-10.

Haenlin, M., Kramatschek, B. and Campos-Ortega, J. A. (1990). The pattern of transcription of the neurogenic gene Delta of Drosophila melanogaster. *Development* 110, 905-914.

Haenlin, M., Kunisch, M., Kramatschek, B. and Campos-Ortega, J. A. (1994). Genomic regions regulating early embryonic expression of the Drosophila neurogenic gene Delta. *Mech. Dev.* 47, 99-110.

Haines, N. and van den Heuvel, M. (2000). A Directed Mutagenesis Screen in Drosophila melanogaster Reveals New Mutants That Influence hedgehog Signalling. *Genetics* 156, 1777-1785.

Halder, G. and Johnson, R. L. (2011). Hippo signalling: growth control and beyond. *Development* 138, 9-22.

Harper, J. A., Yuan, J. S., Tan, J. B., Visan, I. and Guidos, C. J. (2003). Notch signalling in development and disease. *Clin Genet* 64, 461-72.

Harvey, K. and Tapon, N. (2007). The Salvador-Warts-Hippo pathway - an emerging tumour-suppressor network. *Nat Rev Cancer* 7, 182-91.

Hasson, P. and Paroush, Z. (2007). Crosstalk between the EGFR and other signalling pathways at the level of the global transcriptional corepressor Groucho/TLE. *Br J Cancer* 96 Suppl, R21-5.

Hernan, I., Roig, I., Martin, B., Gamundi, M. J., Martinez-Gimeno, M. and Carballo, M. (2004). De novo germline mutation in the serine-threonine kinase STK11/LKB1 gene associated with Peutz-Jeghers syndrome. *Clin Genet* 66, 58-62.

Hietakangas, V. and Cohen, S. M. (2009). Regulation of tissue growth through nutrient sensing. *Annu Rev Genet* 43, 389-410.

Hoeller, D., Volarevic, S. and Dikic, I. (2005). Compartmentalization of growth factor receptor signalling. *Curr Opin Cell Biol* 17, 107-11.

Hoffmans, R. and Basler, K. (2004). Identification and in vivo role of the Armadillo-Legless interaction. *Development* 131, 4393-400.

Hombria, J. C. and Sotillos, S. (2008). Disclosing JAK/STAT links to cell adhesion and cell polarity. *Semin Cell Dev Biol* 19, 370-8.

Horvitz, H. R. and Sternberg, P. W. (1991). Multiple intercellular signalling systems control the development of the Caenorhabditis elegans vulva. *Nature* 351, 535-541.

Hou, S. X., Zheng, Z., Chen, X. and Perrimon, N. (2002). The Jak/STAT pathway in model organisms: emerging roles in cell movement. *Dev Cell* 3, 765-78.

Huang, A. M. and Rubin, G. M. (2000). A Misexpression Screen Identifies Genes That Can Modulate RAS1 Pathway Signalling in Drosophila melanogaster. *Genetics* 156, 1219-1230.

Igaki, T. (2009). Correcting developmental errors by apoptosis: lessons from Drosophila JNK signalling. *Apoptosis* 14, 1021-8.

Inoki, K., Corradetti, M. N. and Guan, K. L. (2005). Dysregulation of the TSC-mTOR pathway in human disease. *Nat Genet* 37, 19-24.

Irish, V. F. and Gelbart, W. M. (1987). The decapentaplegic gene is required for dorsal-ventral patterning of the Drosophila embryo. *Genes Dev* 1, 868-79.

Jackson, S. M., Nakato, H., Sugiura, M., Jannuzi, A., Oakes, R., Kaluza, V., Golden, C. and Selleck, S. B. (1997). dally, a Drosophila glypican, controls cellular responses to the TGF-beta-related morphogen, Dpp. *Development* 124, 4113-4120.

Jacob, L. and Lum, L. (2007). Deconstructing the hedgehog pathway in development and disease. *Science* 318, 66-8.

Jacobs, C. I. (2008). A review of the role of insulin-like growth factor 2 in malignancy and its potential as a modifier of radiation sensitivity. *Clin Oncol (R Coll Radiol)* 20, 345-52.

Jang, A. C., Starz-Gaiano, M. and Montell, D. J. (2007). Modeling migration and metastasis in Drosophila. *J Mammary Gland Biol Neoplasia* 12, 103-14.

Janic, A., Mendizabal, L., Llamazares, S., Rossell, D. and Gonzalez, C. (2010). Ectopic expression of germline genes drives malignant brain tumor growth in Drosophila. *Science* 330, 1824-7.

Janknecht, R., Wells, N. J. and Hunter, T. (1998). TGF-beta-stimulated cooperation of smad proteins with the coactivators CBP/p300. *Genes Dev* 12, 2114-9.

Januschke, J. and Gonzalez, C. (2008). Drosophila asymmetric division, polarity and cancer. *Oncogene* 27, 6994-7002.

Jiang, Z., Li, X., Hu, J., Zhou, W., Jiang, Y., Li, G. and Lu, D. (2006). Promoter hypermethylation-mediated down-regulation of LATS1 and LATS2 in human astrocytoma. *Neurosci Res* 56, 450-8.

Jin, T. (2008). The WNT signalling pathway and diabetes mellitus. *Diabetologia* 51, 1771-80.

Jones, S. M. and Kazlauskas, A. (2001). Growth factor-dependent signalling and cell cycle progression. *Chem Rev* 101, 2413-23.

Kango-Singh, M. and Halder, G. (2004). Drosophila as an emerging model to study metastasis. *Genome Biol* 5, 216.

Kango-Singh, M. and Singh, A. (2009). Regulation of organ size: insights from the Drosophila Hippo signalling pathway. *Dev Dyn* 238, 1627-37.

Karim, F. D., Chang, H. C., Therrien, M., Wassarman, D. A., Laverty, T. and Rubin, G. M. (1996). A Screen for Genes That Function Downstream of Ras1 During Drosophila Eye Development. *Genetics* 143, 315-329.

Kataoka, H. (2009). EGFR ligands and their signalling scissors, ADAMs, as new molecular targets for anticancer treatments. *J Dermatol Sci* 56, 148-53.

Kim, N. C. and Marques, G. (2010). Identification of downstream targets of the bone morphogenetic protein pathway in the Drosophila nervous system. *Dev Dyn* 239, 2413-25.

Kim, E. K. and Choi, E. J. Pathological roles of MAPK signalling pathways in human diseases. *Biochim Biophys Acta* 1802, 396-405.

Kimelman, D. (2006). Mesoderm induction: from caps to chips. *Nat Rev Genet* 7, 360-72.

Kleino, A., Valanne, S., Ulvila, J., Kallio, J., Myllymaki, H., Enwald, H., Stoven, S., Poidevin, M., Ueda, R., Hultmark, D. et al. (2005). Inhibitor of apoptosis 2 and TAK1-binding protein are components of the Drosophila Imd pathway. *EMBO J* 24, 3423-34.

Kuan, C. T., Wikstrand, C. J. and Bigner, D. D. (2001). EGF mutant receptor vIII as a molecular target in cancer therapy. *Endocr Relat Cancer* 8, 83-96.

Kumar, J. P. (2001). Signalling pathways in Drosophila and vertebrate retinal development. *Nat Rev Genet* 2, 846-57.

Lage, P., Jan, Y. N. and Jarman, A. P. (1997). Requirement for EGF receptor signalling in neural recruitment during formation of Drosophila chordotonal sense organ clusters. *Curr Biol* 7, 166-75.

Le Bras, S., Loyer, N. and Le Borgne, R. (2011). The multiple facets of ubiquitination in the regulation of notch signalling pathway. *Traffic* 12, 149-61.

Lecuit, T. and Cohen, S. M. (1998). Dpp receptor levels contribute to shaping the Dpp morphogen gradient in the Drosophila wing imaginal disc. *Development* 125, 4901-7.

Lindquist, R., Ottina, K., Wheeler1, D., Hsu, P., Thoreen, C., Guertin, D., Ali, S., Sengupta, S., Shaul, Y., Lamprecht, M. et al. (2011). Genome-scale RNAi on living-cell microarrays identifies novel regulators of Drosophila melanogaster TORC1–S6K pathway signalling *Genome Res.* 21, 433-446.

Logan, C. Y. and Nusse, R. (2004). The Wnt signalling pathway in development and disease. *Annu Rev Cell Dev Biol* 20, 781-810.

Luo, K., Stroschein, S. L., Wang, W., Chen, D., Martens, E., Zhou, S. and Zhou, Q. (1999). The Ski oncoprotein interacts with the Smad proteins to repress TGFbeta signalling. *Genes Dev* 13, 2196-206.

Lum, L., Yao, S., Mozer, B., Rovescalli, A., Von Kessler, D., Nirenberg, M. and Beachy, P. A. (2003). Identification of Hedgehog pathway components by RNAi in Drosophila cultured cells. *Science* 299, 2039-45.

Lupo, G., Harris, W. A. and Lewis, K. E. (2006). Mechanisms of ventral patterning in the vertebrate nervous system. *Nat Rev Neurosci* 7, 103-14.

Ma, X. M. and Blenis, J. (2009). Molecular mechanisms of mTOR-mediated translational control. *Nat Rev Mol Cell Biol* 10, 307-18.

Mahoney, M. B., Parks, A. L., Ruddy, D. A., Tiong, S. Y. K., Esengil, H., Phan, A. C., Philandrinos, P., Winter, C. G., Chatterjee, R., Huppert, K. et al. (2006). Presenilin-Based Genetic Screens in Drosophila melanogaster Identify Novel Notch Pathway Modifiers. *Genetics* 172, 2309-2324.

Massague, J., Blain, S. W. and Lo, R. S. (2000). TGFbeta signalling in growth control, cancer, and heritable disorders. *Cell* 103, 295-309.

Massague, J. and Wotton, D. (2000). Transcriptional control by the TGF-beta/Smad signalling system. *EMBO J* 19, 1745-54.

Matallanas, D., Romano, D., Hamilton, G., Kolch, W. and O'Neill, E. (2008). A Hippo in the ointment: MST signalling beyond the fly. *Cell Cycle* 7, 879-84.

Matthews, K. A., Kaufman, T. C. and Gelbart, W. M. (2005). Research resources for Drosophila: the expanding universe. *Nat Rev Genet* 6, 179-93.

Mendelsohn, J. and Baselga, J. (2000). The EGF receptor family as targets for cancer therapy. *Oncogene* 19, 6550-65.

Meyers, A. J., Shah, R. R., Gottlieb, P. A. and Zipris, D. (2010). Altered Toll-like receptor signalling pathways in human type 1 diabetes. *J Mol Med* 88, 1221-31.

McNeill, H. and Woodgett, J. R. (2010). When pathways collide: collaboration and connivance among signalling proteins in development. *Nat Rev Mol Cell Biol* 11, 404-13.

Milan, M., Campuzano, S. and Garcia-Bellido, A. (1996). Cell cycling and patterned cell proliferation in the wing primordium of Drosop[hila. *P.N.A.S.* 93, 640-645.

Miller, J. P., Holcomb, J., Al-Ramahi, I., de Haro, M., Gafni, J., Zhang, N., Kim, E., Sanhueza, M., Torcassi, C., Kwak, S. et al. (2010). Matrix metalloproteinases are modifiers of huntingtin proteolysis and toxicity in Huntington's disease. *Neuron* 67, 199-212.

Mills, I. G. (2007). The interplay between clathrin-coated vesicles and cell signalling. *Semin Cell Dev Biol* 18, 459-70.

Miura, G. I., Buglino, J., Alvarado, D., Lemmon, M. A., Resh, M. D. and Treisman, J. E. (2006). Palmitoylation of the EGFR ligand Spitz by Rasp increases Spitz activity by restricting its diffusion. *Dev Cell* 10, 167-76.

Miyazono, K., Kamiya, Y. and Morikawa, M. (2010). Bone morphogenetic protein receptors and signal transduction. *J Biochem* 147, 35-51.

Miyazono, K., Maeda, S. and Imamura, T. (2005). BMP receptor signalling: transcriptional targets, regulation of signals, and signalling cross-talk. *Cytokine Growth Factor Rev* 16, 251-63.

Mok, G. F. and Sweetman, D. (2011). Many routes to the same destination: lessons from skeletal muscle development. *Reproduction* 141, 301-12.

Molnar, C., Lopez-Varea, A., Hernandez, R. and de Celis, J. F. (2006). A gain-of-function screen identifying genes required for vein formation in the Drosophila melanogaster wing. *Genetics* 174, 1635-59.

Moussian, B. and Roth, S. (2005). Dorsoventral axis formation in the Drosophila embryo--shaping and transducing a morphogen gradient. *Curr Biol* 15, R887-99.

Mukherjee, T., Schafer, U. and Zeidler, M. P. (2006). Identification of Drosophila Genes Modulating Janus Kinase/Signal Transducer and Activator of Transcription Signal Transduction. *Genetics* 172, 1683-1697.

Muller, D., Kugler, S. J., Preiss, A., Maier, D. and Nagel, A. C. (2005a). Genetic Modifier Screens on Hairless Gain-of-Function Phenotypes Reveal Genes Involved in Cell Differentiation, Cell Growth and Apoptosis in Drosophila melanogaster. *Genetics* 171, 1137-1152.

Muller, P., Kuttenkeuler, D., Gesellchen, V., Zeidler, M. P. and Boutros, M. (2005b). Identification of JAK/STAT signalling components by genome-wide RNA interference. *Nature* 436, 871-5.

Mummery-Widmer, J. L., Yamazaki, M., Stoeger, T., Novatchkova, M., Bhalerao, S., Chen, D., Dietzl, G., Dickson, B. J. and Knoblich, J. A. (2009). Genome-wide analysis of Notch signalling in Drosophila by transgenic RNAi. *Nature* 458, 987-92.

Neufeld, T., de la Cruz, A., Johnston, L. and Edgar, B. (1998). Coordination of growth and cell division in the Drosophila wing. *Cell* 93, 1183-1193.

Nusse, R. (1999). WNT targets. Repression and activation. *Trends Genet* 15, 1-3.

Nusslein-Volhard, C. and Wieschaus, E. (1980). Mutations affecting segment number and polarity in Drosophila. *Nature* 287, 795-801.

Nybakken, K., Vokes, S. A., Lin, T. Y., McMahon, A. P. and Perrimon, N. (2005). A genome-wide RNA interference screen in Drosophila melanogaster cells for new components of the Hh signalling pathway. *Nat Genet* 37, 1323-32.

O'Neill, L. A. (2003). Therapeutic targeting of Toll-like receptors for inflammatory and infectious diseases. *Curr Opin Pharmacol* 3, 396-403.

O'Sullivan, L. A., Liongue, C., Lewis, R. S., Stephenson, S. E. and Ward, A. C. (2007). Cytokine receptor signalling through the Jak-Stat-Socs pathway in disease. *Mol Immunol* 44, 2497-506.

Overholtzer, M., Zhang, J., Smolen, G. A., Muir, B., Li, W., Sgroi, D. C., Deng, C. X., Brugge, J. S. and Pan, D. (2010). The hippo signalling pathway in development and cancer. *Dev Cell* 19, 491-505.

Pajni-Underwood, S., Wilson, C. P., Elder, C., Mishina, Y. and Lewandoski, M. (2007). BMP signals control limb bud interdigital programmed cell death by regulating FGF signalling *Development* 134, 2359-2368.

Parks, A. L., Turner, F. R. and Muskavitch, M. A. T. (1995). Relationships between complex Delta expression and the specification of retinal cell fates during Drosophila eye development. *Mech. Dev.* 50, 201-216.

Peacock, C. D., Wang, Q., Gesell, G. S., Corcoran-Schwartz, I. M., Jones, E., Kim, J., Devereux, W. L., Peifer, M. and Pham, A. D., Muller, S. and Sauer, F. (1999). Mesoderm-determining transcription in Drosophila is alleviated by mutations in TAF(II)60 and TAF(II)110. *Mech Dev* 84, 3-16.

Perea, D., Terriente, J. and Diaz-Benjumea, F. J. (2009). Temporal and spatial windows delimit activation of the outer ring of wingless in the Drosophila wing. *Dev Biol* 328, 445-55.

Perrimon, N. and McMahon, A. P. (1999). Negative feedback mechanisms and their roles during pattern formation. *Cell* 97, 13-16.

Petcherski, A. G. and Kimble, J. (2000). Mastermind is a putative activator for Notch. *Curr Biol* 10, R471-3.

Pfeifer, A. C., Timmer, J. and Klingmuller, U. (2008). Systems biology of JAK/STAT signalling. *Essays Biochem* 45, 109-20.

Pfeiffer, S. and Vincent, J. P. (1999). Signalling at a distance: transport of Wingless in the embryonic epidermis of Drosophila. *Semin Cell Dev Biol* 10, 303-9.

Pi, H. and Chien, C. T. (2007). Getting the edge: neural precursor selection. *J Biomed Sci* 14, 467-73.

Piddini, E. and Vincent, J. P. (2003). Modulation of developmental signals by endocytosis: different means and many ends. *Curr Opin Cell Biol* 15, 474-81.

Polakis, P. (2000). Wnt signalling in oncogenesis and embryogenesis--a look outside the nucleus. *Science* 287, 1606-9.

Pouponnot, C., Jayaraman, L. and Massague, J. (1998). Physical and functional interaction of SMADs and p300/CBP. *J Biol Chem* 273, 22865-8.

Qi, C., Zhu, Y. T., Hu, L. and Zhu, Y. J. (2009). Identification of Fat4 as a candidate tumor suppressor gene in breast cancers. *Int J Cancer* 124, 793-8.

Raftery, L. A., Twombly, V., Wharton, K. and Gelbart, W. M. (1995). Genetic screens to identify elements of the decapentaplegic signalling pathway in Drosophila. *Genetics* 139, 241-54.

Raftery, L. A. and Sutherland, D. J. (1999). TGF-beta family signal transduction in Drosophila development: from Mad to Smads. *Dev Biol* 210, 251-68.

Rane, S. G. and Reddy, E. P. (2000). Janus kinases: components of multiple signalling pathways. *Oncogene* 19, 5662-79.

Read, R. D., Cavenee, W. K., Furnari, F. B. and Thomas, J. B. (2009). A drosophila model for EGFR-Ras and PI3K-dependent human glioma. *PLoS Genet* 5, e1000374.

Read, R. D., Goodfellow, P. J., Mardis, E. R., Novak, N., Armstrong, J. R. and Cagan, R. L. (2005a). A Drosophila Model of Multiple Endocrine Neoplasia Type 2. *Genetics* 171, 1057-1081.

Rebay, I., Chen, F., Hsiao, F., Kolodziej, P. A., Kuang, B. H., Laverty, T., Suh, C., Voas, M., Williams, A. and Rubin, G. M. (2000). A Genetic Screen for Novel Components of the Ras/Mitogen-Activated Protein Kinase Signalling Pathway That Interact With the yan Gene of Drosophila Identifies split ends, a New RNA Recognition Motif-Containing Protein. *Genetics* 154, 695-712.

Reiter, L. T., Potocki, L., Chien, S., Gribskov, M. and Bier, E. (2001). A systematic analysis of human disease-associated gene sequences in Drosophila melanogaster. *Genome Res* 11, 1114-25.

Resnick, L. and Fennell, M. (2004). Targeting JNK3 for the treatment of neurodegenerative disorders. *Drug Discov Today* 9, 932-9.

Resnik-Docampo, M. and de Celis, J. F. (2011). MAP4K3 is a component of the TORC1 signalling complex that modulates cell growth and viability in Drosophila melanogaster. *PLoS One* 6, e14528.

Rhodes, J. T., Huff, C. A., Beachy, P. A. et al. (2007). Hedgehog signalling maintains a tumor stem cell compartment in multiple myeloma. *Proc Natl Acad Sci U S A* 104, 4048-53.

Ricci, R., Sumara, G., Sumara, I., Rozenberg, I., Kurrer, M., Akhmedov, A., Hersberger, M., Eriksson, U., Eberli, F. R., Becher, B. et al. (2004). Requirement of JNK2 for scavenger receptor A-mediated foam cell formation in atherogenesis. *Science* 306, 1558-61.

Rooke, H. M. and Crosier, K. E. (2001). The smad proteins and TGFbeta signalling: uncovering a pathway critical in cancer. *Pathology* 33, 73-84.

Roose, J., Molenaar, M., Peterson, J., Hurenkamp, J., Brantjes, H., Moerer, P., van de Wetering, M., Destree, O. and Clevers, H. (1998). The Xenopus Wnt effector XTcf-3 interacts with Groucho-related transcriptional repressors. *Nature* 395, 608-12.

Rorth, P., Szabo, K., Bailey, A., Laverty, T., Rehm, J., Rubin, G. M., Weigmann, K., Milan, M., Benes, V., Ansorge, W. et al. (1998). Systematic gain-of-function genetics in Drosophila. *Development* 125, 1049-57.

Rosner, M., Hanneder, M., Siegel, N., Valli, A., Fuchs, C. and Hengstschlager, M. (2008). The mTOR pathway and its role in human genetic diseases. *Mutat Res* 659, 284-92.

Ruiz-Gomez, A., Molnar, C., Holguin, H., Mayor, F., Jr. and de Celis, J. F. (2007). The cell biology of Smo signalling and its relationships with GPCRs. *Biochim Biophys Acta* 1768, 901-12.

Ruiz i Altaba, A., Sanchez, P. and Dahmane, N. (2002). Gli and hedgehog in cancer: tumours, embryos and stem cells. *Nat Rev Cancer* 2, 361-72.

Sang, T. K. and Jackson, G. R. (2005). Drosophila models of neurodegenerative disease. *NeuroRx* 2, 438-46.

Sato, M., Kojima, T., Michiue, T. and Saigo, K. (1999). Bar homeobox genes are latitudinal prepattern genes in the developing Drosophila notum whose expression is regulated by the concerted functions of decapentaplegic and wingless. *Development* 126, 1457-1466.

Schindler, C. W. (2002). Series introduction. JAK-STAT signalling in human disease. *J Clin Invest* 109, 1133-7.

Schwanbeck, R., Martini, S., Bernoth, K. and Just, U. (2010). The Notch signalling pathway: Molecular basis of cell context dependency. *Eur J Cell Biol.*

Schubbert, S., Shannon, K. and Bollag, G. (2007). Hyperactive Ras in developmental disorders and cancer. *Nat Rev Cancer* 7, 295-308.

Seidel, C., Schagdarsurengin, U., Blumke, K., Wurl, P., Pfeifer, G. P., Hauptmann, S., Taubert, H. and Dammann, R. (2007). Frequent hypermethylation of MST1 and MST2 in soft tissue sarcoma. *Mol Carcinog* 46, 865-71.

Seto, E. S. and Bellen, H. J. (2004). The ins and outs of Wingless signalling. *Trends Cell Biol* 14, 45-53.

Shilo, B. Z. (2003). Signalling by the Drosophila epidermal growth factor receptor pathway during development. *Exp Cell Res* 284, 140-9.

Smith, W. W., Gorospe, M. and Kusiak, J. W. (2006). Signalling mechanisms underlying Abeta toxicity: potential therapeutic targets for Alzheimer's disease. *CNS Neurol Disord Drug Targets* 5, 355-61.

So, E. Y. and Ouchi, T. (2010). The application of Toll like receptors for cancer therapy. *Int J Biol Sci* 6, 675-81.

Sorkin, A. and von Zastrow, M. (2009). Endocytosis and signalling: intertwining molecular networks. *Nat Rev Mol Cell Biol* 10, 609-22.

Sotillos, S. and De Celis, J. F. (2005). Interactions between the Notch, EGFR, and decapentaplegic signalling pathways regulate vein differentiation during Drosophila pupal wing development. *Dev Dyn* 232, 738-52.

Stanisic, V., Lonard, D. M. and O'Malley, B. W. (2010). Modulation of steroid hormone receptor activity. *Prog Brain Res* 181, 153-76.

Steinhardt, A. A., Gayyed, M. F., Klein, A. P., Dong, J., Maitra, A., Pan, D., Montgomery, E. A. and Anders, R. A. (2008). Expression of Yes-associated protein in common solid tumors. *Hum Pathol* 39, 1582-9.

Steinhauer, J. and Treisman, J. E. (2009). Lipid-modified morphogens: functions of fats. *Curr Opin Genet Dev* 19, 308-14.

Stern, C. (1954). Two or three bristles. *Am. Scientist*, 213-247.

Steventon, B., Araya, C., Linker, C., Kuriyama, S. and Mayor, R. (2009). Differential requirements of BMP and Wnt signalling during gastrulation and neurulation define two steps in neural crest induction. *Development* 136, 771-9.

Stroschein, S. L., Wang, W., Zhou, S., Zhou, Q. and Luo, K. (1999). Negative feedback regulation of TGF-beta signalling by the SnoN oncoprotein. *Science* 286, 771-4.

Su, G. H., Hilgers, W., Shekher, M. C., Tang, D. J., Yeo, C. J., Hruban, R. H. and Kern, S. E. (1998). Alterations in pancreatic, biliary, and breast carcinomas support MKK4 as a genetically targeted tumor suppressor gene. *Cancer Res* 58, 2339-42.

Su, M. A., Wisotzkey, R. G. and Newfeld, S. J. (2001). A Screen for Modifiers of decapentaplegic Mutant Phenotypes Identifies lilliputian, the Only Member of the Fragile-X/Burkitt's Lymphoma Family of Transcription Factors in Drosophila melanogaster. *Genetics* 157, 717-725.

Sumara, G., Belwal, M. and Ricci, R. (2005). "Jnking" atherosclerosis. *Cell Mol Life Sci* 62, 2487-94.

Sun, Y., Liu, X., Eaton, E. N., Lane, W. S., Lodish, H. F. and Weinberg, R. A. (1999a). Interaction of the Ski oncoprotein with Smad3 regulates TGF-beta signalling. *Mol Cell* 4, 499-509.

Sun, Y., Liu, X., Ng-Eaton, E., Lodish, H. F. and Weinberg, R. A. (1999b). SnoN and Ski protooncoproteins are rapidly degraded in response to transforming growth factor beta signalling. *Proc Natl Acad Sci U S A* 96, 12442-7.

Tabata, T. and Kornberg, T. B. (1994). Hedgehog is a signalling protein with a key role in patterning Drosophila imaginal discs. *Cell* 76, 89-102.

Taguchi, A., Sawamoto, K. and Okano, H. (2000). Mutations Modulating the Argos-Regulated Signalling Pathway in Drosophila Eye Development. *Genetics* 154, 1639-1648.

Taipale, J. and Beachy, P. A. (2001). The Hedgehog and Wnt signalling pathways in cancer. *Nature* 411, 349-54.

Tartaglia, M. and Gelb, B. D. (2005). Noonan syndrome and related disorders: genetics and pathogenesis. *Annu Rev Genomics Hum Genet* 6, 45-68.

Tazi-Ahnini, R., Cork, M. J., Wengraf, D., Wilson, A. G., Gawkrodger, D. J., Birch, M. P., Messenger, A. G. and McDonagh, A. J. (2003). Notch4, a non-HLA gene in the MHC is strongly associated with the most severe form of alopecia areata. *Hum Genet* 112, 400-3.

ten Dijke, P. and Arthur, H. M. (2007). Extracellular control of TGFbeta signalling in vascular development and disease. *Nat Rev Mol Cell Biol* 8, 857-69.

Thompson, B. J. (2010). Developmental control of cell growth and division in Drosophila. *Curr Opin Cell Biol* 22, 788-94.

Tomoyasu, Y., Nakamura, M. and Ueno, N. (1998). Role of Dpp signalling in prepattern formation of the dorsocentral mechanosensory organ in Drosophila melanogaster. *Development* 125, 4215-4224.

Towers, M. and Tickle, C. (2009). Generation of pattern and form in the developing limb. *Int J Dev Biol* 53, 805-12.

Turenchalk, G. S., St John, M. A., Tao, W. and Xu, T. (1999). The role of lats in cell cycle regulation and tumorigenesis. *Biochim Biophys Acta* 1424, M9-M16.

Tyler, D. M., Li, W., Zhuo, N., Pellock, B. and Baker, N. E. (2007). Genes affecting cell competition in Drosophila. *Genetics* 175, 643-57.

Urban, S., Lee, J. R. and Freeman, M. (2002). A family of Rhomboid intramembrane proteases activates all Drosophila membrane-tethered EGF ligands. *EMBO J* 21, 4277-86.

Ujike, H., Takehisa, Y., Takaki, M., Tanaka, Y., Nakata, K., Takeda, T., Kodama, M., Fujiwara, Y., Yamamoto, A. and Kuroda, S. (2001). NOTCH4 gene polymorphism and susceptibility to schizophrenia and schizoaffective disorder. *Neurosci Lett* 301, 41-4.

Valanne, S., Wang, J. H. and Ramet, M. (2011). The Drosophila Toll signalling pathway. *J Immunol* 186, 649-56.

van Der Heide, L. P., Hoekman, M. F. and Smidt, M. P. (2004). The ins and outs of FoxO shuttling: mechanisms of FoxO translocation and transcriptional regulation. *Biochem J* 380, 297-309.

van Slegtenhorst, M., de Hoogt, R., Hermans, C., Nellist, M., Janssen, B., Verhoef, S., Lindhout, D., van den Ouweland, A., Halley, D., Young, J. et al. (1997). Identification of the tuberous sclerosis gene TSC1 on chromosome 9q34. *Science* 277, 805-8.

Vargesson, N., Patel, K., Lewis, J. and Tickle, C. (1998). Expression patterns of Notch1, Serrate1, Serrate2 and Delta1 in tissues of the developing chick limb. *Mech Dev* 77, 197-9.

Verheyen, E. M., Purcell, K. J., Fortini, M. E. and Artavanis-Tsakonas, S. (1996). Analysis of Dominant Enhancers and Suppressors of Activated Notch in Drosophila. *Genetics* 144, 1127-1141.

Vidal, M. and Cagan, R. L. (2006). Drosophila models for cancer research. *Curr Opin Genet Dev* 16, 10-6.

Vivekanand, P., Tootle, T. L. and Rebay, I. (2004). MAE, a dual regulator of the EGFR signalling pathway, is a target of the Ets transcription factors PNT and YAN. *Mech Dev* 121, 1469-79.

Vu Manh, T. P., Mokrane, M., Georgenthum, E., Flavigny, J., Carrier, L., Semeriva, M., Piovant, M. and Roder, L. (2005). Expression of cardiac myosin-binding protein-C (cMyBP-C) in Drosophila as a model for the study of human cardiomyopathies. *Hum Mol Genet* 14, 7-17.

Wackerhage, H. and Ratkevicius, A. (2008). Signal transduction pathways that regulate muscle growth. *Essays Biochem* 44, 99-108.

Waeber, G., Delplanque, J., Bonny, C., Mooser, V., Steinmann, M., Widmann, C., Maillard, A., Miklossy, J., Dina, C., Hani, E. H. et al. (2000). The gene MAPK8IP1, encoding islet-brain-1, is a candidate for type 2 diabetes. *Nat Genet* 24, 291-5.

Waite, K. A. and Eng, C. (2003). From developmental disorder to heritable cancer: it's all in the BMP/TGF-beta family. *Nat Rev Genet* 4, 763-73.

Waltzer, L. and Bienz, M. (1998). Drosophila CBP represses the transcription factor TCF to antagonize Wingless signalling. *Nature* 395, 521-5.

Waltzer, L. and Bienz, M. (1999). A function of CBP as a transcriptional co-activator during Dpp signalling. *EMBO J* 18, 1630-41.

Wechsler-Reya, R. and Scott, M. P. (2001). The developmental biology of brain tumors. *Annu Rev Neurosci* 24, 385-428.

Wei, J. and Hemmings, G. P. (2000). The NOTCH4 locus is associated with susceptibility to schizophrenia. *Nat Genet* 25, 376-7.

Wesley, C. S. (1999). Notch and wingless regulate expression of cuticle patterning genes. *Mol Cell Biol* 19, 5743-58.

Whitworth, A. J. and Russell, S. (2003). Temporally dynamic response to Wingless directs the sequential elaboration of the proximodistal axis of the Drosophila wing. *Dev Biol* 254, 277-88.

Wright, V. M., Vogt, K. L., Smythe, E. and Zeidler, M. P. (2011). Differential activities of the Drosophila JAK/STAT pathway ligands Upd, Upd2 and Upd3. *Cell Signal* 23, 920-7.

Wu, J. and Cohen, S. M. (2002). Repression of Teashirt marks the initiation of wing development. *Development* 129, 2411-8.

Wu, M., Pastor-Pareja, J. C. and Xu, T. (2010). Interaction between Ras(V12) and scribbled clones induces tumour growth and invasion. *Nature* 463, 545-8.

Yang, M., Nelson, D., Funakoshi, Y. and Padgett, R. W. (2004). Genome-wide microarray analysis of TGFbeta signalling in the Drosophila brain. *BMC Dev Biol* 4, 14.

Zavadil, J. and Böttinger, E. P. (2005). TGF-beta and epithelial-to-mesenchymal transitions. *Oncogene* 24, 5764-5774.

Zecca, M. and Struhl, G. (2002). Subdivision of the Drosophila wing imaginal disc by EGFR-mediated signaling. *Development* 129, 1357-1368.

Zender, L., Spector, M. S., Xue, W., Flemming, P., Cordon-Cardo, C., Silke, J., Fan, S. T., Luk, J. M., Wigler, M., Hannon, G. J. et al. (2006). Identification and validation of oncogenes in liver cancer using an integrative oncogenomic approach. *Cell* 125, 1253-67.

Zeng, Q. and Hong, W. (2008). The emerging role of the hippo pathway in cell contact inhibition, organ size control, and cancer development in mammals. *Cancer Cell* 13, 188-92.

Zhou, S., Fujimuro, M., Hsieh, J. J., Chen, L., Miyamoto, A., Weinmaster, G. and Hayward, S. D. (2000). SKIP, a CBF1-associated protein, interacts with the ankyrin repeat domain of NotchIC To facilitate NotchIC function. *Mol Cell Biol* 20, 2400-10.

Zhu, H. and Lo, H. W. The Human Glioma-Associated Oncogene Homolog 1 (GLI1) Family of Transcription Factors in Gene Regulation and Diseases. *Curr Genomics* 11, 238-45.

Zhu, H. J. and Burgess, A. W. (2001). Regulation of transforming growth factor-beta signalling. *Mol Cell Biol Res Commun* 4, 321-30.

Zhu, J. and Mohan, C. (2010). Toll-like receptor signalling pathways--therapeutic opportunities. *Mediators Inflamm* 2010, 781235.

Zirin, J. D. and Mann, R. S. (2007). Nubbin and Teashirt mark barriers to clonal growth along the proximal-distal axis of the Drosophila wing. *Dev Biol* 304, 745-58.

Zoncu, R., Efeyan, A. and Sabatini, D. M. (2011). mTOR: from growth signal integration to cancer, diabetes and ageing. *Nat Rev Mol Cell Biol* 12, 21-35.

2

The FGF Family in Humans, Mice, and Zebrafish: Development, Physiology, and Pathophysiology

Sayaka Sasaki, Hiroya Ohta, Yoshiaki Nakajima,
Morichika Konishi, Ayumi Miyake and Nobuyuki Itoh
Kyoto University Graduate School of Pharmaceutical Sciences
Japan

1. Introduction

In vertebrates, various signaling pathways are activated in a highly coordinated manner to ensure proper development and morphogenesis. Secreted signaling molecules such as FGFs (Fibroblast growth factors), BMPs (Bone morphogenetic factors), WNTs (Wingless/int), and Hedgehogs play crucial roles in development and morphogenesis by acting over variable distances to influence intracellular signaling events in neighboring cells. FGFs are polypeptide growth factors with diverse biological functions. The human FGF family comprises twenty-two members. The mouse and zebrafish are widely used vertebrate models for studying gene function *in vivo*. The mouse and zebrafish FGF families comprise twenty-two and twenty-eight members, respectively. These FGFs can be classified as paracrine, endocrine, and intracrine FGFs by their mechanisms of action (Itoh & Ornitz, 2008). Paracrine FGFs (canonical FGFs) mediate biological responses by binding to and activating cell surface tyrosine kinase FGFRs. They act as local paracrine signaling molecules and function in multiple developmental processes including differentiation, cell proliferation, and migration (Itoh & Ornitz, 2008; Beenken & Mohammadi, 2009). Endocrine FGFs are thought to mediate biological responses in an FGFR-dependent manner. However, they function over long distances as endocrine hormones (Kharitonenkov, 2009; Itoh, 2010). In contrast, intracrine FGFs act as FGFR-independent intracellular molecules that regulate the function of voltage-gated sodium channels (Goldfarb et al., 2007; Laezza et al., 2009).

Targeted mutagenesis of *Fgf* genes in mice has elucidated their functions in development and metabolism. Studies with zebrafish *Fgf* mutant and knockdown embryos also have revealed their functions in development. In addition, evidence for the involvement of FGF signaling in hereditary, paraneoplastic, and metabolic diseases has also accumulated. FGF signaling disorders contribute to pathological conditions. In this article, we provide a succinct review of the FGF family in humans, mice, and zebrafish and their developmental physiological and pathophysiological roles.

2. The human/mouse FGF family

FGF1 and FGF2 are prototypic FGFs originally isolated from the brain and pituitary as mitogens for cultured fibroblasts (Gospodarowicz, 1975; Gospodarowicz, et al., 1978). New

FGF proteins have since been isolated as growth factors for cultured cells or been identified as oncogene products. In addition, new *Fgf* genes have been identified by homology-based PCR/DNA database searching and as genes responsible for hereditary diseases or cancer (Itoh & Ornitz, 2008; Beenken & Mohammadi, 2009; Itoh, 2007; Krejci et al., 2009; Turner & Grose, 2010). The human/mouse *Fgf* family comprises twenty-two members, *Fgf1-Fgf23*. No other *Fgf* genes have been identified in the human/mouse genome.

Human/mouse FGFs are proteins of ~150-300 amino acids and have a conserved core of ~120-amino acids with ~30-60% identity. *Fgf15* has not been identified in humans. *Fgf19* has not been identified in mice. *Fgf15* and *Fgf19* are likely to be orthologous genes in vertebrates. Except for rodents, the orthologs are named *Fgf19* in vertebrates (Itoh & Ornitz, 2004; Itoh & Ornitz, 2008). In this review, we refer to these genes as *Fgf15/19*. Phylogenetic analysis indicates potential evolutionary relationships in the gene family. However, this alone is not sufficient to determine the relationships. Analyzing gene loci on chromosomes gives a more precise indication of the evolutionary relationships in a gene family. The gene location analysis of the human/mouse *Fgf* family has identified seven subfamilies; *Fgf/1/2/5*, *Fgf3/4/6*, *Fgf7/10/22*, *Fgf8/17/18*, *Fgf9/16/20*, *Fgf11/12/13/14*, and *Fgf15/19/21/23* (Itoh & Ornitz, 2004; Itoh & Ornitz, 2008). FGFs can also be classified as paracrine, endocrine, and intracrine FGFs based on their mechanisms of action (Fig. 1). Paracrine FGFs comprise members of the FGF/1/2/5, FGF3/4/6, FGF7/10/22, FGF8/17/18, and FGF9/16/20 subfamilies. They are secreted proteins, which mediate biological responses in a paracrine manner. Endocrine FGFs, FGF15/19, FGF21, and FGF23, are also secreted proteins. However, they mediate biological responses in an endocrine manner. Intracrine FGFs, FGF11-FGF14, are intracellular proteins, which mediate biological responses in an intracrine manner (Fig. 2).

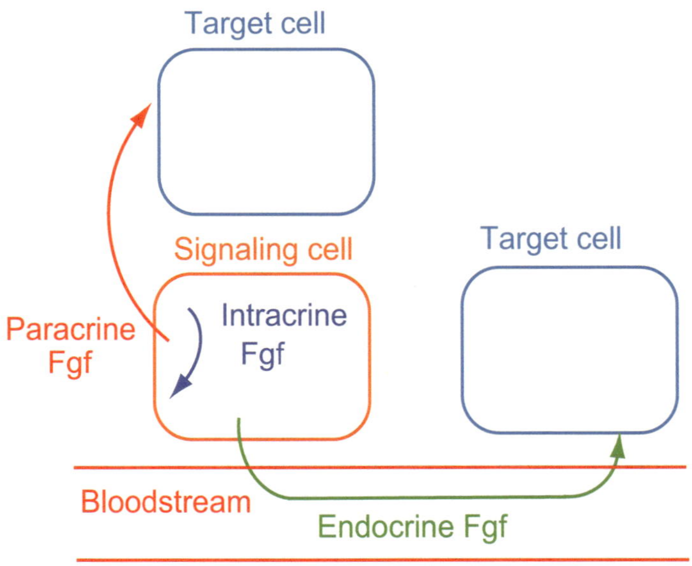

Fig. 1. Action mechanisms of Fgfs. Fgfs act on target cells in a paracrine, endocrine , or intracrine manner.

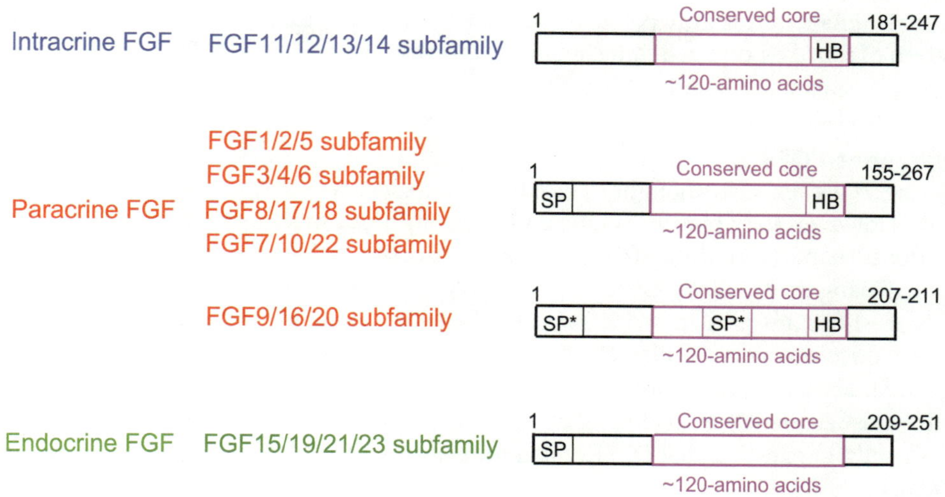

Fig. 2. Schematic representations of structure. Schematic diagrams of intracrine, paracrine, and endocrine FGFs are shown. SP, SP* and HB indicate a cleavable secreted signal sequence, an uncleaved bipartite secreted signal sequence, and a heparin-binding site, respectively.

3. Mechanisms of action

3.1 Paracrine FGFs

Most paracrine FGFs are secreted proteins with cleavable N-terminal secreted signal peptides. However, FGF9, FGF16, and FGF20 have uncleaved bipartite secreted signal sequences (Revest et al., 2000). By contrast, FGF1 and FGF2 without N-terminal signal sequences are not typical secreted proteins. They might be released from damaged cells or by an exocytotic mechanism that is independent of the endoplasmic reticulum-Golgi pathway (Mohan et al., 2010; Nickel, 2010). Paracrine FGFs mediate biological responses as extracellular proteins by binding to and activating cell surface tyrosine kinase FGFR receptors (FGFRs) with heparin/heparan sulfate as a cofactor.

The human/mouse *Fgfr* gene family comprises four *Fgfr* genes, *Fgfr1*–*Fgfr4* (Beenken & Mohammadi, 2009; Turner & Grose, 2010). All FGFR proteins are receptor tyrosine kinases of ~800 amino acids with an extracellular ligand-binding domain with three immunoglobulin-like domains (I, II, and III). *Fgfr1*–*Fgfr3* encode two major versions of immunoglobin-like domain III (IIIb and IIIc) generated by alternative splicing that utilizes one of two unique exons. The immunoglobulin-like domain III is an essential determinant of ligand-binding specificity (Zhang et al., 2006). Thus, seven major FGFR proteins (FGFRs 1b, 1c, 2b, 2c, 3b, 3c, and 4) with differing ligand-binding specificity are generated from four *Fgfr* genes.

Paracrine FGFs have a heparin-binding site and interaction with heparin-like molecules is necessary for their stable interaction with FGFRs and local signaling (Goetz et al., 2007). Paracrine FGFs function in development by influencing the intracellular signaling events of neighboring cells from a distance. The range of FGF signaling is regulated in part by affinity for extracellular matrix heparan sulfate proteoglycans (Kalinina et al., 2009) and in part by the dimerization of some FGFs (Kalinina et al., 2009; Harada et al., 2009). The binding of FGFs to FGFRs induces functional dimerization, receptor transphosphorylation, and the activation of four key downstream signaling pathways: RAS-RAF-MAPK, PI3K-AKT, STAT, and PLCγ (Beenken & Mohammadi, 2009; Turner & Grose, 2010).

3.2 Endocrine FGFs

Endocrine FGFs are also thought to mediate biological responses in an FGFR-dependent manner. However, they bind to FGFRs and heparin/heparan sulfate with very low affinity. The reduced heparin-binding affinity enables endocrine FGFs to function in an endocrine manner (Zhang et al., 2006; Goetz et al., 2007). αKlotho is a single-pass transmembrane protein of ~1,000 amino acids with a short cytoplasmic domain. The phenotypes of *αKlotho* knockout mice are very similar to those of *Fgf23* knockout mice (Shimada et al., 2004), indicating that FGF23 and αKlotho may function in a common signal transduction pathway. αKlotho most efficiently binds to and activates FGFR1c among several isoforms of FGFRs in cultured cells, suggesting that FGFR1c can transduce an FGF23/αKlotho signal(Urakawa et al., 2006).

βKlotho is a protein that shares structural similarity and characteristics with αKlotho. The phenotypes of *βKlotho* knockout mice overlap those of *Fgfr4* knockout mice and *Fgf15/19* knockout mice (Ito et al., 2005; Inagaki et al., 2005). FGF15/19 can bind to a βKlotho-FGFR4 complex in cultured cells. FGF15/19 also activates FGF signaling in hepatocytes that primarily express *Fgfr4* (Kurosu et al., 2007). These results indicate FGFR4 to be the primary receptor for transduction of an FGF15/19/βKlotho signal. βKlotho is also essential for FGF21 signaling in cultured cells (Kharitonenkov et al., 2008). However, *Fgf21* knockout mouse phenotypes are distinct from *βKlotho* knockout mouse phenotypes (Ito et al., 2005; Hotta et al., 2009). In addition, the administration of recombinant human FGF21 to *βKlotho* knockout mice demonstrated that FGF21 signals can be transduced in the absence of βKlotho (Tomiyama et al., 2010). These results indicate the existence of a βKlotho-independent FGF21 signaling pathway in which undefined cofactors might be involved.

3.3 Intracrine FGFs

Intracrine FGFs interact with intracellular domains of voltage-gated sodium channels and with a neuronal MAPK scaffold protein, islet-brain-2 (Schoorlemmer & Goldfarb, 2002; Goldfarb et al., 2007). The only known role for intracrine FGFs is in regulating the electrical excitability of neurons and possibly other cell types (Goldfarb et al., 2007; Xiao et al., 2007; Shakkottai et al., 2009; Dover et al., 2010).

4. Evolutionary history of the human/mouse *Fgf* gene family

The FGF signaling system has been conserved throughout metazoan evolution. Two *Fgf-like* genes have been identified in the nematode, *C. elegans* (Huang & Stern, 2005). Six *Fgf-like* genes, which are potential ancestral genes of the human/mouse *Fgf* subfamilies, have been identified in the ascidian, *C. intestinalis* (Satou et al., 2002). Ascidians belong to the Subphylum Urochordata, the earliest branch in the Phylum Chordata. These results indicate that most ancestral genes of the human/mouse *Fgf* subfamilies were generated by gene duplication after the diversion of protostomes and deuterostomes. The evolutionary history of the mouse *Fgf* family has been proposed (Fig. 3) (Itoh & Ornitz, 2008). The ancestral gene of the *Fgf* family is an ancestral intracrine *Fgf* gene, *Fgf13-like*, with a heparin-binding site but no secreted signal sequence. An ancestral gene of paracrine *Fgfs*, *Fgf4-like*, was generated from *Fgf13-like* by gene duplication during the early stages of metazoan evolution. During this evolution, *Fgf4-like* acquired a secreted signal sequence, thus allowing it to function as a paracrine *Fgf*. Ancestral genes, *Fgf5-like, Fgf8-like, Fgf9-like*, and *Fgf10-like*, of paracrine *Fgf* subfamilies were also generated from *Fgf4-like* by gene duplication after the separation of protostomes and deuterostomes. Secreted signal sequences were conserved in *Fgf5-like, Fgf8-like*, and *Fgf10-like*. A cleavable secreted signal sequence also evolved into an uncleaved bipartite signal sequence in *Fgf9-like*. These FGFs with heparin-binding sites function in a paracrine manner. In contrast, no ancestral gene of endocrine *Fgfs* has been identified in *Ciona intestinalis*. The ancestral gene of endocrine *Fgfs*, *Fgf15/19-like*, appears to have arisen from *Fgf4-like* by local gene duplication early in vertebrate evolution. During this evolution, *Fgf15/19-like* lost its high affinity heparin-binding capacity, thus allowing it to function in an endocrine manner. Conserved gene orders are observed among members of each *Fgf* subfamily, indicating that each subfamily further expanded into three or four members via two large-scale genome duplication events (R1 and R2) during the evolution of early vertebrates.

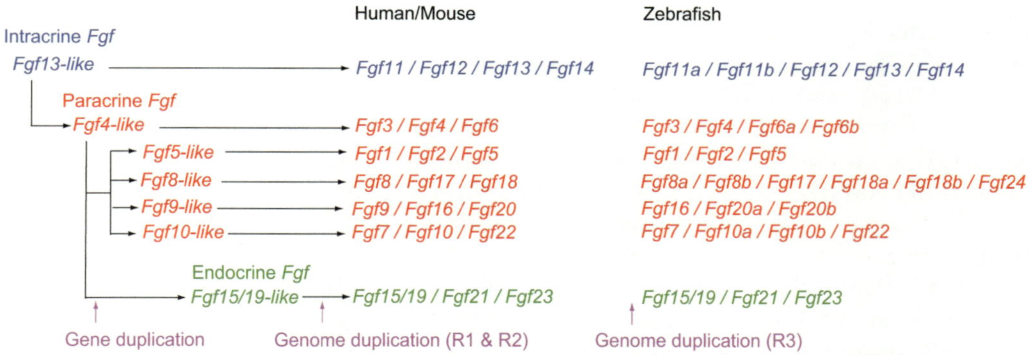

Fig. 3. The functional evolutionary history of the human/mouse/zebrafish *Fgf* gene family. *Fgf13-like* is the ancestral gene of the *Fgf* family. *Fgf4-like* was generated from *Fgf13-like* by gene duplication during the early stages of metazoan evolution. *Fgf5-like, Fgf8-like, Fgf9-like*, and *Fgf10-like* were generated from *Fgf4-like* by gene duplication. *Fgf15/19-like* was also generated from *Fgf4-like* by local gene duplication. Each subfamily further expanded into three or four members via two genome duplication events (R1 &R2) during the evolution of early vertebrates. The zebrafish *Fgf* family further expanded via an additional genome duplication event (R3) shortly after the teleost radiation.

5. The zebrafish FGF family

Almost all zebrafish orthologs of human/mouse *Fgf* genes except for *Fgf9* have been identified. In addition, *Fgf24* has been identified in zebrafish as well as all teleosts examined including the stickleback, medaka, and puffer fish. However, *Fgf24* has not been identified in all tetrapods examined. These results indicate that *Fgf9* and *Fgf24* were lost in the teleost lineage and tetrapod lineage during evolution, respectively. Zebrafish also has six additional *Fgf* genes including *Fgf6b, Fgf8b, fgf10b, fgf13b, fgf18b*, and *fgf20b*. The zebrafish *Fgf* family comprises twenty-eight members. Analysis of the location of the additional genes indicates that they are paralogs (Fig. 3) (Itoh & Konsihi, 2007). Comparisons of mammalian genes with genes of teleost fish have shown that in teleosts, including zebrafish, there are often two homologs of the mammalian equivalent. This suggests that there has been an additional genome duplication event (R3) shortly after the teleost radiation. This duplication must have been either a partial or a whole genome duplication followed by rapid gene loss because gene duplications account for only ~20% of the zebrafish genes examined (Nusslein-Volhard et al., 2002). Zebrafish *Fgf* paralogs were also generated by genome duplication.

6. Physiological roles of FGFs indicated by *Fgf* knockout mouse phenotypes

The mouse is a widely used mammalian model for studying functions of genes. Gene functions can be effectively blocked in mice by targeted disruption of genes. Gene knockout mouse phenotypes have indicated their physiological functions. Most *Fgf* genes have been disrupted in mice. Phenotypes range from early embryonic lethality to changes in adult physiology (Table 1). Paracrine, endocrine, and intracrine FGFs mostly play roles in development, and metabolism, and neuronal functions, respectively.

6.1 Paracrine Fgfs

Paracrine FGFs are a major FGF group, canonical FGFs, including FGF1-FGF10, FGF16-FGF18, FGF20, and FGF22. Knockout mouse phenotypes mostly indicate roles as growth/differentiation factors. *Fgf1* knockout mice are viable and normal (Miller, et al., 2000). *Fgf2* knockout mice are also viable, but have decreased vascular tone and reduced numbers of neurons in deep cortical layers (Raballo et al., 2000; Zhou et al., 1998; Dono et al., 1998). In addition, *Fgf2* knockout mice show impaired recovery from ischemic injury to the heart (House et al., 2003; Virag et al., 2007). *Fgf3* knockout mice are viable, but have phenotypes that include inner ear agenesis and dysgenesis, microtia, and microdontia (Mansour et al., 1993; Alvarez et al., 2003; Tekin et al., 2007)). *Fgf4* and *Fgf8* knockout mice die at early embryonic stages. *Fgf4* and *Fgf8* have essential roles in blastocyst formation and gastrulation, respectively (Feldman et al., 1995; Sun et al., 1999). Conditional inactivation of *Fgf8* has identified additional roles in limb bud development and organogenesis. *Fgf5*, *Fgf6*, and *Fgf7* knockout mice are viable. Abnormal long hair is observed in *Fgf5* knockout mice (Hébert et al., 1994). *Fgf6* knockout mice have defects in muscle regeneration (Floss et al., 1997). *Fgf7* knockout mice have impaired hair and kidney development (Guo et al., 1996; Qiao et al., 1999). *Fgf9*, *Fgf10*, and *Fgf18* knockout mice die shortly after birth. *Fgf10* is critical for epithelial-mesenchymal interactions necessary for the development of epithelial components of multiple organs (Min et al., 1998; Sekine et al., 1999; Ohuchi et al., 2000; Sakaue et al., 2002). *Fgf9* and *Fgf18* have essential roles in the development of mesenchymal components of multiple organs (Colvin et al., 2001a,b; Colvin et al., 2001; Ohbayashi et al., 2002; Liu et ,al. 2002; Usui et al., 2004; Hung et al., 2007). *Fgf16* knockout mice on a C57BL/6 genetic background are viable, but have impaired embryonic cardiomyocyte proliferation (Hotta et al., 2008). *Fgf16* knockout phenotypes may be more severe on a Black Swiss genetic background where they die at embryonic day (E) 10.5 with severely impaired cardiac and facial development (Lu et al., 2008; Lu et al., 2010). *Fgf17* and *Fgf22* knockout mice are viable, but show impaired hindbrain development and impaired synaptic differentiation, respectively (Xu et al., 2000; Terauchi et al., 2010). In addition, *Fgf22* knockout mice also show a clear delay in weight gain upon sexual maturity (Grose et al., unpublished data).

Fgf20 knockout mice are viable but have profound hearing loss (Ornitz et al., unpublished data).

FGF	Physiological roles
FGF1	None identified
FGF2	Loss of vascular tone, slight loss of cortical neurons, defects in heart repair
FGF3	Inner ear agenesis, microtia, microdontia
FGF4	Defects in blastocyst formation
FGF5	Abnormal long hair
FGF6	Defective muscle regeneration
FGF7	Impaired hair and kidney development
FGF8	Defects in gastrulation, limb development, organogenesis
FGF9	Impaired multiple organ development
FGF10	Impaired multiple organ development
FGF11	-
FGF12	None identified, functional redundancy with *Fgf14*
FGF13	-
FGF14	Ataxia, paraoxysmal hyperkinetic movement disorder
FGF15/19 *	Impaired cardiac outflow tract morphogenesis and bile acid metabolism
FGF16	Impaired cardiac and facial development Impaired embryonic cardiomyocte proliferation
FGF17	Impaired hindbrain development
FGF18	Impaired multiple organ development
FGF20	Impaired inner ear development
FGF21	Impaired lipid metabolism
FGF22	Impaired synapse differentiation and delay in weight gain
FGF23	Impaired phosphate and vitamin D metabolism

Table 1. Physiological roles of FGFs indicated by *Fgf* knockout mice Phenotypes of most *Fgf* knockout mice have been published. Phenotypes of *Fgf11*, *Fgf13*, and *Fgf20* knockout mice have not been published. **Fgf15* is referred to as *Fg15/19*.

Although roles of paracrine FGFs in embryogenesis have been revealed from knockout mouse phenotypes, their contributions to adult physiology remain relatively unexplored. The widespread expression of paracrine *Fgf* genes in adult tissues suggests multiple roles in tissue homeostasis and repair (Fon Tacer et al., 2010). Emerging reports indicate homeostatic and regenerative roles for paracrine FGF signaling (Böhm et al., 2010; Yang et al., 2010).

6.2 Endocrine Fgfs

Endocrine FGFs, FGF15/19, FGF21, and FGF23, are hormone-like FGFs. Hormones are usually responsible for communication between tissues in an endocrine manner. However, several hormones are produced in developing tissues that are unrelated to the endocrine gland of origin in adults. These hormones are synthesized locally, and serve as differentiation factors in embryos (Sanders & Harvey, 2008). Endocrine FGFs also act as differentiation factors in embryos and as hormones in adults (Itoh, 2010).

Fgf15/19 knockout mice develop normally until E10.5, but then gradually die. The phenotype indicates that FGF15/19 is required for proper morphogenesis of the cardiac outflow tract at embryonic stages (Vincentz et al., 2005). Although most *Fgf15/19* knockout mice die by postnatal day (P) 7, a few survive and appear phenotypically normal. However, fecal bile acid excretion was found to be increased in surviving *Fgf15/19* knockout mice, indicating that intestinal FGF15/19 plays a crucial role in regulating hepatic bile acid synthesis (Inagaki et al., 2005). *Fgf21* knockout mice are seemingly normal, but show hypertrophy and decreased lipolysis in adipocytes. In contrast, *Fgf21* knockout mice fasted for 24 h show increased lipolysis in adipocytes and increased serum nonesterified fatty acid levels. Their phenotypes indicate that *Fgf21* is important for the metabolic regulation of lipolysis in white adipose tissue (Hotta et al., 2009). *Fgf21* knockout mice fed a ketogenic diet show partial impairments in ketogenesis (Badman et al., 2009). However, we have observed that ketogenesis is not impaired in *Fgf21* knockout mice fed a ketogenic diet (Itoh et al., unpublished data). *Fgf23* knockout mice survive until birth, but then gradually die, usually by 12 weeks of age (Shimada et al., 2004). The mice show hyperphosphatemia and increased active vitamin D levels. *Fgf23,* which is expressed in osteocytes, signals to the kidney where it regulates serum phosphate and active vitamin D levels. FGF23 may have other targets including the parathyroid gland and osteoblasts (Ben-Dov et al., 2007; Tang et al., 2010).

6.3 Intracrine Fgfs

Intracrine FGFs, FGF11-FGF14, are intracellular proteins. *Fgf14* knockout mice are viable. However, they develop ataxia and a paraoxysmal hyperkinetic movement disorder (Goldfarb et al., 2007; Xiao et al., 2007; Shakkottai et al., 2009). In contrast, *Fgf12* knockout mice are apparently normal. *Fgf12*/*Fgf14* double knockout mice show severe ataxia and other neurological deficits (Goldfarb et al., 2007). Phenotypes of *Fgf11* and *Fgf13* knockout mice have not been reported.

7. Roles of FGFs indicated by *Fgf* mutated or knockdown zebrafish phenotypes

The zebrafish is also a widely used vertebrate model for studying functions of genes. Because zebrafish embryos are small, the fertilization and subsequent embryonic development occur externally, and the development is rapid (Nusslein-Volhard et al., 2002), phenotypes of zebrafish embryos in which the functions of genes are blocked–the knockout of which is lethal at early embryonic stages in mice–can be potentially analyzed. In a large-scale screening, many zebrafish mutants, which were mutagenized with ethylnitrosourea, displaying distinct phenotypes in embryos were generated (Haffter et al., 1996). Furthermore, antisense morpholino oligonucleotides can easily block the functions of multiple genes in zebrafish embryos (Nasevicius & Ekker, 2000). Therefore the zebrafish is expected to be a useful vertebrate model for studying physiological functions of *Fgf* genes *in vivo*.

7.1 Paracrine FGFs

Several zebrafish paracrine *Fgf* mutants have been generated by mutagenesis with ethylnitrosourea. *acerebellar* is a mutation of *Fgf8*. *acerebellar* embryos lack a cerebellum and the midbrain-hindbrain boundary organizer (Reifers et al., 1998). *ikarus* is a mutation of *Fgf24*. *ikarus* embryos lack pectoral fin buds (Fischer et al., 2003). *daedalus* is a mutation of *Fgf10*. *Daedalus* embryos have no pectoral fin buds either and a severely dysmorphic hepatopancreatic ductal system (Norton et al., 2005; Dong et al., 2007). *devoid of blastema* is a mutation of *Fgf20a*. *devoid of blastema* embryos have no pectoral fin buds (Whitehead et al., 2005). These results indicate that zebrafish fgfs also play crucial roles in development.
Several paracrine *Fgf* knockdown zebrafish embryos were generated using antisense morpholino oligonucleotides. Phenotypes of these embryos indicate roles of Fgfs in zebrafish. FGF1 is required for normal differentiation of erythrocytes (Songhet et al., 2007). FGF3 and FGF8 are required together for formation of the otic placode and vesicle (Maroon et al., 2002). FGF4 is required for left-right patterning of visceral organs (Yamauchi et al., 2009). In addition, FGF16 is also required for the fin buds to form (Nomura et al., 2006).

7.2 Endocrine FGFs

Fgf15/19 and *Fgf21* knockdown zebrafish embryos were generated using antisense morpholino oligonucleotides. FGF15/19 and FGF21 are required for the forebrain and eye to develop (Miyake et al., 2005; Nakayama et al., 2008), and hematopoiesis (Yamauchi et al., 2006).

8. FGF signaling disorders in human diseases

As described above, FGF signaling is crucial to development, metabolism, and neuronal functions as paracrine, endocrine, and intracrine factors. In addition, FGF signaling disorders also result in human hereditary, paraneoplastic, and metabolic diseases.

8.1 Paracrine FGFs

Michel aplasia is a unique autosomal recessive syndrome characterized by type I microtia, microdontia, and profound congenital deafness associated with a complete absence of inner ear structures. Michel aplasia is caused by mutations in *Fgf3* (Tekin et al., 2007). Nonsense mutations in *Fgf8* are found in familial isolated hypogonadotropic hypogonadism with variable degrees of gonadotropin-releasing hormone deficiency and olfactory phenotypes. These findings confirm that loss-of-function mutations in *Fgf8* cause human gonadotropin-releasing hormone deficiency (Trarbach et al., 2010). Cleft lip and/or palate (CLP) appear when the two halves of the palatal shelves fail to fuse completely. A missense mutation in *Fgf8* was found in a patient with CLP. This mutation is predicted to cause loss-of-function by destabilizing the N-terminal conformation, which is important for FGFR binding affinity and specificity (Riley et al., 2007). Aplasia of lacrimal and salivary glands (ALSG) is an autosomal dominant congenital anomaly characterized by aplasia, atresia, or hypoplasia of the lacrimal and salivary systems. Lacrimo-auriculo-dento-digital syndrome (LADD) is an autosomal-dominant multiple congenital anomaly disorder characterized by aplasia, atresia, or hypoplasia of the lacrimal and salivary systems, cup-shaped ears, hearing loss, and dental and digital anomalies. Both ALSG and LADD are caused by *Fgf10* mutations (Entesarian et al., 2007; Rohmann et al., 2006). *Fgf20* was originally identified as a neurotrophic factor preferentially expressed in dopaminergic neurons within the substantia nigra pars compacta of rat brain (Ohmachi et al., 2003). Parkinson disease (PD) is caused by a pathogenic process responsible for the loss of dopaminergic neurons within the substantia nigra pars compacta. A pedigree disequilibrium test and a case-control association study indicated that *Fgf20* is potentially a risk factor for PD (Gao et al., 2008).

8.2 Endocrine FGFs

Serum FGF15/19 levels are markedly increased in patients with extrahepatic cholestasis caused by a pancreatic tumor. FGF15/19 is abundantly expressed in the liver of cholestatic patients, but not in the normal liver. FGF15/19 signaling may be involved in some of the adaptations that protect the liver against bile salt toxicity (Schaap et al., 2009). Serum FGF15/19 levels are also significantly increased in patients on chronic hemodialysis (Reiche et al., 2010). Nonalcoholic fatty liver disease (NAFLD) is a hepatic manifestation of metabolic syndrome, and ranges from simple fatty liver to nonalcoholic steatohepatitis. Its prevalence has increased dramatically over recent years in developed countries (Morris-Stiff & Feldstein, 2010). The pathophysiological hallmark of NAFLD is insulin resistance. NAFLD may increase the risk of type 2 diabetes and atheroclerosis (Bugianesi et al., 2010). Hepatic lipid metabolism is disturbed in patients with NAFLD. The hepatic response to FGF15/19 is impaired in NAFLD patients with insulin resistance. This impaired response may contribute to the disturbance of lipid homeostasis in NAFLD (Schreuder et al., 2010).

Serum FGF21 levels are significantly increased in NAFLD (Yilmaz et al., 2010; Dushay et al., 2010; Li et al., 2010). Serum FGF21 levels are positively correlated with intrahepatic triglyceride levels (Li et al., 2010). As NAFLD is now recognized as a major public health problem, reliable biomarkers for NEFLD are needed. Serum FGF21 levels might be useful as a biomarker for NEFLD (Morris-Stiff & Feldstein, 2010). Type 2 diabetes connected with visceral obesity and insulin resistance has become a global health concern. Serum FGF21 levels are increased in patients with type 2 diabetes, gestational diabetes, and obesity, indicating FGF21 to be a potential new marker in patients with type 2 diabetes (Table 1) (Chen et al., 2008; Zhang et al., 2008; Chavez et al., 2009; Mraz et al., 2009; Stein et al., 2010; Matuszek et al., 2010). Serum FGF21 levels are independently associated with markers of insulin resistance and an adverse lipid profile (Chen et al., 2008; Stein et al., 2010). The up-regulation of serum FGF21 levels might be a compensatory mechanism to improve glucose metabolism when insulin resistance is present. Impaired glucose tolerance (IGT) is an important category of prediabetes. Serum FGF21 levels were also increased in Chinese subjects with IGT, however, they did not correlate with insulin resistance (Li et al., 2009). Cushing's syndrome is a hormone disorder caused by high levels of cortisol (hypercortisolism) in the blood. Patients with Cushing's syndrome frequently suffer from visceral obesity, insulin resistance/diabetes, and other abnormalities similarly to patients with metabolic syndrome. Serum FGF21 levels are also increased in patients with Cushing's syndrome. The increased FGF21 levels are due to excessive fat accumulation and related metabolic abnormalities rather than a direct effect of cortical on FGF21 production (Durovcová et al., 2010). Lipodystrophy is a common alteration in HIV-1-infected patients under anti-retroviral treatment. This syndrome is usually associated with peripheral lipoatrophy, central adiposity, and, in some cases, lipomatosis, as well as systemic insulin resistance and hyperlipidemia (Villarroya et al., 2007). Serum FGF21 levels are increased in

HIV-1-infected patients with lipodystrophy. This increase is closely associated with insulin resistance, metabolic syndrome, and markers of liver damage. FGF21 might be a biomarker of altered metabolism in HIV-1-infected, antiretroviral-treated patients (Domingo et al., 2010). Serum FGF21 levels correlate with renal function and are markedly increased in chronic kidney disease patients receiving hemodialysis, suggesting a possible link between their FGF21 levels and renal function (Stein et al., 2009). Patients with end-stage renal disease (ESRD) show insulin resistance. Serum FGF21 levels are also markedly increased in patients with ESRD, suggesting FGF21 to play a role in insulin resistance in these patients (Han et al., 2010).

Autosomal dominant hypophosphatemic rickets (AHDR) is caused by gain-of-function mutations of *Fgf23* (ADHR Consortium, 2000). FGF23 is partially cleaved by intracellular proteolysis. The cleaved forms lose their biological activity. *Fgf23* mutations in ADHR result in impaired proteolysis of FGF23 and increased serum levels of active FGF23 (White et al., 2001). Reduced FGF23 signaling also causes human hereditary diseases. Familial tumoral calcinosis (FTC) is characterized by ectopic calcification and hyperphosphatemia. Loss-of-function mutations of *Fgf23* result in FTC. These mutations destabilize the tertiary structure of FGF23 and increase its susceptibility to degradation (Benet-Pagès et al., 2005). Tumors that over-produce FGF23 also cause tumor-induced osteomalacia, which is a paraneoplasitc disease characterized by hypophosphatemia caused by renal phosphate wasting (Shimada et al., 2001). Serum FGF23 levels are also greatly increased in patients with renal failure, partly owing to decreased renal clearance. These results suggest that FGF23 has a compensatory role in the disease (Larsson et al., 2003).

8.3 Intracrine FGFs

Börjeson-Forssman-Lehmann syndrome (BFLS) is a syndromic X-linked mental retardation disease. *Fgf13* is a candidate causative gene for BFLS (Gecz et al., 1999). Hereditary spinocerebellar ataxias (SCAs) are a clinically and genetically heterogeneous group of neurodegenerative disorders. One SCA with early-onset tremors, dyskinesia, and slowly progressive cerebellar ataxia is caused by *Fgf14* mutations (van Swieten et al., 2003; Brusse et al., 2006; Misceo et al., 2009).

9. Conclusion

The human/mouse FGF family comprises twenty-two members, which were generated by gene duplication after the diversion of protostomes and deuterostomes and two genome duplication events (R1 and R2) during the evolution of early vertebrates. In contrast, the zebrafish FGF family comprises twenty-eight members including several paralogs, which were generated by an additional genome duplication event (R3) in the teleost lineage during evolution. FGFs are now recognized as proteins with diverse biological functions and act as extracellular signaling molecules in a paracrine or endocrine manner or as intracellular signaling molecules. Experiments with *Fgf* knockout mice indicate that FGFs play vital roles in development, metabolism, and neuronal functions. Studies with *Fgf* mutated or knockdown zebrafish also indicate that FGFs are crucial to development. In addition, research on human diseases indicates that FGF signaling disorders contribute to pathological conditions. Secreted signaling molecules such as BMPs, WNTs, and Hedgehogs also play crucial roles in development by influencing the intracellular signaling events of their neighbors from a distance. FGFs, along with these signaling molecules, have roles in diverse biological processes in multicellular organisms. However, the interaction/cooperation of FGFs with BMPs, WNTs, and Hedgehogs mostly remain unclear. Further understanding of the roles of FGFs will provide clues to their mechanisms of interaction/cooperation.

10. Acknowledgements

This work was supported by a Grant-in-aid for Scientific Research from the Ministry of Education, Science, Culture and Sports of Japan and the Takeda Science Foundation, Japan.

11. References

ADHR Consortium (2000). Autosomal dominant hypophosphataemic rickets is associated with mutations in FGF23. *Nature Genetics*, Vol. 26, No. 3, pp. 345-348

Alvarez, Y.; Alonso, M.T.; Vendrell V.; Zelarayan, L.C.; Chamero, P.; Theil, T.; Bösl, M.R.; Kato, S.; Maconochie, M.; Riethmacher, D. & Schimmang, T. (2003). Requirements for FGF3 and FGF10 during inner ear formation. *Development*, Vol. 130, No. 25, pp. 6329-6338

Badman, M.K.; Koester, A.; Flier, J.S.; Kharitonenkov, A. & Maratos-Flier, E. (2009). Fibroblast growth factor 21-deficient mice demonstrate impaired adaptation to ketosis. *Endocrinology*, Vol. 150, No. 11, pp. 4931-4940

Beenken, A. & Mohammadi, M. (2009). The FGF family: biology, pathophysiology and therapy. *Nature Review Drug Discovery*, Vol. 8, No. 3, pp. 235-253

Ben-Dov, I.Z.; Galitzer, H.; Lavi-Moshayoff, V.; Goetz, R.; Kuro-o, M.; Mohammadi, M.; Sirkis, R.; Naveh-Many, T. & Silver, J. (2007). The parathyroid is a target organ for FGF23 in rats. *Journal of Clinical Investigation*, Vol. 117, No. 12, pp. 4003-4008

Benet-Pagès, A.; Orlik, P.; Strom, T.M. & Lorenz-Depiereux, B. (2005). An FGF23 missense mutation causes familial tumoral calcinosis with hyperphosphatemia. *Human Molecular Genetics*, Vol. 14, No. 3, pp. 385-390

Böhm, F.; Speicher, T.; Hellerbrand, C.; Dickson, C.; Partanen, J.M.; Ornitz, D.M. & Werner, S. (2010). FGF Receptors 1 and 2 Control Chemically Induced Injury and Compound Detoxification in Regenerating Livers of Mice. *Gastroenterology*, Vol. 139, No. 4, pp. 1385-1396

Brusse, E.; de Koning, I.; Maat-Kievit, A.; Oostra, B.A.; Heutink, P. & van Swieten, J.C. (2006). Spinocerebellar ataxia associated with a mutation in the fibroblast growth factor 14 gene (SCA27): A new phenotype. *Movement Disorders*, Vol. 21, No. 3, pp. 396-401

Bugianesi, E.; Moscatiello, S.; Ciaravella, M.F. & Marchesini, G. (2010). Insulin resistance in nonalcoholic fatty liver disease. *Current Pharmaceutical Design*, Vol. 16, No. 17, pp. 1941-1951

Chen, W.W.; Li, L.; Yang, G.Y.; Li, K.; Qi, X.Y.; Zhu, W.; Tang, Y.; Liu, H. & Boden, G. (2008). Circulating FGF-21 levels in normal subjects and in newly diagnose patients with Type 2 diabetes mellitus. *Experimental and Clinical Endocrinology Diabetes*, Vol. 116, No. 1, pp. 65-68

Chavez, A.O.; Molina-Carrion, M.; Abdul-Ghani, M.A.; Folli, F.; Defronzo, R.A. & Tripathy, D. (2009). Circulating fibroblast growth factor-21 is elevated in impaired glucose tolerance and type 2 diabetes and correlates with muscle and hepatic insulin resistance. *Diabetes Care*, Vol. 32, No. 8, pp. 1542-1546

Colvin, J.S.; Green, R.P.; Schmahl, J.; Capel, B. & Ornitz, D.M. (2001a). Male-to-female sex reversal in mice lacking fibroblast growth factor 9. *Cell*, Vol. 104, No. 6, pp. 875-889
Colvin, J.S.; White, A.C.; Pratt, S.J. & Ornitz, D.M. (2001b). Lung hypoplasia and neonatal death in Fgf9-null mice identify this gene as an essential regulator of lung mesenchyme. *Development*, Vol. 128, No. 11, pp. 2095-2106
Domingo, P.; Gallego-Escuredo, J.M.; Domingo, J.C.; Gutiérrez Mdel, M.; Mateo, M.G.; Fernández, I.; Vidal, F.; Giralt, M. & Villarroya, F. (2010). Serum FGF21 levels are elevated in association with lipodystrophy, insulin resistance and biomarkers of liver injury in HIV-1-infected patients. *AIDS*, Vol. 24, No. 17, pp. 2629-2637
Dong, P.D.; Munson, C.A.; Norton, W.; Crosnier, C.; Pan, X.; Gong, Z.; Neumann, C.J. & Stainier, D.Y. (2007). Fgf10 regulates hepatopancreatic ductal system patterning and differentiation. *Nature Genetics*, Vol. 39, No. 3, pp. 397-402
Dono, R.; Texido, G.; Dussel, R.; Ehmke, H. & Zeller, R. (1998). Impaired cerebral cortex development and blood pressure regulation in FGF-2-deficient mice. *EMBO Journal*, Vol. 17, No. 15, pp. 4213-4225
Dover, K.; Solinas, S.; D'Angelo, E. & Goldfarb, M. (2010). Long-term inactivation particle for voltage-gated sodium channels. *Journal of Physiology*, Vol. 588, No. 19, pp. 3695-3711
Durovcová, V.; Marek, J.; Hána, V.; Matoulek, M.; Zikán, V.; Haluzíková, D.; Kaválková, P.; Lacinová, Z.; Krsek, M. & Haluzík, M. (2010). Plasma concentrations of fibroblast growth factors 21 and 19 in patients with Cushing's syndrome. *Physiological Research*, Vol. 59, No. 3, pp. 415-422
Dushay, J.; Chui, P.C.; Gopalakrishnan, G.S.; Varela-Rey, M.; Crawley, M.; Fisher, F.M.; Badman, M.K.; Martinez-Chantar, M.L. & Maratos-Flier, E. (2010). Increased fibroblast growth factor 21 in obesity and nonalcoholic fatty liver disease. *Gastroenterology*, Vol. 139, No. 2, pp. 456-463
Entesarian, M.; Dahlqvist, J.; Shashi, V.; Stanley, C.S.; Falahat, B.; Reardon, W. & Dahl, N. (2007). FGF10 missense mutations in aplasia of lacrimal and salivary glands (ALSG). *European Journal of Human Genetics*, Vol. 15, No. 3, pp. 379-382
Feldman, B.; Poueymirou, W.; Papaioannou, V.E.; DeChiara, T.M. & Goldfarb, M. (1995). Requirement of FGF-4 for postimplantation mouse development. *Science*, Vol. 267, No. 5195, pp. 246-249
Fischer, S.; Draper, B.W. & Neumann, C.J. (2003). The zebrafish fgf24 mutant identifies an additional level of Fgf signaling involved in vertebrate forelimb initiation. *Development*, Vol. 130, No. 15, pp. 3515-3524
Floss, T.; Arnold, H.H. & Braun, T. (1997). A role for FGF-6 in skeletal muscle regeneration. *Genes & Development*, Vol. 11, No. 16, pp. 2040-2051
Fon Tacer, K.; Bookout, A.L.; Ding, X.; Kurosu, H.; John, G.B.; Wang, L.; Goetz, R.; Mohammadi, M.; Kuro-o, M.; Mangelsdorf, D.J. & Kliewer, S.A. (2010). Research Resource: Comprehensive Expression Atlas of the Fibroblast Growth Factor System in Adult Mouse. *Molecular Endocrinology*, Vol. 24, No. 10, pp. 2050-2064
Gao, X.; Scott, W.K.; Wang, G.; Mayhew, G.; Li, Y.J.; Vance, J.M. & Martin, E.R. (2008). Gene-gene interaction between FGF20 and MAOB in Parkinson disease. *Annals of Human Genetics*, Vol. 72, No. 2, pp. 157-162
Goetz, R.; Beenken, A.; Ibrahimi, O.A.; Kalinina, J.; Olsen, S.K.; Eliseenkova, A.V.; Xu, C.; Neubert, T.A.; Zhang, F.; Linhardt, R.J.; Yu, X.; White, K.E.; Inagaki, T.; Kliewer, S.A.; Yamamoto, M.; Kurosu, H.; Ogawa, Y.; Kuro-o, M.; Lanske, B.; Razzaque, M.S. & Mohammadi, M. (2007). Molecular insights into the klotho-dependent, endocrine mode of action of fibroblast growth factor 19 subfamily members. *Molecular and Cellular Biology*, Vol. 27, No. 9, pp. 3417-3428

Gecz, J.; Baker, E.; Donnelly, A.; Ming, J.E.; McDonald-McGinn, D.M.; Spinner, N.B.; Zackai, E.H.; Sutherland, G.R. & Mulley, J.C. (1999). Fibroblast growth factor homologous factor 2 (FHF2): gene structure, expression and mapping to the Börjeson-Forssman-Lehmann syndrome region in Xq26 delineated by a duplication breakpoint in a BFLS-like patient. *Human Genetics*, Vol. 104, No. 1, pp. 56-63

Goldfarb, M.; Schoorlemmer, J.; Williams, A.; Diwakar, S.; Wang, Q.; Huang, X.; Giza, J.; Tchetchik, D.; Kelley, K.; Vega, A.; Matthews, G.; Rossi, P.; Ornitz, D.M. & D'Angelo, E. (2007). Fibroblast growth factor homologous factors control neuronal excitability through modulation of voltage-gated sodium channels. *Neuron*, Vol. 55, No. 3, pp. 449-463

Gospodarowicz, D. (1975). Purification of a fibroblast growth factor from bovine pituitary. *Journal of Biological Chemistry*, Vol. 250, No. 7, pp. 2515-2520

Gospodarowicz, D.; Bialecki, H. & Greenburg, G. (1978). Purification of fibroblast growth factor activity from bovine brain. *Journal of Biological Chemistry*, Vol. 253, No. 10, pp. 3736-3743

Guo, L.; Degenstein, L. & Fuchs, E. (1996). Keratinocyte growth factor is required for hair development but not for wound healing. *Genes & Development*, Vol. 10, No. 2, pp. 165-175

Haffter, P.; Granato, M.; Brand, M.; Mullins, M.C.; Hammerschmidt, M.; Kane, D.A.; Odenthal, J.; van Eeden, F.J.; Jiang, Y.J.; Heisenberg, C.P.; Kelsh, R.N.; Furutani-Seiki, M.; Vogelsang, E.; Beuchle, D.; Schach, U.; Fabian, C. & Nüsslein-Volhard, C. (1996). The identification of genes with unique and essential functions in the development of the zebrafish, Danio rerio. *Development*, Vol. 123, No. 1, pp. 1-36

Han, S.H.; Choi, S.H.; Cho, B.J.; Lee, Y.; Lim, S.; Park, Y.J.; Moon, M.K.; Lee, H.K.; Kang, S.W.; Han, D.S.; Kim, Y.B.; Jang, H.C. & Park, K.S. (2010). Serum fibroblast growth factor-21 concentration is associated with residual renal function and insulin resistance in end-stage renal disease patients receiving long-term peritoneal dialysis. *Metabolism*, Vol. 59, No. 11, pp. 1656-1562

Harada, M.; Murakami, H.; Okawa, A.; Okimoto, N.; Hiraoka, S.; Nakahara, T.; Akasaka, R.; Shiraishi, Y.; Futatsugi, N.; Mizutani-Koseki, Y.; Kuroiwa, A.; Shirouzu, M.; Yokoyama, S.; Taiji, M.; Iseki, S.; Ornitz, D.M. & Koseki, H. (2009). FGF9 monomer-dimer equilibrium regulates extracellular matrix affinity and tissue diffusion. *Nature Genetics*, Vol. 41, No. 3, pp. 289-298

Hébert, J.M.; Rosenquist, T.; Götz, J. & Martin, G.R. (1994). FGF5 as a regulator of the hair growth cycle: evidence from targeted and spontaneous mutations. *Cell*, Vol. 78, No. 6, pp. 1017-1025

Hotta,Y.; Sasaki, S.; Konishi, M.; Kinoshita, H.; Kuwahara, K.; Nakao, K. & Itoh, N. (2008). Fgf16 is required for cardiomyocyte proliferation in the mouse embryonic heart. *Developmental Dynamics*, Vol. 237, No. 10, pp. 2947-2954

Hotta, Y.; Nakamura, H.; Konishi, M.; Murata, Y.; Takagi, H.; Matsumura, S.; Inoue, K.; Fushiki, T. & Itoh, N. (2009). Fibroblast growth factor 21 regulates lipolysis in white adipose tissue but is not required for ketogenesis and triglyceride clearance in liver. *Endocrinology*, Vol. 150, No. 10, pp. 4625-4633

House, S.L.; Bolte, C.; Zhou, M.; Doetschman, T.; Klevitsky, R.; Newman, G. & Schultz Jel, J. (2003). Cardiac-specific overexpression of fibroblast growth factor-2 protects against myocardial dysfunction and infarction in a murine model of low-flow ischemia. *Circulation*, Vol. 108, No. 25, pp. 3140-3148

Huang, P. & Stern, M.J. (2005). FGF signaling in flies and worms: more and more relevant to vertebrate biology. *Cytokine & Growth Factor Reviews*, Vol. 16, No. 2, pp. 151-158

Hung, I.H.; Yu, K.; Lavine, K.J. & Ornitz, D.M. (2007). FGF9 regulates early hypertrophic chondrocyte differentiation and skeletal vascularization in the developing stylopod. *Developmental Biology*, Vol. 307, No. 2, pp. 300-313

Inagaki, T.; Choi, M.; Moschetta, A.; Peng, L.; Cummins, C.L.; McDonald, J.G.; Luo, G.; Jones, S.A.; Goodwin, B.; Richardson, J.A.; Gerard, R.D.; Repa, J.J.; Mangelsdorf, D.J. & Kliewer, S.A. (2005). Fibroblast growth factor 15 functions as an enterohepatic signal to regulate bile acid homeostasis. *Cell Metabolism*, Vol. 2, No. 4, pp. 217-225

Ito, S.; Fujimori, T.; Furuya, A.; Satoh, J.; Nabeshima, Y. & Nabeshima, Y. (2005). Impaired negative feedback suppression of bile acid synthesis in mice lacking betaKlotho. *Journal of Clinical Investigation*, Vol. 115, No. 8, pp. 2202-2208

Itoh, N. & Ornitz, D.M. (2004). Evolution of the Fgf and Fgfr gene families. *Trends in Genetics*, Vol. 20, No. 11, pp. 563-569

Itoh, N. (2007). The Fgf families in humans, mice, and zebrafish: their evolutional processes and roles in development, metabolism, and disease. *Biological & Pharmaceutical Bulletin*, Vol. 30, No. 10, pp. 1819-1825

Itoh, N. & Konishi, M. (2007). The zebrafish fgf family. *Zebrafish*, Vol. 4, No. 3, pp. 179-186

Itoh, N. & Ornitz, D.M. (2008). Functional evolutionary history of the mouse Fgf gene family. *Developmental Dynamics*, Vol. 237, No. 1, pp. 18-27

Itoh, N. (2010). Hormone-like (endocrine) Fgfs: their evolutionary history and roles in development, metabolism, and disease. *Cell and Tissue Research*, Vol. 342, No. 1, pp. 1-11

Kalinina, J.; Byron, S.A.; Makarenkova, H.P.; Olsen, S.K.; Eliseenkova, A.V.; Larochelle, W.J.; Dhanabal, M.; Blais, S.; Ornitz, D.M.; Day, L.A.; Neubert, T.A.; Pollock, P.M. & Mohammadi, M. (2009). Homodimerization controls the fibroblast growth factor 9 subfamily's receptor binding and heparan sulfate-dependent diffusion in the extracellular matrix. *Molecular and Cellular Biology*, Vol. 29, No. 17, pp. 4663-4678

Kharitonenkov, A. (2009). FGFs and metabolism. *Current Opinion in Pharmacology*, Vol. 9, No. 6, pp. 805-810

Kharitonenkov, A.; Dunbar, J.D.; Bina, H.A.; Bright, S.; Moyers, J.S.; Zhang, C.; Ding, L.; Micanovic, R.; Mehrbod, S.F.; Knierman, M.D.; Hale, J.E.; Coskun, T. & Shanafelt, A.B. (2008). FGF-21/FGF-21 receptor interaction and activation is determined by betaKlotho. *Journal of Cellular Physiology*, Vol. 215, No. 1, pp. 1-7

Kurosu, H.; Choi, M.; Ogawa, Y.; Dickson, A.S.; Goetz, R.; Eliseenkova, A.V.; Mohammadi, M.; Rosenblatt, K.P.; Kliewer, S.A. & Kuro-o, M. (2007). Tissue-specific expression of betaKlotho and fibroblast growth factor (FGF) receptor isoforms determines metabolic activity of FGF19 and FGF21. *Journal of Biological Chemistry*, Vol. 282, No. 37, pp. 26687-2695

Krejci, P.; Prochazkova, J.; Bryja, V.; Kozubik, A. & Wilcox, W.R. (2009). Molecular pathology of the fibroblast growth factor family. *Human Mutation*, Vol. 30, No. 9, pp. 1245-1255

Laezza, F.; Lampert, A.; Kozel, M.A.; Gerber, B.R.; Rush, A.M.; Nerbonne, J.M.; Waxman, S.G.; Dib-Hajj, S.D. & Ornitz, D.M. (2009). FGF14 N-terminal splice variants differentially modulate Nav1.2 and Nav1.6-encoded sodium channels. *Molecular and Cellular Neuroscience*, Vol. 42, No. 2, pp. 90-101

Larsson, T.; Nisbeth, U.; Ljunggren, O.; Jüppner, H. & Jonsson, K.B. (2003). Circulating concentration of FGF-23 increases as renal function declines in patients with chronic kidney disease, but does not change in response to variation in phosphate intake in healthy volunteers. *Kidney International*, Vol. 64, No. 6, pp. 2272-2279

Li, H.; Bao, Y.; Xu, A.; Pan, X.; Lu, J.; Wu, H.; Lu, H.; Xiang, K. & Jia, W. (2009). Serum fibroblast growth factor 21 is associated with adverse lipid profiles and gamma-glutamyltransferase but not insulin sensitivity in Chinese subjects. *Journal of Clinical Endocrinology and Metabolism*, Vol. 94, No. 6, pp. 2151-2156

Li, H.; Fang, Q.; Gao, F.; Fan, J.; Zhou, J.; Wang, X.; Zhang, H.; Pan, X.; Bao, Y.; Xiang, K.; Xu, A. & Jia, W. (2010). Fibroblast growth factor 21 levels are increased in nonalcoholic fatty liver disease patients and are correlated with hepatic triglyceride. *Journal of Hepatology*, Vol. 53, No. 5, pp. 934-940

Liu, Z.; Xu, J.; Colvin, J.S. & Ornitz, D.M. (2002). Coordination of chondrogenesis and osteogenesis by fibroblast growth factor 18. *Genes & Development*, Vol. 16, No. 7, pp. 859-869

Lu, S.Y.; Sheikh, F.; Sheppard, P.C.; Fresnoza, A.; Duckworth, M.L.; Detillieux, K.A. & Cattini, P.A. (2008). FGF-16 is required for embryonic heart development. *Biochemical and Biophysical Research Communication*, Vol. 373, No. 2, pp. 270-274

Lu, S.Y.; Jin, Y.; Li, X.; Sheppard, P.; Bock, M.E.; Sheikh, F.; Duckworth, M.L. & Cattini, P.A. (2010). Embryonic survival and severity of cardiac and craniofacial defects are affected by genetic background in fibroblast growth factor-16 null mice. *DNA and Cell Biology*, Vol. 29, No. 8, pp. 407-415

Mansour, S.L.; Goddard, J.M. & Capecchi, M.R. (1993). Mice homozygous for a targeted disruption of the proto-oncogene int-2 have developmental defects in the tail and inner ear. *Development*, Vol. 117, No. 1, pp. 13-28

Maroon, H.; Walshe, J.; Mahmood, R.; Kiefer, P.; Dickson, C. & Mason, I. (2002). Fgf3 and Fgf8 are required together for formation of the otic placode and vesicle. *Development*, Vol. 129, No. 9, pp. 2099-2108

Matuszek, B.; Lenart-Lipińska, M.; Duma, D.; Solski, J. & Nowakowski, A. (2010). Evaluation of concentrations of FGF-21 - a new adipocytokine in type 2 diabetes. *Endokrynolgia Polska*, Vol. 61, No. 1, pp. 50-54

Miller, D.L.; Ortega, S.; Bashayan, O.; Basch, R. & Basilico, C. (2000). Compensation by fibroblast growth factor 1 (FGF1) does not account for the mild phenotypic defects observed in FGF2 null mice. *Molecular and Cellular Biology*, Vol. 20, No. 6, pp. 2260-2268

Min, H.; Danilenko, D.M.; Scully, S.A.; Bolon, B.; Ring, B.D.; Tarpley, J.E.; DeRose, M. & Simonet, W.S. (1998). Fgf-10 is required for both limb and lung development and exhibits striking functional similarity to Drosophila branchless. *Genes & Development*, Vol. 12, No. 20, pp. 3156-3161

Miyake, A.; Nakayama, Y.; Konishi, M. & Itoh, N. (2005). Fgf19 regulated by Hh signaling is required for zebrafish forebrain development. *Developmental Biology*, Vol. 288, No. 1, pp. 259-275

Misceo, D.; Fannemel, M.; Barøy, T.; Roberto, R.; Tvedt, B.; Jaeger, T.; Bryn, V.; Strømme, P. & Frengen, E. (2009). SCA27 caused by a chromosome translocation: further delineation of the phenotype. *Neurogenetics*, Vol. 10, No. 4, pp. 371-374

Mohan, S.K.; Rani, S.G. & Yu, C. (2010). The heterohexameric complex structure, a component in the non-classical pathway for fibroblast growth factor 1 (FGF1) secretion. *Journal of Biological Chemistry*, Vol. 285, No. 20, pp. 15464-15475

Morris-Stiff, G. & Feldstein, A.E. (2010). Fibroblast growth factor 21 as a biomarker for NAFLD: integrating pathobiology into clinical practice. *Journal of Hepatology*, Vol. 53, No. 5, pp. 795-796

Mraz, M.; Bartlova, M.; Lacinova, Z.; Michalsky, D.; Kasalicky, M.; Haluzikova, D.; Matoulek, M.; Dostalova, I.; Humenanska, V. & Haluzik, M. (2009). Serum concentrations and tissue expression of a novel endocrine regulator fibroblast growth factor-21 in patients with type 2 diabetes and obesity. *Clinical Endocrinology,* Vol. 71, No. 3, pp. 369-375

Nakayama, Y.; Miyake, A.; Nakagawa, Y.; Mido, T.; Yoshikawa, M.; Konishi, M. & Itoh, N. (2008). Fgf19 is required for zebrafish lens and retina development. *Developmental Biology,* Vol. 313, No. 2, pp. 752-766

Nasevicius, A. & Ekker, S.C. (2000). Effective targeted gene 'knockdown' in zebrafish. *Nature Genetics,* Vol. 26, No. 2, pp. 216-220

Nickel, W. (2010). Pathways of unconventional protein secretion. *Current Opinion in Biotechnology,* Vol. 21, No. 5, pp. 621-626

Nomura, R.; Kamei, E.; Hotta, Y.; Konishi, M.; Miyake, A. & Itoh, N. (2006). Fgf16 is essential for pectoral fin bud formation in zebrafish. *Biochemical and Biophysical Research Communications,* Vol. 347, No. 1, pp. 340-346

Norton, W.H.; Ledin, J.; Grandel, H. & Neumann, C.J. (2005). HSPG synthesis by zebrafish Ext2 and Extl3 is required for Fgf10 signalling during limb development. *Development,* Vol. 132, No. 22, pp. 4963-4973

Nusslein-Volhard, C.; Gilmour, D.T. & Dahm, R. (2002). Zebrafish eds. Nusslein-Volhard, C. & Dahm, R., *Oxford University Press,* London, pp. 1–6

Ohbayashi, N.; Shibayama, M.; Kurotaki, Y.; Imanishi, M.; Fujimori, T.; Itoh, N. & Takada, S. (2002). FGF18 is required for normal cell proliferation and differentiation during osteogenesis and chondrogenesis. *Genes & Development,* Vol. 16, No. 7, pp. 870-879

Ohmachi, S.; Mikami, T.; Konishi, M.; Miyake, A. & Itoh, N. (2003). Preferential neurotrophic activity of fibroblast growth factor-20 for dopaminergic neurons through fibroblast growth factor receptor-1c. *Journal of Neuroscience Research,* Vol. 72, No. 4, pp. 436-443

Ohuchi, H.; Hori, Y.; Yamasaki, M.; Harada, H.; Sekine, K.; Kato, S. & Itoh, N. (2000). FGF10 acts as a major ligand for FGF receptor 2 IIIb in mouse multi-organ development. *Biochemical and Biophysical Research Communication,* Vol. 277, No. 3, pp. 643-649

Qiao, J.; Uzzo, R.; Obara-Ishihara, T.; Degenstein, L.; Fuchs, E. & Herzlinger, D. (1999). FGF-7 modulates ureteric bud growth and nephron number in the developing kidney. *Development,* Vol. 126, No. 3, pp. 547-554

Raballo, R.; Rhee, J.; Lyn-Cook, R.; Leckman, J.F.; Schwartz, M.L. & Vaccarino, F.M. (2000). Basic fibroblast growth factor (Fgf2) is necessary for cell proliferation and neurogenesis in the developing cerebral cortex. *Journal of Neuroscience,* Vol. 20, No. 13, pp. 5012-5023

Reiche, M.; Bachmann, A.; Lössner, U.; Blüher, M.; Stumvoll, M. & Fasshauer, M. (2010). Fibroblast growth factor 19 serum levels: relation to renal function and metabolic parameters. *Hormone and Metabolic Research,* Vol. 42, No. 3, pp. 178-181

Reifers, F.; Böhli, H.; Walsh, E.C.; Crossley, P.H.; Stainier, D.Y. & Brand, M. (1998). Fgf8 is mutated in zebrafish acerebellar (ace) mutants and is required for maintenance of midbrain-hindbrain boundary development and somitogenesis. *Development,* Vol. 125, No. 13, pp. 2381-2395

Revest, J.M.; DeMoerlooze, L. & Dickson, C. (2000). Fibroblast growth factor 9 secretion is mediated by a non-cleaved amino-terminal signal sequence. *Journal of Biological Chemistry,* Vol. 275, No. 11, pp. 8083-8090

Riley, B.M.; Mansilla, M.A.; Ma, J.; Daack-Hirsch, S.; Maher, B.S.; Raffensperger, L.M.; Russo, E.T.; Vieira, A.R.; Dodé, C.; Mohammadi, M.; Marazita, M.L. & Murray, J.C. (2007). Impaired FGF signaling contributes to cleft lip and palate. *Proceedings of*

Natural Academy Sciences of the United State of America, Vol. 104, No. 11, pp. 4512-4517

Rohmann, E.; Brunner, H.G.; Kayserili, H.; Uyguner, O.; Nürnberg, G.; Lew, E.D.; Dobbie, A.; Eswarakumar, V.P.; Uzumcu, A.; Ulubil-Emeroglu, M.; Leroy, J.G.; Li, Y.; Becker, C.; Lehnerdt, K.; Cremers, C.W.; Yüksel-Apak, M.; Nürnberg, P.; Kubisch, C.; Schlessinger, J.; van Bokhoven, H. & Wollnik, B. (2006). Mutations in different components of FGF signaling in LADD syndrome. *Nature Genetics*, Vol. 38, No. 4, pp. 414-417

Sakaue, H.; Konishi, M.; Ogawa, W.; Asaki, T.; Mori, T.; Yamasaki, M.; Takata, M.; Ueno, H.; Kato, S.; Kasuga, M. & Itoh, N. (2002). Requirement of fibroblast growth factor 10 in development of white adipose tissue. *Genes & Development*, Vol. 16, No. 8, pp. 908-912

Satou, Y.; Imai, K.S. & Satoh, N. (2002). Fgf genes in the basal chordate Ciona intestinalis. *Development Genes and Evolution*, Vol. 212, No. 9, pp. 432-438

Sanders, E.J. & Harvey, S. (2008). Peptide hormones as developmental growth and differentiation factors. *Developmental Dynamics*, Vol. 237, No. 6, pp. 1537-1552

Schaap, F.G.; van der Gaag, N.A.; Gouma, D.J. & Jansen, P.L. (2009). High expression of the bile salt-homeostatic hormone fibroblast growth factor 19 in the liver of patients with extrahepatic cholestasis. *Hepatology*, Vol. 49, No. 4, pp. 1228-1235

Schreuder, T.C.; Marsman, H.A.; Lenicek, M.; van Werven, J.R.; Nederveen, A.J.; Jansen, P.L. & Schaap, F.G. (2010). The hepatic response to FGF19 is impaired in patients with nonalcoholic fatty liver disease and insulin resistance. *Americal Journal of Physiology. Gastrointestinal and Liver Physiology*, Vol. 298, No. 3, pp. 440-445

Schoorlemmer, J. & Goldfarb, M. (2002). Fibroblast growth factor homologous factors and the islet brain-2 scaffold protein regulate activation of a stress-activated protein kinase. *Journal of Biological Chemistry*, Vol. 277, No. 51, pp. 49111-49119

Sekine, K.; Ohuchi, H.; Fujiwara, M.; Yamasaki, M.; Yoshizawa, T.; Sato, T.; Yagishita, N.; Matsui, D.; Koga, Y.; Itoh, N. & Kato, S. (1999). Fgf10 is essential for limb and lung formation. *Nature Genetics*, Vol. 21, No. 1, pp. 138-141

Shakkottai, V.G.; Xiao, M.; Xu, L.; Wong, M.; Nerbonne, J.M.; Ornitz, D.M. & Yamada, K.A. (2009). FGF14 regulates the intrinsic excitability of cerebellar Purkinje neurons. *Neurobiology of Disease*, Vol. 33, No. 1, pp. 81-88

Shimada, T.; Mizutani, S.; Muto, T.; Yoneya, T.; Hino, R.; Takeda, S.; Takeuchi, Y.; Fujita, T.; Fukumoto, S. & Yamashita, T. (2001). Cloning and characterization of FGF23 as a causative factor of tumor-induced osteomalacia. *Proceedings of Natural Academy Sciences of the United State of America*, Vol. 98, No. 11, pp. 6500-6505

Shimada, T.; Kakitani, M.; Yamazaki, Y.; Hasegawa, H.; Takeuchi, Y.; Fujita, T.; Fukumoto, S.; Tomizuka, K. & Yamashita, T. (2004). Targeted ablation of Fgf23 demonstrates an essential physiological role of FGF23 in phosphate and vitamin D metabolism. *Journal of Clinical Investigation*, Vol. 113, No. 4, pp. 561-568

Songhet, P.; Adzic, D.; Reibe, S. & Rohr, K.B. (2007). fgf1 is required for normal differentiation of erythrocytes in zebrafish primitive hematopoiesis. *Developmental Dynamics*, Vol. 236, No. 3, pp. 633-643

Stein, S.; Bachmann, A.; Lössner, U.; Kratzsch, J.; Blüher, M.; Stumvoll, M. & Fasshauer, M. (2009). Serum levels of the adipokine FGF21 depend on renal function. *Diabetes Care*, Vol. 32, No. 1, pp. 126-128

Stein, S.; Stepan, H.; Kratzsch, J.; Verlohren, M.; Verlohren, H.J.; Drynda, K.; Lössner, U.; Blüher, M.; Stumvoll, M. & Fasshauer, M. (2010). Serum fibroblast growth factor 21 levels in gestational diabetes mellitus in relation to insulin resistance and dyslipidemia. *Metabolism*, Vol. 59, No. 1, pp. 33-37

Sun, X.; Meyers, E.N.; Lewandoski, M. & Martin, G.R. (1999). Targeted disruption of Fgf8 causes failure of cell migration in the gastrulating mouse embryo. *Genes & Development*, Vol. 13, No. 14, pp. 1834-1846

Tang, W.J.; Wang, L.F.; Xu, X.Y.; Zhou, Y.; Jin, W.F.; Wang, H.F. & Gao, J. (2010). Autocrine/paracrine action of vitamin D on FGF23 expression in cultured rat osteoblasts. *Calcified Tissue International*, Vol. 86, No. 5, pp. 404-410

Tekin, M.; Hişmi, B.O.; Fitoz, S.; Ozdağ, H.; Cengiz, F.B.; Sirmaci, A.; Aslan, I.; Inceoğlu, B.; Yüksel-Konuk, E.B.; Yilmaz, S.T.; Yasun, O. & Akar, N. (2007). Homozygous mutations in fibroblast growth factor 3 are associated with a new form of syndromic deafness characterized by inner ear agenesis, microtia, and microdontia. *American Journal of Human Genetics*, Vol. 80, No. 2, pp. 338-344

Terauchi, A.; Johnson-Venkatesh, E.M.; Toth, A.B.; Javed, D.; Sutton, M.A. & Umemori, H. (2010). Distinct FGFs promote differentiation of excitatory and inhibitory synapses. *Nature*, Vol. 465, No. 7299, pp. 783-737

Tomiyama, K.; Maeda, R.; Urakawa, I.; Yamazaki, Y.; Tanaka, T.; Ito, S.; Nabeshima, Y.; Tomita, T.; Odori, S.; Hosoda, K.; Nakao, K.; Imura, A. & Nabeshima, Y. (2010). Relevant use of Klotho in FGF19 subfamily signaling system in vivo. *Proceedings of Natural Academy Sciences of the United State of America*, Vol. 107, No. 4, pp. 1666-1671

Trarbach, E.B.; Abreu, A.P.; Silveira, L.F.; Garmes, H.M.; Baptista, M.T.; Teles, M.G.; Costa, E.M.; Mohammadi, M.; Pitteloud, N.; Mendonca, B.B. & Latronico, A.C. (2010). Nonsense mutations in FGF8 gene causing different degrees of human gonadotropin-releasing deficiency. *Journal of Clinical Endocrinology and Metabolism*, Vol. 95, No. 7, pp. 3491-3496

Turner, N. & Grose, R. (2010). Fibroblast growth factor signalling: from development to cancer. *Nature Reviews Cancer*, Vol. 10, No. 2, pp. 116-129

Usui, H.; Shibayama, M.; Ohbayashi, N.; Konishi, M.; Takada, S. & Itoh, N. (2004). Fgf18 is required for embryonic lung alveolar development. *Biochemical and Biophysical Research Communication*, Vol. 322, No. 3, pp. 887-892

Urakawa, I.; Yamazaki, Y.; Shimada, T.; Iijima, K.; Hasegawa, H.; Okawa, K.; Fujita, T.; Fukumoto, S. & Yamashita, T. (2006). Klotho converts canonical FGF receptor into a specific receptor for FGF23. *Nature*, Vol. 444, No. 7120, pp. 770-774

van Swieten, J.C.; Brusse, E.; de Graaf, B.M.; Krieger, E.; van de Graaf, R.; de Koning, I.; Maat-Kievit, A.; Leegwater, P.; Dooijes, D.; Oostra, B.A. & Heutink, P. (2003). A mutation in the fibroblast growth factor 14 gene is associated with autosomal dominant cerebellar ataxia. *American Journal of Human Genetics*, Vol. 72, No. 1, pp. 191-199

Villarroya, F.; Domingo, P. & Giralt, M. (2007). Lipodystrophy in HIV 1-infected patients: lessons for obesity research. *International Journal of Obesity*, Vol. 31, No. 12, pp. 1763-1776

Vincentz, J.W.; McWhirter, J.R.; Murre, C.; Baldini, A. & Furuta, Y. (2005). Fgf15 is required for proper morphogenesis of the mouse cardiac outflow tract. *Genesis*, Vol. 41, No. 4, pp. 192-201

Virag, J.A.; Rolle, M.L.; Reece, J.; Hardouin, S.; Feigl, E.O. & Murry, C.E. (2007). Fibroblast growth factor-2 regulates myocardial infarct repair: effects on cell proliferation, scar contraction, and ventricular function. *American Journal of Pathology*, Vol. 171, No. 5, pp. 1431-1440

White, K.E.; Carn, G.; Lorenz-Depiereux, B.; Benet-Pages, A.; Strom, T.M. & Econs, M.J. (2001). Autosomal-dominant hypophosphatemic rickets (ADHR) mutations stabilize FGF-23. *Kidney International*, Vol. 60, No. 6, pp. 2079-2086

Whitehead, G.G.; Makino, S.; Lien, C.L. & Keating, M.T. (2005). fgf20 is essential for initiating zebrafish fin regeneration. *Science*, Vol. 310, No. 5756, pp. 1957-1960

Xiao, M.; Xu, L.; Laezza, F.; Yamada, K.; Feng, S. & Ornitz, D.M. (2007). Impaired hippocampal synaptic transmission and plasticity in mice lacking fibroblast growth factor 14. *Molecular and Cellular Neurosciences*, Vol. 34, No. 3, pp. 366-377

Xu, J.; Liu, Z. & Ornitz, D.M. (2000). Temporal and spatial gradients of Fgf8 and Fgf17 regulate proliferation and differentiation of midline cerebellar structures. *Development*, Vol. 127, No. 9, pp. 1833-1843

Yamauchi, H.; Miyakawa, N.; Miyake, A. & Itoh, N. (2009). Fgf4 is required for left-right patterning of visceral organs in zebrafish. *Developmental Biology*, Vol. 332, No. 1, pp. 177-185

Yamauchi, H.; Hotta, Y.; Konishi, M.; Miyake, A.; Kawahara, A. & Itoh, N. (2006). Fgf21 is essential for haematopoiesis in zebrafish. *EMBO Reports*, Vol. 7, No. 6, pp. 649-654

Yang, J.; Meyer, M.; Müller, A.K.; Böhm, F.; Grose, R.; Dauwalder, T.; Verrey, F.; Kopf, M.; Partanen, J.; Bloch, W.; Ornitz, D.M. & Werner, S. (2010). Fibroblast growth factor receptors 1 and 2 in keratinocytes control the epidermal barrier and cutaneous homeostasis. *Journal of Cell Biology*, Vol. 188, No. 6, pp. 935-952

Yilmaz, Y.; Eren, F.; Yonal, O.; Kurt, R.; Aktas, B.; Celikel, C.A.; Ozdogan, O.; Imeryuz, N.; Kalayci, C. & Avsar, E. (2010). Increased serum FGF21 levels in patients with nonalcoholic fatty liver disease. *European Journal of Clinical Investigation*, Vol. 40, No. 10, pp. 887-892

Zhang, X.; Ibrahimi, O.A.; Olsen, S.K.; Umemori, H.; Mohammadi, M. & Ornitz, D.M. (2006). Receptor specificity of the fibroblast growth factor family. The complete mammalian FGF family. *Journal of Biological Chemistry*, Vol. 281, No. 23, pp. 15694-15700

Zhang, X.; Yeung, D.C.; Karpisek, M.; Stejskal, D.; Zhou, Z.G.; Liu, F.; Wong, R.L.; Chow, W.S.; Tso, A.W.; Lam, K.S. & Xu, A. (2008). Serum FGF21 levels are increased in obesity and are independently associated with the metabolic syndrome in humans. *Diabetes*, Vol. 57, No. 5, pp. 1246-1253

Zhou, M.; Sutliff, R.L.; Paul, R.J.; Lorenz, J.N.; Hoying, J.B.; Haudenschild, C.C.; Yin, M.; Coffin, J.D.; Kong, L.; Kranias, E.G.; Luo, W.; Boivin, G.P.; Duffy, J.J.; Pawlowski, S.A. & Doetschman, T. (1998). Fibroblast growth factor 2 control of vascular tone. *Nature Medicine*, Vol. 4, No. 2, pp. 201-207

3

Osteoclast Genetic Diseases

Andrea Del Fattore[1] and Anna Teti[2]
[1]*Ospedale Pediatrico Bambino Gesù, Rome*
[2]*University of L'Aquila, L'Aquila*
Italy

1. Introduction

Bone is a specialized connective tissue that performs many important functions: (i) mechanical, supporting the whole body and allowing the movements; (ii) protective, shielding many vital organs, such as brain, lung, heart and bone marrow; (iii) metabolic, regulating the homeostasis of calcium and phosphate (Baron, 1999); (iv) endocrine, regulating kidney function (Fukumoto & Martin, 2009; Mazzaferro et al., 2010) and contributing to global energy balance (Ducy et al., 1996; Ferron et al., 2010; Lee et al., 2007) and male fertility (Oury et al., 2011). Bone is a dynamic tissue, subjected to a continuous process of renewal and remodelling in which bone resorption by osteoclasts and bone formation by osteoblasts occur at the same site along the bone surface (Pogoda et al., 2005). About 10% of bone is replaced each year, with complete skeletal renewal every 10 years. An imbalance between osteoblast and osteoclast activities can cause serious consequences: if bone formation is enhanced or bone resorption is impaired, bone mass is increased, and *vice versa* (Parfitt, 1982; Pogoda et al., 2005). Often osteoclast diseases are monogenic, and in many of them the responsible gene and the respective function have been identified, while for other osteoclast diseases the causative gene has not been isolated or the exact function of the matching protein still remains unknown. In this review, a brief description of osteoclast biology will be provided and examples of genetic osteoclast diseases, including osteopetrosis, pycnodysostosis and Paget's disease of bone, will be discussed.

2. Osteoclast

The osteoclast is the unique cell that is able to destroy the tissue to which it belongs (Teitelbaum, 2007). It is a giant cell with a diameter of 20-100 μm containing 4 to 50 nuclei, depending on the species (Roodman, 1996). The multinuclearity of osteoclast derives from the fusion of monocyte-macrophage mononuclear cells (Figure 1). In histological sections, osteoclasts appear variable in shape and size, adherent to the bone, within a small depression, called Howship's lacuna, that is the result of their bone resorbing activity (Roodman, 1996). Osteoclasts are polarized cells (Takahashi et al., 2007). In fact, it is possible to identify a zone facing the bone matrix presenting a particular area of the plasma membrane, named ruffled border, composed by deep and irregular foldings that increase the size of the membrane located in front of the bone that will be resorbed (Stenbeck, 2002). The peripheral domain, named "sealing membrane", represents the adhesion area by which the osteoclast attaches to the bone matrix around the site where it will be degraded. The remaining membrane constitutes the basolateral domain containing proteins important for ion balance and response to regulatory stimuli. Opposite to the ruffled border domain, there is the apical domain, that is thought to be important for the transcytosis of bone resorption products from the resorbing lacuna to the extracellular fluids (Coxon & Taylor, 2008; Nesbitt & Horton, 1997; Peruzzi & Teti, 2011; Salo et al., 1996; Takahashi et al., 2007). Underneath the apical domain there are the nuclei that, under the light microscope, appear different in shape: some are round and euchromatic, others are irregular and more heterochromatic (Baron, 1989).

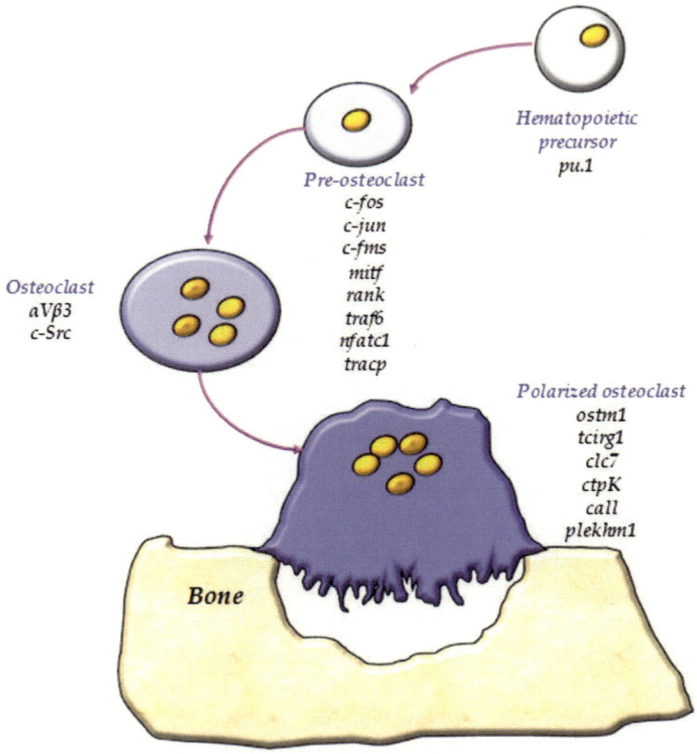

Fig. 1. Osteoclast differentiation. The cartoon illustrates the different phases of osteoclast differentiation, from the hematopoietic precursor to the mature multinuclear osteoclast. Some of the genes implicated in this process are indicated.

Moreover, ultrastructural studies showed Golgi complexes associated with each nucleus, many mitochondria and lysosomes (Baron et al., 1988; Stembeck, 2002). These latter organelles, approximately 0.5 µm in diameter, contain acid hydrolases, such as cathepsin K and Tartrate Resistant Acid Phosphatase (TRAcP), representing markers of the osteoclast phenotype (Garnero, 1998; Sakigiyama et al., 2001). Mitochondria are very abundant, correlating with the high energy expenditure that is required for the degradation of bone matrix (Miyazaki et al., 2006).

2.1 The molecular mechanisms of bone resorption

Bone resorption is a complex process requiring two different phases, the acidification of the extracellular lacuna to dissolve the inorganic bone matrix and the secretion of proteolytic enzymes to digest the organic components (Blair et al., 1986; Vaananen et al., 1998) (Figure 2). To achieve the acidification of the resorption lacunae and begin the process of bone demineralization, Carbonic Anhydrase II (CAII) generates carbonic acid from the hydration of CO_2. Carbonic acid spontaneously dissociates in proton and bicarbonate (Bothwick et al., 2003; Boyle et al., 2003). The protons so generated are actively released in the resorbing lacuna through an osteoclast-specific vacuolar-type (V)-H^+-ATPase (Nishi & Forgac, 2002; Teitelbaum & Patrick, 2003). The excess of bicarbonate is removed by a bicarbonate/chloride exchanger, localised in the basolateral membrane (Baron, 1989; Teti et al., 1989). The chloride ion is then released in the bone resorption lacuna by a Cl^-/H^+ antiport, ClC7, that, coupling with the proton pump activity, balances the ion charge across the membrane (Boyle et al., 2003; Graves et al., 2008; Teitelbaum & Patrick, 2003). The final goal of this process is to demineralise the bone and uncover the organic matrix ready to be digested by proteolytic enzymes, such as the metalloproteinase MMP9 released by endosomal vesicles, and the cathepsin K released by lysosomes (Blair et al., 1986; Bossard et al., 1996; Everts et al., 1992).

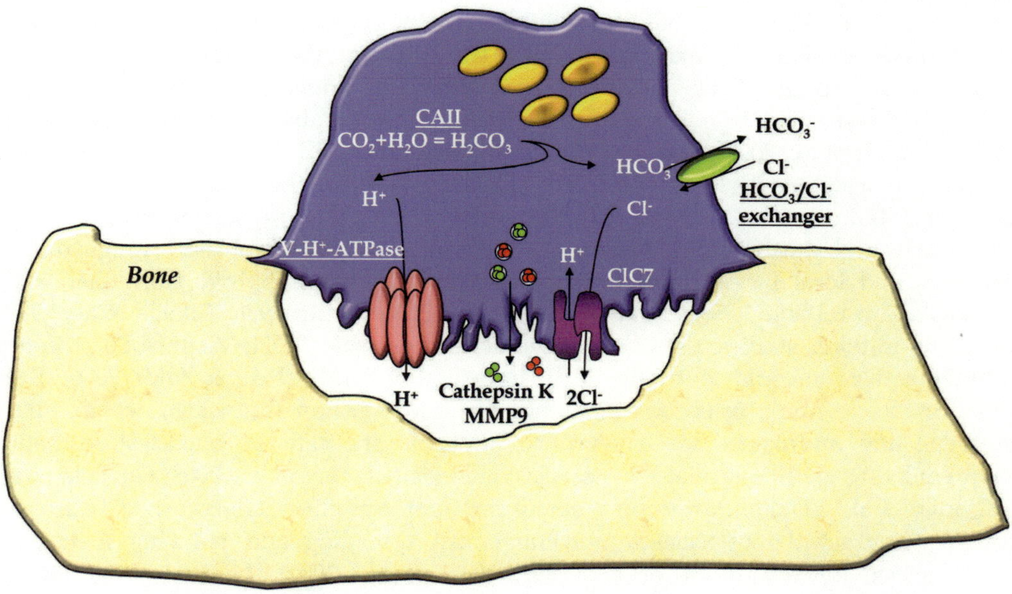

Fig. 2. The bone resorption process. The cartoon illustrates the molecular patterns involved in bone resorption by osteoclasts. See text for detailed description.

2.2 Osteoclastogenesis and regulation of osteoclast activity

Osteoclasts are cells that belong to the monocyte/macrophage lineage and derive from the fusion of monocuclear precursors (Teitelbaum, 2007) (Figure 1). In 1981, Marks and Walker showed, by experiments with parabiotic animals, that circulating blood contains cells able to differentiate into osteoclasts, thus identifying their haematogenous origin (Marks & Walker, 1981). Subsequently, in vitro studies with bone marrow-derived cells (Burger et al., 1989) suggested that osteoclasts arise from the differentiation of precursor cells of the CFU-M (Colony Forming Unit-Macrophage) lineage. This evidence suggested that osteoclasts present the same haematopoietic origin of antigen presenting cells and tissue macrophages. The pathway of osteoclast differentiation is now well characterized (Teitelbaum et al., 1997).

The PU.1 transcription factor is essential for the earliest phase of osteoclast differentiation, regulating the expression of the *c-fms* gene (Hayashi et al., 1998). *c-fms* encodes for the receptor of M-CSF (Macrophage-Colony Stimulating Factor), a cytokine crucial for the survival and the proliferation of early progenitors since it stimulates the cyclinD/CDK4 (Cyclin-Dependent Kinase 4) pathway (Mundy, 1993; So et al., 2003). Moreover, c-fms is able to stimulate the expression of PU.1 itself, establishing an amplification loop (Mundy, 1993). The essential role of PU.1 during osteoclast commitment is even due to its ability to regulate the expression of RANK (Receptor Activator of NF-κB) that, upon interaction of its ligand RANKL, is able to initiate the differentiation and the fusion of osteoclast precursors (Kwon et al., 2005). In fact, subsequent to RANKL-RANK interaction, TRAF6 (TNF Receptor-Associated Factor 6) is recruited and activates IκB and MAP kinases (Takayanagi et al., 2005), causing the nuclear translocation of NF-κB and of other transcription factors, including ATF2 (Activating Transcription Factor 2), c-fos and c-jun, required for the progression of osteoclast differentiation (Wada et al., 2006). Other two transcription factors important for osteoclast differentiation are MITF (MIcrophthalmia-associated Transcription Factor) (So et al., 2003) and NFATc1 (Nuclear Factor of Activated T-cells, cytoplasmic, calcineurin-dependent 1) (Takayanagi, 2007) that regulate the expression of osteoclast specific genes, like *TRAcP, OSCAR* (OSteoClast-Associated immunoglobulin-like Receptor), *CTSK, CLC7* and *OSTM1* (OSteopetrosis associated TransMembrane protein) (Takayanagi, 2007; Meadows et al., 2007). The activation of RANK by RANKL is counterbalanced by the expression of a soluble decoy receptor, OPG (OsteoProteGerin), that is able to bind RANKL, preventing its interaction with RANK (Kong et al., 1999). The expression of RANKL by stromal cells and, during inflammation, by T cells and synovial fibroblasts, is regulated by hormones and local factors as it is stimulated by PTH (ParaThyroid Hormone), PGE_2 (ProstaGlandin E_2) and 1,25$(OH)_2$Vitamin D_3 (Lips, 2006; Parfitt, 1976; Takeda et al., 1999). According to other studies, osteoclast progenitors express 1,25$(OH)_2$Vitamin D_3 receptors and their activation could contribute to the induction of RANK (Blair & Zaidi, 2006). Even sex hormones regulate osteoclast differentiation and function (Manolagas et al., 2002). Estrogens and androgens are believed to attenuate the rate of osteoclast formation downregulating genes essential for osteoclastogenesis (Cheung et al., 2003; Girasole et al., 1992; Imai et al., 2009) and exerting a potent pro-apoptotic effect. Glucocorticoids are also thought to target the osteoclasts, preventing cell spreading and reducing their bone resorbing activity (Dempster et al., 1997; Kim et al., 2007). However, the use of glucocorticoids leads to a reduction of bone mass due to a direct negative effect on osteoblast activity and to inhibition of osteoclasts, that result in the interruption of the bone remodeling cycle (Dovio et al., 2004). Furthermore, osteoclasts are very sensitive to pH levels as it is known that systemic acidosis has detrimental effects on the skeleton and local acidosis is associated with bone destruction (Arnett, 2003; Krieger et al., 2004; Muzylak et al., 2007). It has been shown that the Ovarian cancer G-protein-coupled Receptor 1 (OGR1 or GPR68), a proton sensing receptor, is essential for osteoclast formation inducing RANKL-dependent osteoclastogenesis and activating NFATc1 (Iwai et al., 2007).

3. Osteopetrosis

Osteopetrosis is a rare (>1:100.000) genetic disorder characterized by an impaired osteoclast function that leads to pathological increase of bone mass and skeletal fragility. It was identified for the first time in 1904 by Albers-Scönberg, who described a patient with generalized sclerosis of the skeleton, suffering from several fractures (Albers-Schönberg, 1904). Subsequently, in 1926, Karshner denominated the syndrome "marble bone disease" or "osteopetrosis" (Karshner, 1926). Impaired bone resorption causes persistence of old bone, increase of bone mass and obstruction of cavities containing vital organs such as the bone marrow and the nervous system. Osteopetrotic patients usually suffer from pathological fractures, short stature and haematological and neural failures (Balemans et al.; 2005; Del Fattore et., 2008; Frattini et.; 2003; Loria-Cortes et al., 1977). Osteopetrosis is a heterogeneous disorder which includes several forms that differ on the basis of inheritance, severity and secondary clinical features (Balemans et al., 2005). So far, there is no effective cure for osteopetrosis (Del Fattore et al., 2010). Haematopoietic Stem Cell Transplantation (HSCT) is indicated only for some severe forms; however a large rate of unsuccessful engraftment and persistence of irreversible symptoms are frequently observed (Driesses et al., 2003).

3.1 Clinical features and genetic inheritance

The various forms of osteopetrosis are classified on the basis of clinical, radiological and inheritance features into three major groups (Balemans et al., 2005; Whyte, 2002): the Autosomal Recessive Osteopetrosis (ARO), the Intermediate autosomal Recessive Osteopetrosis (IRO) and the Autosomal Dominant Osteopetrosis (ADO). Although these forms display different symptoms, they share common clinical traits such as increase of bone density, spontaneous fractures and haematological failures (Del Fattore et al., 2008). ARO is the most severe form and it is commonly diagnosed soon after birth or within the first years of life. Patients display a generalised osteosclerosis, especially in skull, pelvis, spine and long bones (Frattini et al., 2000; Kornak et al., 2000; Loria-Cortes et al., 1977), which display the so-called "bone in bone" appearance (Figure 3). The poor development and/or compression of the bone marrow and the nervous system leads to severe anaemia, pancytopenia, hepatosplenomegaly, visual impairment, optic atrophy and deafness. Less common features are hydrocephaly, macrocephaly and strabismus. In a subtype of ARO primary degeneration of brain and retina are observed (Askmyr et al., 2008). Unfortunately, a fatal outcome generally occurs in 75% of ARO patients, who die at 3-4 years of age because of haematological failure and recurrent infections (Balemans et al., 2005).

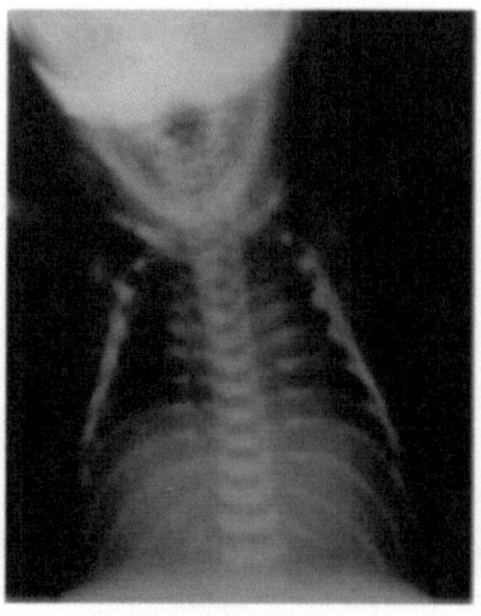

Fig. 3. X-ray analysis illustrating generalized osteosclerosis in an ARO patient. The picture shows the extensive sclerosis of spine, ribs and skull.

IRO is milder than ARO and life expectancy is much longer. Typical symptoms of this form are generalized increase of bone density, osteomyelitis, short stature, dental malformations, and mild to moderate anaemia (Balemans et al., 2005; Bolt et al., 2005; Del Fattore et al., 2010; Sly et al., 1983). The Autosomal Dominant Osteopetrosis, also called Albers-Schönberg disease (Albers-Schönberg, 1904), was previously described inappropriately as the "benign form" but it is now accepted as an extremely heterogeneous osteopetrosis, ranging from asymptomatic to severe (Del Fattore et al., 2006; Frattini et al., 2003; Waguespack et al., 2007). This phenotypic variability is even observed within the same family (Letizia et al., 2004). ADO patients usually present with sclerosis of skull base, pelvis, and vertebral end-plates (Figure 4) (sandwich vertebrae or rugger-jersey spine), bone pain, osteomyelitis and frequent pathological fractures. Life expectancy is generally normal, but in some cases complications due to cranial nerve compression, a rather poor quality of life and death have been reported (Albers-Schönberg, 1904; Balemans et al., 2005; Del Fattore et al., 2006).

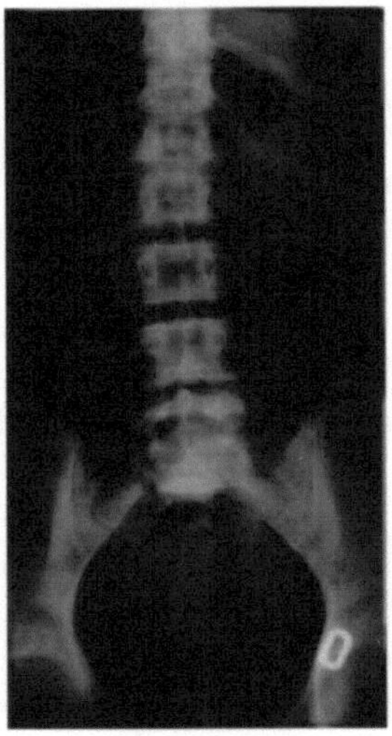

Fig. 4. X-ray analysis of an ADO patient showing sclerosis of vertebral end-plates (sandwich vertebrae) and pelvis.

Besides these classical forms, five male cases have been described so far with X-Linked Osteopetrosis (XLO) associated with lymphedema, anhidrotic ectodermal dysplasia, and immunodeficiency (so-called OL-EDA-ID syndrome). They died very young for severe phenotype and infection complications (Smahi et al., 2002).

3.2 Genetic features

The extreme phenotypic variability of osteopetrosis arises from the genetic heterogeneity. As shown in Table 1, in osteopetrotic patients mutations in genes encoding proteins essential for correct bone resorption or for osteoclast differentiation have been observed. As discussed above, these mutations can be inherited in an autosomal recessive, autosomal dominant or X-linked manner (Del Fattore et al., 2010). ARO, the most severe form, is due in more than 50% of cases to loss-of-function mutations of the *TCIRG1* gene, encoding for the osteoclast-specific a3 subunit of V-H^+-ATPase (Del Fattore et al., 2006; Frattini et al., 2000; Kornak et al., 2000; Taranta el al., 2003).

Gene	Protein	Type of mutation	Form of osteopetrosis
TCIRG1	a3 subunit of vacuolar H^+-ATPase	Loss-of-function	ARO
TCIRG1/ATP6V1B1	a3/B1 subunits of vacuolar H^+-ATPase	Loss-of-function	ARO
CLC7	Chloride/proton antiport	Loss-of-function	ARO
		Dominant negative	ADO
OSTM1	Trasmembrane protein associated with ClC7 function	Loss-of-function	ARO
PLEKHM1	Protein with undefined function, probably associated with vesicular trafficking and acidification	Loss-of-function	IRO
CAII	Carbonic anhydrase type II	Loss-of-function	IRO
NEMO	Regulatory subunit of IKK	Loss-of-function	XLO
TNFSF11	Receptor activator of NF-kB ligand (RANKL)	Loss-of-function	ARO
TNFRSF11A	RANK	Loss-of-function	ARO

Table 1. Genetic defects in human osteopetroses

The V-H^+-ATPase is central to the mechanism of bone resorption because it is located in the osteoclast ruffled border membrane where it releases protons in the underneath resorbing lacuna (Nishi & Forgac, 2002). In rare cases, double mutations of the *TCIRG1* gene and the *ATP6V1B1* genes, this latter encoding the B1 subunit of V-H^+-ATPase, were described (Bothwick et al., 2003). As shown in Table 1, other four genes are associated with ARO. About 10-15% of patients harbours mutations of the *CLC7* gene (Frattini et al., 2003; Kasper et al., 2005; Kornak et al., 2001), encoding for the so called chloride channel type 7, recently reclassified as a Cl^-/H^+ antiport (Graves et al., 2008). This dimeric protein is located in lysosomes and osteoclast ruffled membrane where, as previously described, it is essential to restore the correct electrical potential altered by proton flux (Graves et al., 2008). So far, only 5 patients affected by ARO were found to harbour loss-of-function mutations of the *OSTM1* gene, encoding for a protein whose role in bone resorption is still unknown (Chalhoub et al., 2003; Pangrazio et al., 2006). Ostm1 function is probably important for Cl^- conductance, because it was recently shown that the protein is involved in the stabilization and correct localization of the Cl^-/H^+ antiport (Lange et al., 2006). The correlated functions of ClC7 and Ostm1 proteins are demonstrated by the similar clinical features of patients harbouring mutations of the respective genes (Pangrazio et al., 2006). Primary retinal degeneration and lysosomal storage disease are observed in these patients, who are believed not to benefit from HSCT because it cannot cure the neural defects. Beside the types of AROs described above, so-called "osteoclast-rich" osteopetroses because in these forms osteoclasts form normally or are even increased in number, there is also a particularly rare form of ARO where the osteoclasts are absent (Helfrich, 2005). The patients affected by this "osteoclast-poor" osteopetrosis present mutations of the *TNFSF11* (Sobacchi et al., 2007) or the *TNFRSF11A* (Guerrini et al., 2008) genes (Table 1), encoding the RANKL and its receptor

RANK, respectively. Both proteins are required for osteoclast differentiation. So far, only 6 patients have been described to carry mutations of the *TNFSF11* gene. The importance of this discovery relies on the fact the these patients could not be effectively treated with HSCT, because the genetic defect is not osteoclast-autonomous but rather relies on the inability of stromal/osteoblastic cells to produce RANKL. ADO, the most frequent osteopetrosis, is caused in about 70% of patients by heterozygous dominant negative mutations of the *CLC7* gene (Bollerslev et al., 1988; Del Fattore et al., 2005; Frattini et al., 2003; Letizia et al., 2004; Waguespack et al., 2007). *CLC7* gene mutations tend to affect the entire length of the gene, even if the most frequent mutations have been described in the regions encoding the C-terminal CBS (Cystathionine Beta Synthase) domains of the protein (Del Fattore et al., 2006; Waguespack et al., 2007). As described above, ADO is characterized by a phenotypic variability probably due to the incomplete penetrance of the mutant gene (Frattini et al., 2003; Letizia et al., 2004). No other genes are known so far to be correlated with ADO and about 30% of patients still lacks a genetic diagnosis (Del Fattore et al., 2010). As in ADO, also in IRO a considerable clinical heterogeneity is observed. Presently, the two genes known to be associated with IRO are *CAII* (Bolt et al., 2005) and *PLEKHM1* (Van Wesenbeeck et al., 2007), encoding the carbonic anhydrase type II and the Plekhm1 protein, respectively. Patients harbouring loss of function mutations of the *CAII* gene display, besides osteopetrosis, tubular acidosis, cerebral calcifications and mental retardation (Balemans et al., 2005). The novel gene recently associated with osteopetrosis, *PLEKHM1*, has been identified as the human homolog of the gene responsible of the *incisor absent* (ia) rat phenotype (Van Wesenbeeck et al., 2007). To date, only one female patient affected by IRO has been identified to harbour a mutation of the *PLEKHM1* gene. The clinical features described in this patient were increased bone density, Erlenmeyer flask' deformity of the distal femora and a chondrolysis of the left hip. The exact function of the Plekhm1 protein is not completely elucidated, but recent findings suggest that it is a member of Rab7-regulated proteins involved in late endosomal trafficking (Del Fattore et., 2008; Van Wesenbeeck et al., 2007), vesicular acidification and TRAcP release by osteoclasts (Del Fattore et al., 2008). As previously described, there is a XLO osteopetrosis, due to mutations of the *NEMO* (NF-κB Essential Modulator) gene, encoding the IκB regulatory subunit of IKK. The mutations described in the only 5 so far known patients cause the replacement of the *NEMO* stop codon with tryptophan, leading to the addition of 27 irrelevant residues that strongly destabilize the protein (Smahi et al., 2002). All other forms of osteopetrosis, about 30% of patients, still lack of a recognized gene involved and much effort should be made to identify new genes associated with this disease.

4. Pycnodysostosis

Pycnodysostosis is a skeletal disorder also known as Toulouse-Lautrec disease because it is believed that the famous French painter Henri Toulouse-Lautrec (1864-1901) suffered from this syndrome (Maroteaux & Lamy, 1965). It is a rare monogenic disease (approximately 150 cases reported in the literature worldwide), first described in 1962 by Maroteaux and Lamy, who coined this term from the word of Greek origin *puknos* meaning "dense", associated with the words *dys* meaning "defective" and *ostosis* meaning "condition of the bone". Pycnodysostosis is characterised by a general osteosclerosis leading to short stature and increased bone mass. In fact, Schilling and coworkers analysed the volumetric bone density in a cohort of pycnodysostosis patients and controls showing a value of 686 mg/cm in the group of patients versus 290 mg/cm in the control group (Shilling et al., 2007). This disease appears to be especially common among the Japanese, but many cases are even described in Europe and United States (Muto et al., 1991).

4.1 Clinical features

The diagnosis of pycnodysostosis is usually performed during infancy or early childhood because of increased bone mass, short stature and cranial dysplasia. Pycnodysostosis could be confused with osteopetrosis, although it has peculiar features such as gracile clavicles with hypoplastic ends, obtuse mandibular angle, enlarged skull with opened anterior fontanel and cranial sutures, and acroosteolysis of distal phalanges (Soliman et al., 2001). Moreover, in pycnodysostosis anaemia and hepatosplenomegaly have not been reported. The exfoliation of deciduous teeth is usually altered, as well as the eruption of the permanent dentition. Endobones and radiodense striations are absent. As in osteopetrosis, pycnodysostosis patients may suffer from frequent fractures since the first year of life. Moreover, fractures of the mandible during tooth extractions have been described. Lower limbs seem to be particularly involved in fractures, resulting in *genu valgu* deformity. About 10% of the patients show mental retardation. Moreover, recurrent respiratory infections and right heart failure have been described (Muto et al., 2005).

4.2 Genetic inheritance

Pycnodysostosis is an autosomal recessive disease caused by mutations of the *CTSK* gene. In 1995, Gelb and coworkers first mapped the disease in a narrow region on chromosome 1q21 with a maximal lod score of 11.72 (Gelb et al., 1996). In 1996, they identified the mutated gene, *CTSK*, encoding the cathepsin K, a cystein proteinase expressed in many tissues such as bone, ovary, colon, skeletal muscle, placenta and small intestine (Zhao et al., 2009). Cathepsin K is synthesized as an inactive precursor of 329 amino acids (aa). The N-terminal pro-peptide of 99 aa is cleaved between Arg 114 and Ala 115 to supply the mature cathepsin K of 215 aa (Bromme & Okamoto, 1995). In the bone, it plays an important role in bone resorption since it cleaves, at acidic pH, collagen type I, osteopontin and other proteins of the bone matrix (McQueney et al., 1997). Particularly, cathepsin K cuts triple-helical collagen into small peptides. Cleavage occurs in its non collagenous termini (N- and C-telopeptide regions). These fragments can be detected in urine and serum as markers of bone resorption (Atley et al., 2000). Cathepsin K-deficient mice generated by inactivation of the *ctsk* gene display an increase of bone mass as well as radiological and histological abnormalities typical of pycnodysostosis (Gowen et al., 1999; Saftig et al., 1998). The analysis of the genomic DNA indicated that the *CTSK* gene is composed by eight exons and seven introns (Rood et al., 1997). Presently, 27 different types of mutations, spread throughout the whole gene, have been described in 34 unrelated families (Helfrich, 2003; Toral-López et al., 2011). According to bio-informatic analyses, all mutations seem to affect the protein folding, destabilizing the whole structure or creating locally structural changes that could affect the conformation of a small part of the protein (Donnarumma et al., 2007).

5. Paget's disease of bone

Paget's disease of bone is a common disorder characterized by increased bone turnover within focal lesions throughout the skeleton. It was described for the first time in 1876 by Sir

James Paget as a disease that "begins in middle age or later . . . affects most frequently the long bones of the lower extremities and the skull". Moreover, he stated that "the bones enlarge and soften, and those bearing weight yield and become unnaturally curved and misshapen" (Paget, 1876). Paget's disease of bone affects both men and woman, with a slight predominance in males (van Staa et al., 2002). Although many patients are often asymptomatic, others have a poor quality of life, with bone pain, skeletal deformities and fractures (Selby et al., 2002). The estimated prevalence of Paget's disease of bone in the world is about 1%, arising up to about 3% in North America, Great Britain, Australia and Western Europe. Conversely, this disease is very rare in Scandinavia and in the Indian subcontinent (Detheridge et al., 1982). These marked geographical differences in the prevalence strengthen the importance of genetic factors involved in the pathogenesis of Paget's disease of bone, but some evidence suggests an important role also for environmental determinants.

5.1 Clinical features

Paget's disease of bone is a disorder of bone remodelling. It is very important to underline the localized nature of the disease. It could affect a single bone or only a portion of it, or it could involve more bones (Ralston, 2008). As described above, many patients affected by Paget's disease of bone are often asymptomatic and the diagnosis is usually performed incidentally on the basis of elevated serum alkaline phosphatase levels not correlated with other diseases, or of abnormal skeletal radiographs (Tiegs et al., 2000). Conversely, other patients suffer from mild to moderate bone ache that characteristically begins late in the clinical course (Ralston et al., 2008). The direct cause of pain could be difficult to explain, requiring a careful analysis. An increase of vascularity and consequent warmth usually occur in pagetic bones, leading to unpleasant sensation perceived by patients (Altman, 1980). Micro-fractures that frequently affect the diseased bone can contribute to discomfort. Another typical sign of the disease is skeletal deformity, usually of the femur or tibia, that could aid in the cause of pain onset (Ralston et al., 2008). Moreover, severe secondary osteoarthritis can be observed at joints close to pagetic bones. Patients affected by Paget's disease of bone suffer from fractures that could be either traumatic or pathologic, particularly involving the long bones. The involvement of the skull in the disease complaints occurs in up to one third of the patients, and is characterized by macrocephaly, frontal bossing and hearing loss. Palsies of cranial nerves II, VI and VII could also be observed. Neoplastic degeneration, particularly osteogenic sarcoma involving the pelvis (although both fibrosarcoma and chondrosarcoma are also observed), develop in less that 1% of patients (Reddy et al., 2001).

5.2 Genetic inheritance

As aforementioned, both genetic and environmental factors can contribute to the pathogenesis of Paget's disease of bone. In less than 15-40% of cases, this disease is inherited in an autosomal dominant manner, even if many patients do not have a family history (Haslam et al., 1998; Hocking et al., 2000). Seven different loci have been identified by locus linkage studies associated with the onset of the disease. They are located on chromosomes 2p36, 5q31, 5q35, 10p13, 18q21 and 18q23 (Good et al., 2002; Haslam et al., 1998; Hocking et al., 2001; Laurin et al., 2001; Tilyard et al., 1982). Other studies confute this linkage association, showing that the analysis may have false positives (Ralston, 2008).

Subsequently, Laurin et al. and Hocking et al. identified, by positional cloning studies on chromosome 5q35, the *SQSTM1* gene as the most important cause of the disease (Hocking et al., 2002; Laurin et al., 2002). The *SQSTM1* gene encodes the p62/sequestosome 1, an ubiquitously expressed adapter protein involved in several cellular activities, including regulation of NF-κB signalling, autophagy, sequestration of ubiquitinated proteins and inhibition of ERK-MAPK signalling (Mosca & Diaz-Meco, 2002) (Figure 5). Particularly, it was shown that p62 is able to bind TRAF6 and K48- and K63-linked ubiquitin chains via the UBA (UBiquitin-Associated) domain (Figure 5) (Seibenhener et al., 2004). It was shown that sequestosome 1 colocalizes with ubiquitinated protein aggregates, and it has been detected in protein aggregates typical of Alzheimer's and Parkinson's diseases (Paine et al., 2005). Moreover, most of the mutations found in Paget's disease of bone are located in the UBA domains, preventing protein aggregation or, conversely, inducing the formation of aggregates larger than normal (Cavey et al., 2005; Cavey et al., 2006; Yip et al., 2006). However, it is not yet clear what role these aggregates might play in the pathogenesis of Paget's disease of bone.

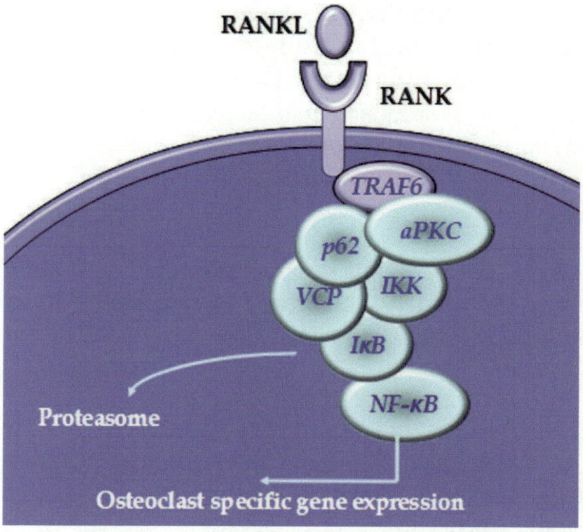

Fig. 5. Sequestosome/p62 pathway in osteoclasts. The binding of RANKL to the receptor RANK results in recruitment of TRAF6, p62 and aPKC (atypical Protein Kinase C). Moreover, the RANKL-RANK interaction leads to the phosphorylation of IKK (Inhibitor of κb kinase), that subsequently phosphorylates IκB (Inhibitor of κB). The phosphorylated IκB is degraded by the proteasome. NF-κB can translocate to the nucleus, inducing the expression of osteoclast specific genes. VCP (Valosin-Containing Protein) is involved in the regulation of IκB degradation by the proteasome.

The first mutation identified in French pagetic patients was the Proline-Leucine mutation affecting codon 392 (P392L) in the UBA domain (Laurin et al., 2002). A transgenic mouse carrying the P392L mutation under the control of the *tracp* promoter was generated and displayed an osteopenic phenotype, with increased number of osteoclasts, but no osteolytic lesions (Kurihara et al., 2000). Another animal model was generated by the group of Ralston, carrying a truncating mutation at serine 409, that developed focal lesions, representing the first true model of the disease (Rojas et al., 2007). Several other genes have been associated with Paget's disease of bone, such as *TNFSF11, TNFRSF11A* and *TNFRSF11B*, this latter particularly in juvenile disease. However, these association studies still lack a sample size large enough to enable to draw definitive conclusions on the involvement of these genes in the disease (Ralston, 2008).

6. Conclusions

Osteopetrosis, pycnodysostosis and Paget's disease of bone are examples of genetic diseases that underlie the essential role of osteoclasts in the regulation of bone homeostasis. They have been instrumental for the understanding of the mechanisms by which osteoclasts form and resorb bone and contributed to shed light on the pathogenesis of more frequent bone diseases, including osteoporosis and bone inflammatory disorders, such as osteoarthritis and rheumatoid arthritis (Tanaka et al., 2005). Further investigation on osteoclast genetic diseases is expected to help increase our knowledge about the recently identified relationships between the bone and other systems, including the immune system (Takayanagi, 2010), the nervous system (Kumar et al., 2010), the endocrine system (Ferron et al., 2010; Fukumoto & Martin, 2009; Karsenty & Oury, 2010), the reproductive system (Oury et., 2011) and the skeletal muscle system (Rufo et al., 2011), in which osteoclasts may be implicated. Therefore, in the next future we are likely to assist to flourishing novel insights into the osteoclast biology, physiology and pathology, which could represent the basis for a better prophylaxis and more effective treatments of bone diseases.

7. Acknowledgments

We gratefully acknowledge the generous support provided by Telethon (grants GGP09018 and GGP06119) to AT and by the 2010 Gideon and Sevgi Rodan Fellowship provided by the International Bone and Mineral Society to ADF.

8. References

Albers-Schönberg, H.E. (1904). Röntgenbilder einer seltenen Knockenerkrankung. *Munch Med Wochenschr*, Vol.5, pp.365-368

Altman, R.D. (1980). Musculoskeletal manifestations of Paget's disease of bone. *Arthritis Rheum*, Vol.23, No.10, (October 1980), pp. 1121-1127

Arnett, T.R. (2008). Extracellular pH regulates bone cell function. *J Nutr*, Vol.138, No.2, (February 2008), pp. 415-418

Askmyr, M.K.; Fasth, A. & Richter, J. (2008). Towards a better understanding and new therapeutic of osteopetrosis. *Br J Haematol.*, Vol.140, No.6, (March 2008), pp. 597-609

Atley, L.M.; Mort, J.S.; Lalumiere, M. & Eyre, D.R. (2000), Proteolysis of human bone collagen by cathepsin K: characterization of the cleavage sites generating by cross-linked N-telopeptide neoepitope. Bone, Vol.26, No.3, (March 2000), pp. 241-247

Balemans, W.; Van Wesenbeeck, L. & Van Hul, W. (2005). A clinical and molecular overview of the human osteopetroses. *Calcif Tissue Int.*, Vol.77, No.5, (November 2005), pp. 263-274

Baron, R. (1989). Polarity and membrane transport in osteoclasts. *Connect Tissue Res.*, Vol.20, pp. 109-12

Baron, R. (1999). Anatomy and Ultrastructure of Bone. In: *Primer on the Metabolic Bone Diseases and Disorders of Mineral Metabolism*. Lippincott Williams & Wilkins, pp. 3-10, Philadelphia, PA

Baron, R.; Neff, L.; Brown, W.; Courtoy, P.J.; Louvard, D. & Farquhar, M.G. (1988). Polarized secretion of lysosomal enzymes: co-distribution of cation-independent mannose-6-phosphate receptors and lysosomal enzymes along the osteoclast exocytic pathway. *J Cell Biol.*, (Jun 1988), Vol.106, No.6, pp. 1863-1872

Blair, H.C.; Kahn, A.J.; Crouch, E.C.; Jeffrey, J.J. & Teitelbaum, S.L. (1986). Isolated osteoclasts resorb the organic and inorganic components of bone. *J Cell Biol.*, Vol.102, No.4, (April 1986), pp. 1164-1172

Blair, H.C. & Zaidi, M. (2006). Osteoclastic differentiation and function regulated by old and new pathways. *Rev Endocr Metab Disord.*, Vol.7, No.1-2, (June 2006), pp. 23-32.

Bolt, R.J.; Wennink, J.M.; Verbeke, J.I.; Shah, G.N.; Sly, W.S. & Bokenkamp, A. (2005). Carbonic anhydrase type II deficiency. *Am J Kidney Dis.*, Vol.46, No.5, (November 2005), pp. 71-73

Bossard, M.J.; Tomaszek, T.A.; Thompson, S.K.; Amegadzie, B.Y.; Hanning, C.R.; Jones, C.; Kurdyla, J.T.; McNulty, D.E.; Drake, F.H.; Gowen, M. & Levy, M.A. (1996). Proteolytic activity of human osteoclast cathepsin K. Expression, purification, activation, and substrate identification. *J Biol Chem.*, Vol.271, No.21, (May 1996), pp. 12517-12524

Bothwick, K.J.; Kandemir, N.; Topaloglu, R.; Kornak, U.; Bakkaloglu, A.; Yordam, N.; Ozen, S.; Mocan, H.; Shah, G.N.; Sly, W.S. & Karet, F.E. (2003). A phenocopy of CAII deficiency: a novel genetic explanation for inherited infantile osteopetrosis with distal renal tubular acidosis. *J Med Genet.*, Vol.40, No.2, (February 2003), pp. 115-121

Boyle, W.J.; Simonet, W.S. & Lacey, D.L. (2003). Osteoclast differentiation and activation. *Nature*, Vol.423, No.6937, (May 2003), pp. 337-342

Bromme, D. & Okamoto, K. (1995). Human cathepsin O2, a novel cysteine protease highly expressed in osteoclastomas and ovary molecular cloning, sequencing and tissue distribution. Biol Chem Hoppe Seyler., Vol.376, No.6 (June 1995), pp. 379-384

Burger, E.H.; Veldhuijzen, J.P.; Nulend, J.K. & Van Loon, J.J. (1989). Osteoclastic invasion and mineral resorption of fetal mouse long bone rudiments are inhibited by culture under intermittent compressive force. Connect Tissue Res., Vol.20, No.1-4, pp. 131-41

Cavey, J.R.; Ralston, S.H.; Hocking, L.J.; Sheppard, P.W.; Ciani, B.; Searle, M.S. & Layfield, R. (2005). Loss of ubiquitin-binding associated with Paget's disease of bone p62 (*SQSTM1*) mutations. *J. Bone Miner. Res.*, Vol.20, No.4, (April 2005), pp. 619-624

Cavey, J.R.; Ralston, S.H.; Sheppard, P.W.; Ciani, B.; Gallagher, T.R.; Long, J.E.; Searle, M.S. & Layfield, R. (2006). Loss of ubiquitin binding is a unifying mechanism by which mutations of *SQSTM1* cause Paget's disease of bone. *Calcif. Tissue Int.*, Vol.78, No.5, (May 2006), pp. 271-277

Chalhoub, N.; Benachenhou, N.; Rajapurohitam, V.; Pata, M.; Ferron, M.; Frattini, A.; Villa, A. & Vacher, J. (2003). Grey-lethal mutation induces severe malignant autosomal recessive osteopetrosis in mouse and human. *Nat Med.*, Vol.9, No.4, (April 2003), pp. 399-406

Cheung, J.; Mak, Y.T.; Papaioannou, S.; Evans, B.A.; Fogelman, I. & Hampson, G. (2003). Interleukin-6(IL-6), IL-1, receptor activator of nuclear factor kappa B ligand

(RANKL) and osteoprotegerin production by human osteoblastic cells: comparison of the effects of 17-beta oestradiol and raloxifene. *J Endocrinol.*, Vol.177, No.3, (June 2003), pp. 423-433

Coxon, FP. & Taylor, A. (2008). Vesicular trafficking in osteoclasts. *Semin Cell Dev Biol.*, Vol.19, No.5, (October 2008), pp. 424-433

Del Fattore, A.; Capannolo, M. & Rucci, N. (2010). Bone and bone marrow: the same organ. Arch Biochem Biophys. Vol.1, No.503, (November 2010), pp 28-34

Del Fattore, A.; Cappariello, A. & Teti, A. (2008). Genetics, Pathogenesis and Complications of Osteopetrosis. *Bone*, Vol.42, No.1, (January 2008), pp. 19-29

Del Fattore, A.; Peruzzi, B.; Rucci, N.; Recchia, I.; Cappariello, A.; Longo, M.; Fortunati, D.; Ballanti, P.; Iacobini, M.; Luciani, M.; Devito, R.; Pinto, R.; Caniglia, M.; Lanino, E.; Messina, C.; Cesaro, S.; Letizia, C.; Bianchini, G.; Fryssira, H.; Grabowski, P.; Shaw, N.; Bishop, N.; Hughes, D.; Kapur, R.P.; Datta, H.K.; Taranta, A.; Fornari, R.; Migliaccio, S. & Teti, A. (2006). Clinical, genetic, and cellular analysis of 49 osteopetrotic patients: implications for diagnosis and treatment. *J Med Genet.*, Vol.43, No.4, (April 2006), pp. 315-325.

Del Fattore, A.; Van Wesenbeeck, L.; Fornari, R.; Peruzzi, B.; Cappariello, A.; Rucci, N.; Spera, G.; Helfrich, M.; Van Hul, M.; Migliaccio, S. & Teti, A. (2008). A new heterozygous mutation (R714C) of the osteopetrosis gene, pleckstrin homolog domain containing family M (with run domain) member 1 (PLEKHM1), impairs vesicular acidification and increases TRACP secretion in osteoclasts. *J Bone Miner Res.*, Vol.23, No.3, (March 2008), pp. 380-391

Dempster, D.W.; Moonga, B.S.; Stein, L.S.; Horbert, W.R. & Antakly, T. Glucocorticoids inhibit bone resorption by isolated rat osteoclasts by enhancing apoptosis. J *Endocrinol.*, Vol.154, No.3, (September 1997), pp. 397-406

Detheridge, F.M.; Guyer, P.B. & Barker, D.J. (1982). European distribution of Paget's disease of bone. *Br Med J.*, Vol.285, No.6347 (October 1982), pp. 1005-1008

Donnarumma, M.; Regis, S.; Tappino, B.; Rosano, C.; Assereto, S.; Corsolini, F.; Di Rocco, M. & Filocamo, M. (2007). Molecular analysis and characterization of nine novel CTSK mutations in twelve patients affected by pycnodysostosis. Mutation in brief #961. Online. *Hum Mutat.*, Vol.28, No.5, (May 2007), pp. 524

Dovio, A.; Perazzolo, L.; Osella, G.; Ventura, M.; Termine, A.; Milano, E.; Bertolotto, A. & Angeli, A. (2004). Immediate fall of bone formation and transient increase of bone resorption in the course of high-dose, short-term glucocorticoid therapy in young patients with multiple sclerosis. *J Clin Endocrinol Metab.*, Vol.89, No.10, (October 2004), pp. 4923-4928

Driessen, G.J.; Gerritsen, E.J.; Fischer, A.; Fasth, A.; Hop, W.C.; Veys, P.; Porta, F.; Cant, A.; Steward, C.G.; Vossen, J.M.; Uckan, D. & Friedrich, W. (2003). Long-term outcome of haematopoietic stem cell transplantation in autosomal recessive osteopetrosis: an EBMT report. *Bone Marrow Transplant.*, Vol.32, No.7, (October 2003), pp. 657-663

Ducy, P.; Desbois, C.; Boyce, B.; Pinero, G.; Story, B.; Dunstan, C.; Smith, E.; Bonadio, J.; Goldstein, S.; Gundberg, C.; Bradley, A. & Karsenty, G. (1996). Increased bone formation in osteocalcin-deficient mice. *Nature*, Vol.1, No.382, (August 1996), pp. 448-452

Everts, V.; Delaisse, J.M.; Korper, W.; Niehof, A.; Vaes, G. & Beertsen, W. (1992). Degradation of collagen in the bone-resorbing compartment underlying the osteoclast involves both cysteine-proteinases and matrix metalloproteinases. *J Cell Physiol.*, Vol.150, No.2, (February 1992), pp. 221-231

Ferron, M.; Wei, J.; Yoshizawa, T.; Del Fattore, A.; DePinho, R.A.; Teti, A.; Ducy, P. & Karsenty, G. (2010). Insulin signaling in osteoblasts integrates bone remodeling and energy metabolism. *Cell.*, Vol.23, No.142, (July 2010), pp. 296-308

Frattini, A.; Orchard, P.J.; Sobacchi, C.; Giliani, S.; Abinun, M.; Mattsson, J.P.; Keeling, D.J.; Andersson, A.K.; Wallbrandt, P.; Zecca, L.; Notarangelo, L.D.; Vezzoni, P. & Villa, A. (2000). Defects in TCIRG1 subunit of the vacuolar proton pump are responsible for a subset of human autosomal recessive osteopetrosis. *Nat Genet.*, Vol.25, No.3, (July 2000), pp. 343-346

Frattini, A.; Pangrazio, A.; Susani, L.; Sobacchi, C.; Mirolo, M.; Abinum, M.; Andolina, M.; Flanagan, A.; Horwitz, E.M.; Mihci, E.; Notarangelo, L.D.; Ramenghi, U.; Teti, A.; Van Hove, J.; Vujic, D.; Young, T.; Albertini, A.; Orchard, P.J.; Vezzoni, P. & Villa, A. (2003). Chloride channel ClCN7 mutations are responsible for severe recessive, dominant, and intermediate osteopetrosis. *J Bone Miner Res.*, Vol.18, No.10, (October 2003), pp. 1740-1747

Fukumoto, S. & Martin, T.J. (2009). Bone as an endocrine organ. *Trends Endocrinol Metab.*, Vol.20, No.5 (July 2009), pp. 230-236

Garnero, P.; Borel, O.; Byrjalsen, I.; Ferreras, M.; Drake, FH.; McQueney, MS.; Foged, NT.; Delmas, PD. & Delaisse, JM. (1998). The collagenolytic activity of cathepsin K is unique among mammalian proteinases. *J Biol Chem.*, Vol.273, No.48, (November 1998), pp. 32347-32352

Gelb, B.D.; Shi, G.P.; Chapman, H.A. & Desnick, R.J. Pycnodysostosis, a lysosomal disease caused by cathepsin K deficiency. *Science*, Vol.273, No.5279, (August 1996), pp. 1236-1238.

Girasole, G.; Jilka, R.L.; Passeri, G.; Boswell, S.; Boder, G.; Williams, D.C. & Manolagas, S.C. (1992). 17 β-estradiol inhibits interleukin-6 production by bone marrow-derived stromal cells and osteoblasts in-vitro: a potential mechanism for the antiosteoporotic effect of estrogens. *J Clin Invest.*, Vol.89, No.3, (March 1992), pp. 883-891

Good, D.A.; Busfield, F.; Fletcher, B.H.; Duffy, D.L.; Kesting, J.B.; Andersen, J. & Shaw, J.T. (2002). Linkage of Paget disease of bone to a novel region on human chromosome 18q23. *Am J Hum Genet.*, Vol.70, No2, (February 2002), pp. 517-525

Gowen, M.; Lazner, F.; Dodds, R.; Kapadia, R.; Feild, J.; Tavaria, M.; Bertoncello, I.; Drake, F.; Zavarselk, S.; Tellis, I.; Hertzog, P.; Debouck, C. & Kola, I. (1999). Cathepsin K knockout mice develop osteopetrosis due to a deficit in matrix degradation but not demineralization. *J Bone Miner Res.*, Vol.14, No.10, (October 1999), pp. 1654-1663

Graves, A.R.; Curran, P.K.; Smith, C.L. & Mindell, J.A. (2008). The Cl-/H+ antiporter ClC-7 is the primary chloride permeation pathway in lysosomes. *Nature*, Vol.453, No.7196, (June 2008), pp. 788-792

Guerrini, M.M.; Sobacchi, C.; Cassani, B.; Abinun, M.; Kilic, S.S.; Pangrazio, A.; Moratto, D.; Mazzolari, E.; Clayton-Smith, J.; Orchard, P.; Coxon, F.P.; Helfrich, M.H.; Crockett, J.C.; Mellis, D.; Vellodi, A.; Tezcan, I.; Notarangelo, L.D.; Rogers, M.J.; Vezzoni, P.; Villa, A. & Frattini, A. (2008). Human osteoclast-poor osteopetrosis with hypogammaglobulinemia due to TNFRSF11A (RANK) mutations. *Am J Hum Genet.*, Vol.83, No.1, (July 2008), pp. 64-76

Haslam, S.I.; Van Hul, W.; Morales-Piga, A.; Balemans, W.; San-Millan, J.L.; Nakatsuka, K.; Willems, P.; Haites, N.E. & Ralston, S.H. (1998). Paget's disease of bone: evidence for a susceptibility locus on chromosome 18q and for genetic heterogeneity. *J Bone Miner Res.*, Vol.13, No.6, (June 1998), pp. 911-917

Hayashi, S.; Yamane, T.; Miyamoto, A.; Hemmi, H.; Tagaya, H.; Tanio, Y.; Kanda, H.; Yamazaki, H. & Kunisada, T. (1998). Commitment and differentiation of stem cells to the osteoclast lineage. *Biochem Cell Biol.*, Vol.76, No.6, pp. 911-922

Helfrich, M.H. (2003). Osteoclast diseases. Microsc Res Tech., Vol. 61, No.15, (August 2003), pp. 514-32

Hocking, L.; Slee, F.; Haslam, S.I.; Cundy, T.; Nicholson, G.; Van Hul, W. & Ralston, S.H. (2000). Familial Paget's disease of bone: patterns of inheritance and frequency of linkage to chromosome 18q. Bone, Vol.26, No.6, (June.2000), pp. 577-580

Hocking, L.J.; Herbert, C.A.; Nicholls, R.K.; Williams, F.; Bennett, S.T.; Cundy, T.; Nicholson, G.C.; Wuyts, W.; Van Hul, W. & Ralston, S.H. (2001). Genomewide search in familial Paget disease of bone shows evidence of genetic heterogeneity with candidate loci on chromosomes 2q36, 10p13, and 5q35. *Am J Hum Genet.*, Vol.69, No.5, (November 2001), pp. 1055-1061

Hocking, L.J.; Lucas, G.J.; Daroszewska, A.; Mangion, J.; Olavesen, M.; Cundy, T.; Nicholson, G.C.; Ward, L.; Bennett, S.T.; Wuyts, W.; Van Hul, W. & Ralston SH. (2002). Domain-specific mutations in sequestosome 1 (SQSTM1) cause familial and sporadic Paget's disease. *Hum Mol Genet.*, Vol.11, No.22, (October 2002), pp. 2735-2739

Imai, Y.; Youn, M.Y.; Kondoh, S.; Nakamura, T.; Kouzmenko, A.; Matsumoto, T.; Takada, I.: Takaoka, K. & Kato, S. Estrogens maintain bone mass by regulating expression of genes controlling function and life span in mature osteoclasts. *Ann N Y Acad Sci.* Vol.1173, No.1, (September 2009), pp. 31-39

Iwai, K.; Koike, M.; Ohshima, S.; Miyatake, K.; Uchiyama, Y.; Saeki, Y. & Ishii, M. (2007). RGS18 acts as a negative regulator of osteoclastogenesis by modulating the acid-sensing OGR1/NFAT signaling pathway. *J Bone Miner Res.*, Vol.22, No.10, (October 2007), pp. 1612-1620

Karsenty, G. & Oury, F. (2010). The central regulation of bone mass, the first link between bone remodeling and energy metabolism. *J Clin Endocrinol Metab.*, Vol.95, No.11, (November 2010), pp. 4795-4801

Karshner, R.G. (1926). Osteopetrosis, *Amer. J. Roentg.*, Vol.16, No.403

Kasper, D.; Planells-Cases, R.; Fuhrmann, J.C.; Scheel, O.; Zeitz, O.; Ruether, K.; Schmitt, A.; Poet, M.; Steinfeld, R.; Schweizer, M.; Kornak, U. & Jentsch, T.J. (2005). Loss of the chloride channel ClC-7 leads to lysosomal storage disease and neurodegeneration. *EMBO J.*, Vol.24, No.5, (March 2005), pp.1079-1091

Kim, H.J.; Zhao, H.; Kitaura, H.; Bhattacharyya, S.; Brewer, J.A.; Muglia, L.J.; Patrick, R.F. & Teitelbaum, S.L. (2007). Glucocorticoids and the osteoclast. Ann N Y Acad Sci., Vol.1116, (November 2007), pp. 335-339

Kong, Y.Y.; Yoshida, H.; Sarosi, I.; Tan, H.L.; Timms, E.; Capparelli, C.; Morony, S.; Oliveira-dos-Santos, A.J.; Van, G.; Itie, A.; Khoo, W.; Wakeham, A.; Dunstan, C.R.; Lacey, D.L.; Mak, T.W.; Boyle, W.J. & Penninger, J.M. (1999). OPGL is a key regulator of osteoclastogenesis, lymphocyte development and lymph-node organogenesis. *Nature*, Vol.397, No.6717, (January 1999), pp. 315-323

Kornak, U.; Kasper, D.; Bosl, M.R.; Kaiser, E.; Schweizer, M.; Schulz, A.; Friedrich, W.; Delling, G. & Jentsch, T.J. (2001). Loss of the ClC-7 chloride channel leads to osteopetrosis in mice and man. *Cell*, Vol.104, No.2, (January 2001), pp. 205-215

Kornak, U.; Schulz, A.; Friedrich, W.; Uhlhaas, S.; Kremens, B.; Voit, T.; Hasan, C.; Bode, U.; Jentsch, T.J. & Kubish, C. (2000). Mutations in the a3 subunit of the vacuolar H^+-ATPase cause infantile malignant osteopetrosis. *Hum Mol Genet.*, Vol.9, No.13, (August 2000), pp. 2059-2063

Krieger, N.S.; Frick, K.K. & Bushinsky, D.A. (2004). Mechanism of acidinduced bone resorption. *Curr Opin Nephrol Hypertens.*, Vol.13, No.4, (July 2004), pp. 423-436

Kumar, K.K.; Tung, S. & Iqbal, J. (2010). Bone loss in anorexia nervosa: leptin, serotonin, and the sympathetic nervous system. Ann N Y Acad Sci., Vol.1211, (November 2010), pp. 51-65

Kurihara, N.; Hiruma, Y.; Zhou, H.; Subler, M.A.; Dempster, D.W.; Singer, F.R.; Reddy, S.V.; Gruber, H.E.; Windle, J.J. & Roodman, G.D. Mutation of the sequestosome 1 (p62) gene increases osteoclastogenesis but does not induce Paget disease. *J Clin Invest.*, Vol.117, No.1, (January 2007), pp. 133-142

Kwon, O.H.; Lee, C.K.; Lee, Y.I.; Paik, S.G. & Lee, H.J. (2005). The hematopoietic transcription factor PU.1 regulates RANK gene expression in myeloid progenitors. *Biochem Biophys Res Commun.*, Vol.335, No.2, (September 2005), pp. 437-446

Lange, P.F.; Wartosch, L.; Jentsch, T.J. & Fuhrmann, J.C. (2006). ClC-7 requires Ostm1 as a beta-subunit to support bone resorption and lysosomal function. *Nature*, Vol.440, No.7081, (March 2006), pp. 220-223

Laurin, N.; Brown, J.P.; Lemainque, A.; Duchesne, A.; Huot, D.; Lacourcière, Y. ; Drapeau, G.; Verreault, J.; Raymond, V. & Morissette, J. (2001). Paget disease of bone: mapping of two loci at 5q35-qter and 5q31. Am J Hum Genet., Vol.69, No3, (September 2001), pp. 528-543.

Laurin, N.; Brown, J.P.; Morissette, J. & Raymond, V. (2002). Recurrent mutation of the gene encoding sequestosome 1 (SQSTM1/p62) in Paget disease of bone. *Am J Hum Genet.*, Vol.70, No.6, (Jun 2002), pp. 1582-1588

Lee, N.K.; Sowa, H.; Hinoi, E.; Ferron, M.; Ahn, J.D.; Confavreux, C.; Dacquin, R.; Mee, P.J.; McKee, M.D.; Jung, D.Y.; Zhang, Z.; Kim, J.K.; Mauvais-Jarvis, F.; Ducy, P. & Karsenty, G. (2007). Endocrine regulation of energy metabolism by the skeleton. *Cell.* Vol.10, No.3, (August 2010), pp. 456-469

Letizia, C.; Taranta, A.; Migliaccio, S.; Caliumi, C.; Diacinti, D.; Delfini, E.; D'Erasmo, E.; Iacobini, M.; Roggini, M.; Albagha, O.M.; Ralston, S.H. & Teti A. (2004). Type II Benign Osteopetrosis (Albers-Schönberg Disease) caused by a novel mutation in ClCN7 presenting with unusual clinical manifestations. *Calcif Tissue Int.*, Vol.74, No.1, (January 2004), pp. 42-46

Lips, P. (2006). Vitamin D physiology. *Prog Biophys Mol Biol.*, Vol. 92, No.1, (September 2006), pp. 4-8.

Loria-Cortes, R.; Quesada-Calvo, E. & Cordero-Chavarri, C. (1977). Osteopetrosis in children: a report of 26 cases. *J. Pediatr.*, Vol.91, No.1, (July 1977), pp. 43-47

Manolagas, S.C.; Kousteni, S. & Jilka, R.L. (2002). Sex steroids and bone. *Recent Prog Horm Res.*, Vol.57, pp. 385-409

Marks, S.C. & Jr Walker, D.G. (1981). The hematogenous origin of osteoclasts: experimental evidence from osteopetrotic (microphthalmic) mice treated with spleen cells from beige mouse donors. *Am J Anat.*, Vol.161, No.1, (May 1981), pp. 1-10

Maroteaux, P. & Lamy, M. (1965). The malady of Toulouse-Lautrec. *JAMA.* Vol.191, pp. 715-717

Mazzaferro, S.; Pasquali, M.; Pirrò, G.; Rotondi, S. & Tartaglione L. (2010). The bone and kidney. *Arch Biochem Biophys.*, Vol.503, No.1 (July 2010), pp. 95-102

McQueney, M.S.; Amegadzie, B.Y.; D'Alessio, K.; Hanning, C.R.; McLaughlin, M.M.; McNulty, D.; Carr, S.A.; Ijames, C.; Kurdyla, J. & Jones, C.S. (1997). Autocatalytic activation of human cathepsin K. *J Biol Chem.*, Vol.272, No.21, (May 1997) pp. 13955-13960

Meadows, N.A.; Sharma, S.M.; Faulkner, G.J.; Ostrowski, M.C.; Hume, D.A. & Cassady, A.I. (2006). The expression of Clcn7 and Ostm1 in osteoclasts is coregulated by microphthalmia transcription factor. *J Biol Chem.*, Vol.282, No.3, (January 2006), pp. 1891-1904

Miyazaki, T.; Tanaka, S.; Sanjay, A. & Baron, R. (2006). The role of c-Src kinase in the regulation of osteoclast function. *Mod Rheumatol.*, Vol.16, No.2, (2006), pp. 68-74

Moscat, J. & Diaz-Meco, M.T. (2002). The atypical PKC scaffold protein P62 is a novel target for anti-inflammatory and anti-cancer therapies. *Adv Enzyme Regul.*, Vol.42, (2002), pp. 173-179

Mundy, G.R. (1993). Cytokines and growth factors in the regulation of bone remodeling. *J Bone Miner Res.*, Vol.8, No.2, (December 1993), pp. 505-10

Muto, T.; Michiya, H.; Taira, H. ; Murase, H. & Kanazawa, M. (1991). Pycnodysostosis. Report of a case and review of the Japanese literature, with emphasis on oral and maxillofacial findings. *Oral Surg Oral Med Oral Pathol.*, Vol.72, No.4, (October 1991), pp. 449-55

Muto, T.; Yamazaki, A.; Takeda, S.; Tsuji, Y. & Shibata, T. (2005). Pharyngeal narrowing as a common feature in pycnodysostosis--a cephalometric study. *Int J Oral Maxillofac Surg.*, Vol.34, No.6, (September 2005), pp. 680-685

Muzylak, M.; Arnett, T.R.; Price, J.S. & Horton, M.A. (2007). The in vitro effect of pH on osteoclasts and bone resorption in the cat: implications for the pathogenesis of FORL. J Cell Physiol., Vol.213, No.1, (October 2007), pp. 144-150

Nesbitt, S.A. & Horton, M.A. (1997). Trafficking of matrix collagens through bone-resorbing osteoclasts. *Science.* Vol.11, No.276, (April 1997), pp. 266-269

Nishi, T. & Forgac, M. (2002). The Vacuolar (H^+)-ATPase. Nature's most versatile proton pumps. *Nat Rev Mol Cell Biol.*, Vol.3, No.2, (February 2002), pp. 94-103

Oury, F.; Sumara, G.; Sumara, O.; Ferron, M.; Chang, H.; Smith, C.E.; Hermo, L.; Suarez, S.; Roth, B.L.; Ducy, P. & Karsenty, G. (2011). Endocrine regulation of male fertility by the skeleton. Cell., Vol.144, No.5, (March 2011), pp. 796-809

Paget, J. (1876). On a form of chronic inflammation of bones (osteiti deformans). *Med-Chir Trans* ix:37-38

Paine, M.G.; Babu, J.R.; Seibenhener, M.L. & Wooten, M.W. (2005). Evidence for p62 aggregate formation: role in cell survival. *FEBS Lett.* Vol.579, No.22, (September 2005), pp. 5029-5034

Pangrazio, A.; Poliani, P.L.; Megarbane, A.; Lefranc, G.; Lanino, E.; Di Rocco, M.; Rucci, F.; Lucchini, F.; Ravanini, M.; Facchetti, F.; Abinun, M.; Vezzoni, P.; Villa, A. &

Frattini, A. (2006). Mutations in OSTM1 (grey lethal) define a particularly severe form of autosomal recessive osteopetrosis with neural involvement. *J Bone Miner Res.*, Vol.21, No.7, (July 2006), pp. 1098-1105

Parfitt, A.M. (1976). The actions of parathyroid hormone on bone: relation to bone remodeling and turnover, calcium homeostasis, and metabolic bone diseases. II. PTH and bone cells: bone turnover and plasma calcium regulation. *Metabolism,* Vol.25, No.9, (September 1976), pp. 1033-1069

Parfitt, A.M. (1982). The coupling of bone formation to bone resorption: a critical analysis of the concept and of its relevance to the pathogenesis of osteoporosis. *Metab Bone Dis Relat Res.*, Vol.4, No.1, pp. 1-6

Peruzzi, B. & Teti, A. (2011). The Physiology and Pathophysiology of the Osteoclast. *Clinic Rev Bone Miner Metab.*, (2011)

Pogoda, P.; Priemel, M.; Rueger, J.M. & Amling, M.; (2005). Bone remodeling: new aspects of a key process that controls skeletal maintenance and repair. *Osteoporos Int.*, Vol.16, No.2, (March 2005), pp. 18-24

Ralston, S.H. (2008). Pathogenesis of Paget's disease of bone. *Bone,* Vol.43, No.5, (Novmber 2008), pp. 819-825

Ralston, S.H.; Langston, A.L. & Reid, I.R. Pathogenesis and management of Paget's disease of bone. *Lancet,* Vol.372, No.9633, (July 2008), pp. 155-163

Reddy, S.V.; Kurihara, N.; Menaa, C.; Landucci, G.; Forthal, D.; Koop, B.A.; Windle, J.J. & Roodman, G.D. (2001). Osteoclasts formed by measles virus-infected osteoclast precursors from hCD46 transgenic mice express characteristics of pagetic osteoclasts. *Endocrinology,* Vol. 142, No.7, (July 2001), pp. 2898-2905

Rojas, J.A.; Daroszewska, A.; Helfrich, M.; Layfield, R.; van't Hof, R. & Ralston, S.H. (2007). Mice with a truncation mutation affecting sequestosome 1 exhibit several phenotypic features in common with Paget's disease of bone. *Calcif Tiss Int.,* Vol.81, (2007), p. 149

Rood, J.A.; Van Horn, S.; Drake, F.H.; Gowen, M. & Debouck, C. (1997). Genomic organization and chromosome localization of the human cathepsin K gene (CTSK). *Genomics.* Vol.41, No.2, (April 1997), pp. 169-176

Roodman, G.D. (1996). Advances in bone biology: the osteoclast. *Endocr Rev.*, Vol.14, No.4, (August 1996), pp. 308-332

Rufo, A.; Del Fattore, A.; Capulli, M.; Carvello, F.; De Pasquale, L.; Ferrari, S.; Pierroz, D.; Morandi, L.; De Simone, M.; Rucci, N.; Bertini, E.; Bianchi, M.L.; De Benedetti, F. & Teti, A. (2011). Mechanisms inducing low bone density in Duchenne muscular dystrophy in mice and humans. (August 2011)

Saftig, P.; Hunziker, E.; Wehmeyer, O.; Jones, S.; Boyde, A.; Rommerskirch, W.; Moritz, J.D.; Schu, P. & von Figura, K. (1998). Impaired osteoclastic bone resorption leads to osteopetrosis in cathepsin-K-deficient mice. *Proc Natl Acad Sci USA*, Vol.95, No.23, (November 1998), pp. 13453-13458

Sakiyama, H.; Masuda, R.; Inoue, N.; Yamamoto, K.; Kuriiwa, K.; Nakagawa, K. & Yoshida, K. (2001). Establishment and characterization of macrophage-like cell lines expressing osteoclast-specific markers. *J Bone Miner Metab.*, Vol.19, No.4, pp. 220-227

Salo, J.; Metsikkö, K.; Palokangas, H.; Lehenkari, P. & Väänänen, H.K. (1996). Bone-resorbing osteoclasts reveal a dynamic division of basal plasma membrane into two different domains. *J Cell Sci.*, Vol.109, No.2, (February 1996), pp. 301-317

Schilling, A.F.; Mülhausen, C.; Lehmann, W.; Santer, R.; Schinke, T.; Rueger, J.M. & Amling, M. (2007). High bone mineral density in pycnodysostotic patients with a novel mutation in the propeptide of cathepsin K. *Osteoporos Int.*, Vol.18, No.5, (May 2007), pp. 659-669

Seibenhener, M.L.; Babu, J.R.; Geetha, T.; Wong, H.C.; Krishna, N.R. & Wooten, M.W. (2004). Sequestosome 1/p62 is a polyubiquitin chain binding protein involved in ubiquitin proteasome degradation. *Mol. Cell. Biol.*, Vol.24, No.18, (September 2004), pp. 8055-8068

Selby, P.L.; Davie, M.W.; Ralston, S.H. & Stone, M.D. (2002). Bone and Tooth Society of Great Britain; National Association for the Relief of Paget's Disease. Guidelines on the management of Paget's disease of bone. *Bone*, Vol.31, No.3, (September 2002), pp. 366-373

Sly, W.S.; Hewett-Emmett, D.; Whyte, M.P.; Yu, Y.S. & Tashian, R.E. (1983). Carbonic anhydrase II deficiency identified as the primary defect in the autosomal recessive syndrome of osteopetrosis with renal tubular acidosis and cerebral calcification. *Proc Natl Acad Sci USA*, Vol.80, No.9, (May 1983), pp .2752-2756

Smahi, A.; Courtois, G.; Rabia, S.H. ; Doffinger, R.; Bodemer, C.; Munnich, A.; Casanova, J.L. & Israel, A. (2002). The NF-kappaB signalling pathway in human diseases: from incontinentia pigmenti to ectodermal dysplasias and immune-deficiency syndromes. *Hum Mol Genet.*, Vol.11, No.20, (October 2002), pp. 2371-2375

So, H.; Rho, J.; Jeong, D.; Park, R.; Fisher, D.E.; Ostrowski, M.C.; Choi, Y. & Kim, N. (2003). Microphthalmia transcription factor and PU.1 synergistically induce the leukocyte receptor osteoclast-associated receptor gene expression. *J Biol Chem.*, Vol.278, No.26, (June 2003), pp. 24209-24216

Sobacchi, C.; Frattini, A.; Guerrini, M.M.; Abinun, M.; Pangrazio, A.; Susani, L.; Bredius, R.; Mancini, G.; Cant, A.; Bishop, N.; Grabowski, P.; Del Fattore, A.; Messina, C.; Errigo, G.; Coxon, F.P.; Scott, D.I.; Teti, A.; Rogers, M.J.; Vezzoni, P.; Villa, A. & Helfrich, M.H. (2007). Osteoclast-poor human osteopetrosis due to mutations in the gene encoding RANKL. *Nat Genet.*, Vol.39, No.8, (August 2007), pp. 960-962

Soliman, A.T.; Ramadan, M.A.; Sherif, A.; Aziz Bedair, E.S. & Rizk, M.M. (2001) Pycnodysostosis: clinical, radiologic, and endocrine evaluation and linear growth after growth hormone therapy. *Metabolism*, Vol.50, No.8, (August 2001), pp. 905-911

Stenbeck, G. (2002). Formation and function of the ruffled border in osteoclasts. *Semin Cell Dev Biol.*, Vol.13, No.4, (August 2002), pp. 285-292

Takahashi, N.; Ejiri, S.; Yanagisawa, S. & Ozawa, H. (2007). Regulation of osteoclast polarization. *Odontology*, Vol.95, No.1, (July 2007), pp. 1-9

Takayanagi, H. (2007). The role of NFAT in osteoclast formation. *Ann N Y Acad Sci.*, Vol.1116, (November 2007), pp. 227-37

Takayanagi, H. (2010). New immune connections in osteoclast formation. *Ann N Y Acad Sci.*, Vol.1191, (March), pp. 117-123

Takayanagi, H.; Sato, K.; Takaoka, A. & Taniguchi, T. Interplay between interferon and other cytokine systems in bone metabolism. *Immunol Rev.*, Vol.208, (December 2005), pp. 181-93

Takeda, S.; Yoshizawa, T.; Nagai, Y.; Yamato, H.; Fukumoto, S.; Sekine, K.; Kato, S.; Matsumoto, T. & Fujita, T. (1999) Stimulation of osteoclast formation by 1, 25-dihydroxyvitamin D requires its binding to vitamin D receptor (VDR) in osteoblastic cells: studies using VDR knockout mice. *Endocrinology*, Vol.140, No.2, (February 1999), pp. 1005-1008

Tanaka, Y.; Nakayamada, S. & Okada, Y. Osteoblasts and osteoclasts in bone remodeling and inflammation. *Curr Drug Targets Inflamm Allergy*, Vol.4, No.3 (June 2005), pp. 325-328

Taranta, A.; Migliaccio, S.; Recchia, I.; Caniglia, M.; Luciani, M.; De Rossi, G.; Dionisi-Vici, C.; Pinto, RM.; Francalanci, P.; Boldrini, R.; Lanino, E.; Dini, G.; Morreale, G.; Ralston, SH.; Villa, A.; Vezzoni, P.; Del Principe, D.; Cassini, F.; Palombo, G. & Teti A. (2003) Genotype-Phenotype relationship in Human ATP6i-Dependent Autosomal Recessive Osteopetrosis. *Am J Pathol*, Vol.162, No.1, (January2003), pp. 57-68

Teitelbaum, S.L. & Ross, P. (2003). Genetic regulation of osteoclast development and function. *Nat Rev Genet.*, Vol.4, No.8, (August 2003), pp. 638-649

Teitelbaum, S.L. (2007). Osteoclasts: what do they do and how do they do it? *Am J Pathol.*, Vol.170, No. 2, (February 2008), pp. 427-435

Teitelbaum, S.L.; Tondravi, M.M. & Ross, F.P. (1997). Osteoclasts, macrophages, and the molecular mechanisms of bone resorption. *J Leukoc Biol.*, Vol.61, No.4, (April 1997), pp. 381-388

Teti, A.; Blair, H.C.; Teitelbaum, S.L.; Kahn, A.J.; Koziol, C.; Konsek, J.; Zambonin-Zallone, A. & Schlesinger, P.H. (1989). Cytoplasmic pH regulation and chloride/bicarbonate exchange in avian osteoclasts. *J Clin Invest.*, Vol.83, No.1 (January 1989), pp. 227-233

Tiegs, R.D.; Lohse, CM.; Wollan, P.C. & Melton, L.J. (2000). Long-term trends in the incidence of Paget's disease of bone. *Bone*, Vol.27, No.3, (September 2000), pp. 423-427

Tilyard, MW.; Gardner, R.J.; Milligan, L.; Cleary, T.A. & Stewart R.D. A probable linkage between familial Paget's disease and the HLA loci. *Australian & New Zealand Journal of Medicine*, Vol.12, No.5, (October 1982), pp. 498-500

Toral-López, J.; Gonzalez-Huerta, L.M.; Sosa, B.; Orozco, S.; González, H.P. & Cuevas-Covarrubias, S.A. (2011) Familial pycnodysostosis: identification of a novel mutation in the CTSK gene (cathepsin K). *J Investig Med.*, Vol.59, No.2, (February 2011), pp. 277-280

Vaananen, H.K.; Iu, Y.K.; Lehenkari, P. & Uemara, T. (1998). How do osteoclasts resorb bone? *Mat Sci Eng C.*, Vol.6, pp. 205-209

van Staa, T.P.; Selby, P.; Leufkens, H.G.; Lyles, K.; Sprafka, J.M. & Cooper, C. (2002). Incidence and natural history of Paget's disease of bone in England and Wales. *J Bone Miner Res.*, Vol.17, No.3, (March 2002), pp. 465-471

Van Wesenbeeck, L.; Odgren, P.R.; Coxon, F.P.; Frattini, A.; Moens, P.; Perdu, B.; MacKay, C.A.; Van Hul, E.; Timmermans, J-P.; Vanhoenacker, F.; Jacobs, R.; Peruzzi, B.; Teti, A.; Helfrich, M.H.; Rogers, M.J.; Villa, A. & Van Hul, W. (2007) Involvement of *PLEKHM1* in osteoclastic vesicular transport and osteopetrosis in incisors absent rats and humans. *J Clin Invest.*, Vol.117, No.4, (April 2007), pp. 919-930

Wada, T.; Nakashima, T.; Hiroshi, N. & Penninger, J.M. (2006). RANKLRANK signaling in osteoclastogenesis and bone disease. *Trends Mol Med.*, Vol.12, No.1, (January 2006), pp. 17-25

Waguespack, S.G.; Hui, S.L.; Dimeglio, L.A. & Econs, M.J. (2007) Autosomal dominant osteopetrosis: clinical severity and natural history of 94 subjects with a chloride channel 7 gene mutation. *J Clin Endocrinol Metab.*, Vol.92, No.3, (March 2007), pp. 771-778

Walker, D.G. (1981). Control of bone resorption by hematopoietic tissue. The induction and reversal of congenital osteopetrosis in mice through use of bone marrow and splenic transplants. *Am J Anat.*, Vol.161, No.1, (May 1981), pp. 1-10

Whyte, MP. (2002). Osteopetrosis. In: *Connective Tissue and Its Heritable Disorders: Medical, Genetic, and Molecular Aspects*. Royce, P.M., Steinman, B. New York, Wiley-Liss, Inc, pp. 753-770

Yip, KHM.; Feng, HT.; Pavlos, NJ.; Zheng, MH. & Xu JK. (2006). p62 Ubiquitin binding-associated domain mediated the receptor activator of nuclear factor-κB ligand-induced osteoclast formation – A new insight into the pathogenesis of Paget's disease of bone. *Am. J. Pathol.*, Vol.169, No.2, (August 2006), pp. 503–514

Zhao, Q.; Jia, Y. & Xiao, Y. (2009). Cathepsin K: a therapeutic target for bone diseases. *Biochem Biophys Res Commun.*, Vol.380, No.4, (March 2009), pp. 721-723

4

MRE11A Gene Mutations Responsible for the Rare Ataxia Telangiectasia-Like Disorder

Ghazi Alsbeih
King Faisal Specialist Hospital & Research Centre, Radiation Biology Section, Biomedical Physics Department, KFSHRC, Kingdom of Saudi Arabia

1. Introduction

Ataxia telangiectasia like disorder (ATLD) is a rare variant of ataxia telangiectasia (A-T) that share a number of clinical features and similar cellular characteristics with the hallmark of increased sensitivity to ionizing radiation (Taylor et al., 1975; Taylor, 2001; Tauchi et al., 2002). These conditions are typically diagnosed at young age at about the time the affected children start to walk. A-T and ATLD patients develop progressive cerebellar ataxia which is required for their clinical diagnosis. Although classified as another variant of A-T, Nijmegen breakage syndrome (NBS) is characterized by microcephaly and growth retardation without ataxia. The other major clinical characteristics are variable and include dilated blood vessels (telangiectasia) usually in the eyes, immunodeficiency, high level of spontaneously occurring chromosome abnormalities, and predisposition to cancer particularly lymphoreticular malignancies. Genetically, the A-T is caused by biallelic inactivating mutations in the ATM gene at 11q22-23, the NBS is caused by mutation in the NBS1 gene mapped at 8q21, and the ATLD is caused by mutation in the MRE11A gene located at 11q21.

Therefore, a disorder virtually indistinguishable from A-T is caused by mutation in the MRE11A gene. In view of the fact that the ATM and the MRE11A loci are situated nearby (11q22-23 and 11q21) only a very detailed linkage analysis would have historically separated ATLD from A-T on the basis of genetic data. Assuming that the mutation rate is proportional to the length of the coding sequence of the two genes, about 6% of A-T cases might be expected to have MRE11A mutations (Stewart et al., 1999). Thus, ATLD patients were first recognized as a subset of A-T who does not have mutations in the ATM gene. Hence, Stewart *et al.* had designated this syndrome as ataxia-telagnietasia-like disorder (Stewart et al., 1999). The clinical features are very similar to those of A-T; with the clearest similarity being the progressive cerebellar ataxia. In contrast to A-T, however, ATLD patients show no telangiectasia (Hernandez et al., 1993; Klein et al., 1996). In addition, the patients show later onset of the neurological features, and slower progression of the disorder giving the overall appearance of a milder A-T condition in early years.

The function of Mre11 protein is linked to Nbs1 and both are members of the Mre11/Rad50/Nbs1 (MRN) complex involved in different DNA healing mechanisms due to innate processes or in responses to damage induced by ionizing radiation and radiomimetic chemicals (Carney et al., 1998; Petrini, 2000), including complexing with chromatin and with other damage response proteins, formation of radiation-induced foci, and the induction of cell cycle checkpoints (Figure 1). The MRN complex is among the earliest respondents to DNA damage and acts as sensor of DNA double-strand breaks (DSBs). Upon exposure to ionizing radiation the complex along with ATM becomes rapidly activated and associate with the DNA DSBs (Figure 2). This association holds broken DNA ends until the damage is repaired (Nelms et al., 1998). Loss of functional Nbs1 protein in NBS patients prevents the formation of the radiation-induced Mre11/Rad50 nuclear foci (Carney et al., 1998). In comparison, the loss of function of ATM protein in A-T patients causes abnormal reduction in the formation of MRN foci that is less severe than in NBS cells (Maser et al., 1997). Thus, the function of MRN proteins complex is biochemically linked to ATM, which is a critical component of the cellular response to DNA damage. Since Nbs1 and ATM deficiencies abrogate specific DNA damage-dependent cell cycle checkpoints, the association of MRN complex with DSBs suggests that the DNA damage recognition functions of the complex are linked to the signal transduction pathways required to activate ATM-dependent cell cycle checkpoints. These observations strengthen the molecular connection between DSB recognition by MRN protein complex and the ability of the cell to activate the DNA damage response pathway controlled by ATM.

2. Clinical manifestations of ATLD

ATLD is rare with, at present, only 25 published cases, four in the UK (2 of them from Pakistani origin), two in Italy, 15 in Saudi Arabia and four in Japan (Stewart et al., 1999; Pitts et al., 2001; A.M. Taylor et al., 2004; Fernet et al., 2005; Uchisaka et al., 2009; Bohlega et al., 2011; Matsumoto et al., 2011). The 4 British patients belonged to 2 unrelated families. Although none of the affected individuals from either family exhibited ocular telangiectasia, they presented with many clinical features consistent with the diagnosis of A-T, especially progressive cerebellar degeneration (Stewart et al., 1999). The 2 affected Italian patients were born to non-consanguineous parents. They had both normal psychomotor development until the age of 3 - 6 years when they developed progressive unsteadiness, showed diffuse cerebellar signs, i.e. ataxic gait, delayed speech and writing difficulties, choreoathetoid arm movements and oculomotor apraxia (Delia et al., 2004). The disease progressed slowly till the age of 14 and then stabilized. The latest neurological examination of the elder patient at 36 years of age showed cerebellar dysarthria, oculomotor apraxia, ataxic gait with unaided walk for few steps, choreoathethosis of the superior limbs, jerk nystagmus on horizontal and vertical gaze, dysmetria, dyskinetic movements of mouth and slight dystonia of the hands, diffuse hypotonia, reduced tendon reflexes in the arms, and absent ankle jerks with flexor plantar responses.

The 15 Saudi patients represent the largest set of ATLDs identified to date. Consanguinity is a major feature in all these families with affected children with parents were mostly first cousins. Patients were initially presented with clinical features that fall within the Ataxia Oculomotor Apraxia spectrum and exhibited a combination of early-onset, slowly progressive, ataxia plus ocular apraxia. Age at onset is almost similar to that of AT, but disease progression is slower with the absence of telangiectasia. Pedigrees and further details on these families were described previously (Fernet et al., 2005; Bohlega et al., 2011). Clinical features include progressive ataxia that was noted as early as two years old in some patients. Oculomotor apraxia was variable among the affected individuals with very slow saccadic eye movement and impaired vertical and or horizontal pursuit eye movement with

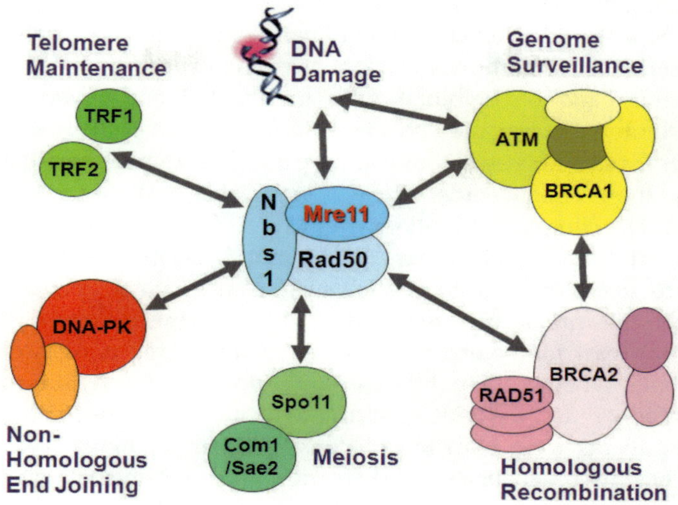

Fig. 1. Role of the Mre11 protein in the cellular response and DNA repair machinery showing the major interacting molecules (Adapted from: www.lmb.uni-muenchen.de/hopfner/research.html with modification).

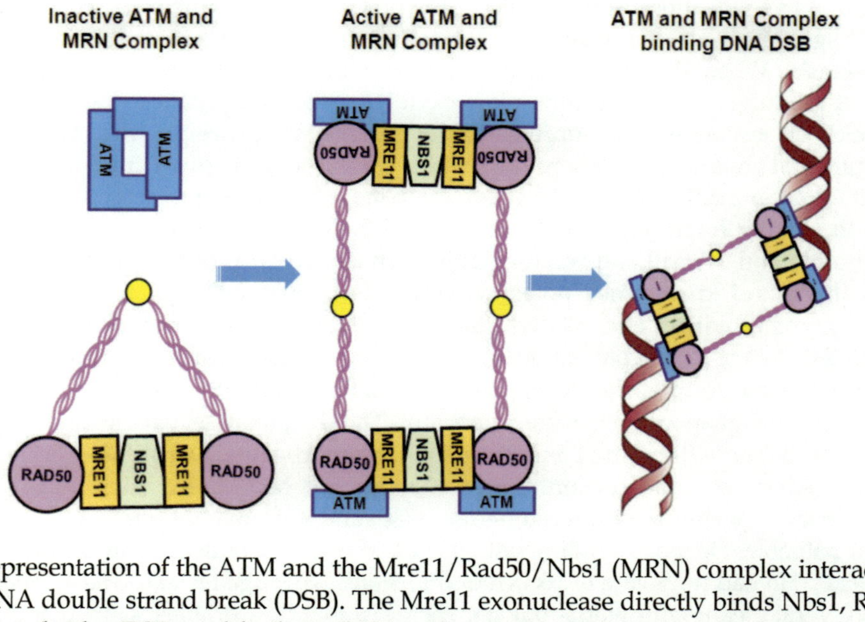

Fig. 2. Representation of the ATM and the Mre11/Rad50/Nbs1 (MRN) complex interacting with a DNA double strand break (DSB). The Mre11 exonuclease directly binds Nbs1, Rad50 and DNA to bridge DSBs and facilitate DNA end processing. The C-terminal of the ataxia telangiectasia mutated (ATM) kinase contributing to MRN regulatory roles in DSB sensing, stabilization, signaling, and effector scaffolding. MRN has 3 coupled critical functions: (1) prompt establishment of protein--nucleic acid tethering scaffolds for the recognition and stabilization of DSBs; (2) initiation of DSB sensing, cell-cycle checkpoint signaling cascades via the ATM kinase; and (3) functional regulation of chromatin remodeling in the vicinity of a DSB (Williams et al., 2007).

head thrusts. Vibration senses were decreased distally and tendon reflexes were absent. Although few patients had no cognitive impairment, others presented cognitive and behavioral problem with forgetfulness, lack of attention, word finding difficulty, emotional liability, impulsivity and disinhibition with fragmented and reversed sleep patterns. Dysarthria in addition to dystonic and choreatic movement were frequently noted. The disease was relentlessly progressive and some patients became wheelchair-bound around age of 18 years. Intra-familial variability was noticeable with some patients were more severely affected. The clinical observations on this set of patients, together with those from previously reported cases, establish that ATLD is not associated with recurrent pulmonary infections due to immune deficiency. However, some patients presented with certain differences with the previously reported ATLD patients, namely the presence of microcephaly in at least four patients, the latter feature being reminiscent of the clinical presentation of NBS. Whether these differences are specific to the W210C mutation found in Saudi patients or only reflect the wide spectrum of the disease needs further investigation.

The 4 Japanese patients were born to non-consanguineous parents. Two sibling patients were born after healthy pregnancies and deliveries. They had characteristic clinical features of short stature, pointy nose, small jaw, atrophy of the lower legs, and equinus foot deformities (Uchisaka et al., 2009). They had cerebellar ataxia, slurred and explosive speech, and ocular apraxia, but did not show any evidence of involuntary movement such as dystonia or dyskinesia. The patients started to speak at 2 years old where ataxic gait was noted. The cerebellar ataxia with atrophy of the cerebellum and mental retardation had progressed and was more severe in the elder patient who became wheelchair bound at 6 years of age. There was no history of serious infection or evidence of skin or conjunctival telangiectasia. When they were 15 and 9 years old, both patients were diagnosed with nonsmall-cell lung cancer with multiple bone metastases. One Japanese patient was born at 37 weeks of gestation after unremarkable pregnancy. However, the patient showed developmental retardation where he could sit alone but could not stand or walk (Matsumoto et al., 2011). At age 13 years, the patient had severe microcephaly, a bird-like face with sloping forehead, a big nose, large and simple ears, short palpebral fissures, a small mouth, and a small and receding chin with decreased range of motion in shoulders, elbows, hips, and knees. Also noted were scoliosis, subluxation of the left elbow joint, bilateral cryptorchidism, and bilateral talipes equinus. His tendon reflexes were slightly exaggerated. At age 33, the patient does not speak meaningful words, but recognizes people, communicates by gesture, shows fondness by touching, does not show ocular apraxia and had neither malignancy nor severe infections. The 4th Japanese patient had intrauterine growth retardation with a small femora and a disproportionately small head (Matsumoto et al., 2011). After caesarian section delivery the patient had severe microcephaly, a bird-headed facial appearance with receding forehead, and a prominent nose. Anterior fontanel was not palpable. He stood holding onto a chair at age 30 months, sat alone and walked at age 3 years. He had no severe or recurrent infections. Now aged 8 years, he is toilet trained, speaks several meaningful words but sentence. He attends a primary school, and is affable and friendly. He is farsighted with astigmatism. He is able to run with a slow pitch and kick a soccer ball. He shows neither ocular apraxia nor cerebellar ataxia.

3. MRE11A gene mutations

The 25 genetically confirmed ATLD patients (4 in the UK, 2 in Italy, 4 in Japan and 15 in Saudi Arabia were either homozygous or compound heterozygous for 10 different mutations (Figure 3). The four British patients were related to two independent families. The two patients of the 1st family were homozygous for a C-to-T transition at nucleotide 1897 (c.1897C>T). This change, CGA>TGA, resulted in an in frame 633R > stop codon, prematurely truncating the Mre11 protein. The two patients of the 2nd family were compound heterozygous for two mutations, an A>G missense mutation at nucleotide 350 (c.350A>G), resulting in a Asn to Ser amino acid change at residue 117 (N117S) and C-to-T transition at nucleotide 1714 (c.1714C>T) resulting in a stop codon (572R> stop) (A.M. Taylor et al., 2004). This mutation is predicted to encode a prematurely truncated protein of 65 kDa that was not detected suggesting that this mutation destabilizes the transcript by nonsense-mediated decay (NMD) surveillance mechanism which eliminates the errors in the biogensis of mRNA (Frischmeyer et al., 2002; Nicholson et al., 2010). The two Italian sibling patients were compound heterozygous for two mutations, a missense mutation at position 1422 (c.1422C>A) resulting in Thr to Lys amino acid change at residue 481 (T481K) and the already known single C>T base change in exon 15, corresponding to nucleotide 1714 in the cDNA sequence (c.1714C>T), which introduces a premature stop codon (Delia et al., 2004).

The four Japanese patients belonged to 3 unrelated families. In two brothers with ATLD with lung cancer, genetic studies had looked at alteration in the 20 exons and the flanking intronic sequences of the MRE11A gene. This revealed a T>C substitution in exon 8 at position 727 (c.727T>C) and a G>C base substitution at nucleotide 24994 situated in intron 10 (g.24994G>A; Figure 3), 5bp downstream from exon 10 (Uchisaka et al., 2009). RT-PCR showed the presence of two products. Sequencing of these cDNA products confirmed the T>C base substitution at nucleotide 727 in exon 8 in 1 of the alleles and uncovered an 81 bp deletion in exon 10 on another allele. The alteration of these DNA sequences predicted a Trp to Arg amino acid substitution at residue 243 (W243R) and the loss of 27 amino acids, respectively. The base substitution in intron 10 might have given rise to an alternative splicing of MRE11A, leading to an in frame 81 bp deletion in exon 10. Thus, the two Japanese sibling patients were compound heterozygous for two novel MRE11A gene mutations that have not been reported before, one in exon 8 (c.727 T>C) and one in intron 10 (g.24994 G>A).

The two other unrelated Japanese patients were presented with NBS-like severe microcephaly, bird-like faces, growth and mental retardation remnant of Nijmegen breakage syndrome (NBS). However, genetic studies revealed no mutation in the NBN gene responsible for NBS. Therefore, the MRE11A gene was sequenced in both patients and found to be compound heterozygous for three different types of mutations: an A-to-C transversion in nucleotide 658 (c.658A>C), a G-to-A transition in nucleotide 16513 (g.16513; i.e. c.659+1G>A) and an A-to-G transition in position 338 (c.338A>G). Patient-1 had c.658A>C substitution plus a g.16513 splicing mutation, and patient-2 had c.658A>C and c.338A>G substitutions. Sequencing analysis demonstrated that g.16513G>A resulted in exon 7 skipping leading to a premature termination codon (p.Ser183ValfsX31). The c.658A>C substitution located within exon 7 did not alter amino acids but affected splicing efficiency that contributed to exon 7 skipping. The c.338A>G situated in exon 5 lead to a missense mutation with an amino acid substitution of Asp to Gly at residue 113 (D113G) located within the highly conserved phosphoesterase domain, which is essential for endonuclease activity. The c.658A>C substitution common to both patients and the c.338A>G substitution resulted in a reduced level of normally functioning Mre11 protein.

The 15 Saudi Arabian patients were related to 5 independent families and represent the largest ATLD cohort (Fernet et al., 2005; Khan et al., 2008; Bohlega et al., 2011). Genetic

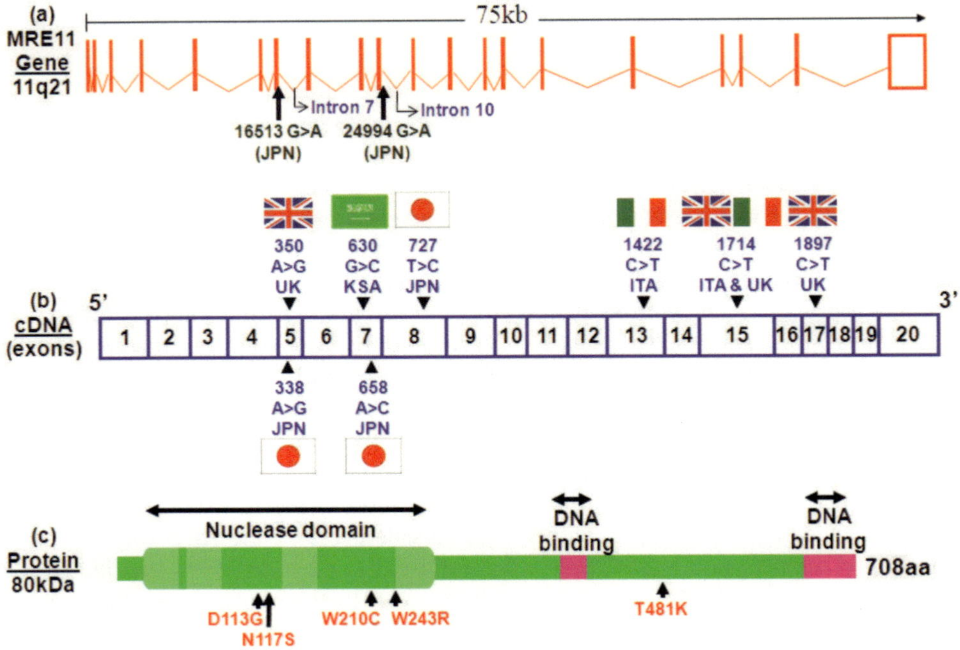

Fig. 3. Representation of the human (a) MRE11A gene, (b) cDNA and (c) protein. Location of the exonic (cDNA) and intronic mutations causing the 25 confirmed cases of ATLD from United Kingdom (UK), Italy (ITA), Japan (JPN) and the Kingdom of Saudi Arabia (KSA), are indicated. Only mutations detectable in a full-length Mre11 protein are indicated at the protein level. (Assembled from *www.ensembl.org* and Taylor et al., 2004 with substantial modifications and update).

studies have identified in all patients the same G to C transversion at position 630 (c.630G>C) located in exon 7, which results in the missense change of Trp to Cys (W210C). No other nucleotide change was identified in the coding sequences or flanking intronic sequences of MRE11A. Tryptophan at position 210 is a highly conserved residue in the Mre11 protein, being invariable from yeast to mammals and its replacement by the small polar residue cysteine is likely to affect the structure or function of the protein. In addition, this residue lies between motifs III and IV of the N-terminal nuclease domain of the Mre11 protein, a region where another missense mutation (N117S) had been identified in ATLD patients (Figure 3). Thus, all patients were homozygous for a novel missense mutation (c.630 G>C) of the MRE11A gene that seems to be specific to Saudi Arabia. The resulting amino acid change (W210C) does not seem to affect the level of Mre11 protein expression but results in an inability of the mutant Mre11 protein to interact with Nbs1 protein leading to destabilization of the MRN complex and the loss of its normal function.

4. Frequency of MRE11A gene mutations

While the frequency of the different mutations in the MRE11A gene is unknown, the high number of Saudi ATLD patients with the 630 G>C particular mutation would suggest noticeable frequency of heterozygous carriers in the Arabic peninsula. This may have impact on premarital and preimplantation screening to limit genetic diseases and to provide informed genetic counseling. Therefore, a study was initiated to assess the allelic frequency of this mutation (Alsbeih et al., 2008). Currently, a cohort of 528 phenotypically normal individuals was included in the study. There were 146 females and 382 males. The methodological procedures to detect the G to C missense mutation at nucleotide 630 of the MRE11A gene and the PCR primers used were described previously (Alsbeih et al., 2008). Briefly, genomic DNA was extracted from 3-5 ml peripheral whole blood or cultured skin fibroblasts, using Puregene DNA Purification Kit (Gentra System, Minneapolis, MN). Relevant segments of DNA were amplified by thermal cycling (95 °C for 15 min, 39 rounds of 95 °C for 1 min, 55 °C for 1 min and 72 °C for 1 min and final extension at 72 °C for 7 min) using HotStarTaq DNA polymerase (Qiagen, Venlo, Netherlands), and 50 ng template DNA in 25 microlitter volume with standard reaction conditions. The quality of the PCR product was checked by running 5 microlitter of the reaction in 1% agarose gel. The amplified fragment was directly sequenced using the DYEnamic ET Dye Terminator Cycle Sequencing Kit (Amersham Biosciences, Piscatway, NJ) according to the manufacturer's instruction, and were run on the MegaBase 1000 sequencer (Applied Biosystems, Fostercity, CA). Sequencing results were aligned to the corresponding reference sequence and the missense mutation was genotyped using SeqManII sequence analysis software (DNASTAR Inc., Madison, WI). Out of the 528 individuals, only two were heterozygous (G630C) for the missense mutation, while the remaining 526 were all wild-type. The genotype and allelic distributions of the missence mutation in the MRE11A are listed in Table 1. This gives a frequency of 99.6 for the G/G wild-type and 0.4% for the heterozygous G/C. In addition, one individual was heterozygous for a new SNP in intron 6, position 18026 (*Ensembl* annotation), 131 nucleotides upstream of the G630C mutation (Alsbeih et al., 2008).

Genotype and allele	Individuals *n*	Frequencies (%)
	MRE11A g.18157 mutation G>C	
G/G	526	99.6
G/C	2	0.4
C/C	0	0
G	1054	99.8
C	2	0.2

Table 1. Genotype and allele frequencies of the MRE11A 630G>C (g.18157, p.210 Trp>Cys) misense mutation in 528 Saudi individuals. Sequence reported on the negative strand as per the gene direction.

The presence of two heterozygous individuals indicates the existence of this rare mutation in the population with an estimated heterozygous genotype G/C of 0.4% and estimated mutant C allele frequency of 0.2%. Therefore, the diagnosis of MRE11A ATLD should be in the mind of physicians whenever they encounter an A-T like disorder and genetic study should be carried out to confirm the diagnosis. This is how the 5 patients reported by Bohlega and colleagues were diagnosed (Bohlega et al., 2011). The fact that the 10 previously described Saudi ATLD patients (Fernet et al., 2005) are from the central region of Saudi Arabia could suggest higher frequency of this mutation in geographically isolated families with high level of consanguineous marriages. However, larger studies with members from different regions are required to precisely estimate the exact frequency of this mutation in Saudi Arabia.

5. ATLD and other ataxia causing disorders

Ataxia occurs when parts of the nervous system that control movement are damaged. Most disorders that result in ataxia cause cells in the cerebellum, and sometimes in the spine or even the peripheral nervous systems, to degenerate or atrophy. Cerebellar and spinocerebellar degeneration have many different causes. Genetic causes form a heterogeneous group with different pattern of inheritance and onset of the symptoms. Currently this group encompasses the following distinct conditions: ataxia telangiectasia (A-T), ataxia telangiectasia-like disorder (ATLD), ataxia oculomotor apraxias (AOA), and the two "A-T variants", Nijmegen breakage syndrome (NBS) with microcephaly but without ataxia, and A-T (Fresno) that combines features of both NBS and A-T. This is in addition to other hereditary ataxia such as Friedreich ataxia (FA) and Machado-Joseph Disease (MJD) caused by triplet repeat expansion, spastic ataxia of the Charlevoix-Saguenay, Autosomal recessive ataxia associated with isolated vitamin E deficiency, Infantile onset spinocerebellar ataxia, ataxia with hearing loss and optic atrophy, spinocerebellar ataxia with axonal neuropathy, Cayman ataxia, cerebellar ataxia with mental retardation optic atrophy and skin abnormalities, Salla syndrome, Marinesco-Sjögren and the childhood spinocerebellar ataxia (Bouhlal et al., 2005). Table 2 summarizes some of the genetic disorders grouped under hereditary ataxias and its variants of relevance to ATLD.

Disorder	Acronym	Inheritance	Chromosomal location	Protein affected	Reference
Ataxia telangiectasia	A-T	Recessive	11q22-23	ATM	(Savitsky et al., 1995)
Ataxia telangiectasia-like disorder	ATLD	Recessive	11q21	Mre11	(Stewart et al., 1999)
Ataxia oculomotor apraxia 1	AOA1	Recessive	9p13	Aprataxin	(Date et al., 2001)
Ataxia oculomotor apraxia 2	AOA2	Recessive	9q34	Senataxin	(Moreira et al., 2004)
Nijmegen breakage syndrome	NBS	Recessive	8q21	Nbs1 (nibrin)	(Varon et al., 1998)
Ataxia telangiectasia Fresno*	A-T Fresno	Recessive	11q23	ATM	(Gilad et al., 1998)
Friedreich ataxia	FRDA	Recessive	9q13-q21	Frataxin	(Campuzano et al., 1996)
Machado-Joseph Disease	MJD	Dominant	14q32	Ataxin-3	(Kawaguchi et al., 1994)

* A-T Fresno combines features of A-T and NBS with mutation in ATM.

Table 2. Genetic disorders grouped under hereditary ataxias and its variants

Diagnosis is usually suggested by the clinical manifestations. Non-specific complementary tests may be done to differentiate between them or to exclude other disorders or conditions that may cause ataxia. The molecular characterization of these different disorders allows genetic tests to confirm a clinically suggested diagnosis. In general, there are no specific treatments available for most of the inherited ataxia disorders. Symptoms are treated with physical and occupational therapy, assistive devices, and medication for muscle pain or spasms that may occur. Genetic counseling provides education to parents of individuals with an inherited ataxia disorder to be aware that they may pass the disorder on to their children. Some affected families may choose to test members to see if they have inherited the gene responsible for the disorder.

6. Conclusions

Hereditary ataxias are a heterogeneous group of cerebellar degeneration causing failure of muscle control, resulting in a lack of coordination, imbalance and ataxic gait. ATLD is a rare variant of A-T with only 25 confirmed cases worldwide, 4 in the UK, 2 in Italy, 4 in Japan and 15 in Saudi Arabia. The patients were either homozygous or compound heterozygous for 10 different hypomorphic mutations in exons and splice sites. The 15 Saudi Arabian patients were related to 5 independent families and represent the largest ATLD cohort which would suggest the presence of a noticeable frequency of heterozygous carriers of MRE11A gene mutation in the population. Therefore, the diagnosis of ATLD should be in the mind of physicians whenever they encounter an A-T like disorder and genetic study should be carried out to confirm the diagnosis. Testing for MRE11A gene mutations could ultimately be incorporated to premarital, pre-implementation or prenatal screening to reduce the risk of transmission of genetic diseases.

7. Acknowledgments

I wish to thank Mr. Khaled Al-Hadyan and Ms. Najla Al-Harbi for their help and assistance. This work was funded by KFSHRC grants # 2000 031.

8. References

Alsbeih, G., Al-Hadyan, K. & Al-Harbi, N. (2008). Assessment of carriers' frequency of a novel MRE11 mutation responsible for the rare ataxia telangiectasia-like disorder. *Genet Test*, Vol. 12, No. 3, (Sep), pp. 387-389, 1090-6576

Bohlega, S.A., Shinwari, J.M., Al Sharif, L.J., Khalil, D.S., Alkhairallah, T.S. & Al Tassan, N.A. (2011). Clinical and molecular characterization of ataxia with oculomotor apraxia patients in saudi arabia. *BMC Med Genet*, Vol. 12, No. pp. 27, 1471-2350

Bouhlal, Y., El-Euch-Fayeche, G., Amouri, R. & Hentati, F. (2005). Distinct phenotypes within autosomal recessive ataxias not linked to already known loci. *Acta Myol*, Vol. 24, No. 2, (Oct), pp. 155-161, 1128-2460

Campuzano, V., Montermini, L., Molto, M.D., Pianese, L., Cossee, M., Cavalcanti, F., Monros, E., Rodius, F., Duclos, F., Monticelli, A., Zara, F., Canizares, J., Koutnikova, H., Bidichandani, S.I., Gellera, C., Brice, A., Trouillas, P., De Michele, G., Filla, A., De Frutos, R., Palau, F., Patel, P.I., Di Donato, S., Mandel, J.L., Cocozza, S., Koenig, M. & Pandolfo, M. (1996). Friedreich's ataxia: autosomal recessive disease caused by an intronic GAA triplet repeat expansion. *Science*, Vol. 271, No. 5254, (Mar 8), pp. 1423-1427,

Carney, J.P., Maser, R.S., Olivares, H., Davis, E.M., Le Beau, M., Yates, J.R., 3rd, Hays, L., Morgan, W.F. & Petrini, J.H. (1998). The hMre11/hRad50 protein complex and Nijmegen breakage syndrome: linkage of double-strand break repair to the cellular DNA damage response. *Cell*, Vol. 93, No. 3, pp. 477-486,

Date, H., Onodera, O., Tanaka, H., Iwabuchi, K., Uekawa, K., Igarashi, S., Koike, R., Hiroi, T., Yuasa, T., Awaya, Y., Sakai, T., Takahashi, T., Nagatomo, H., Sekijima, Y., Kawachi, I., Takiyama, Y., Nishizawa, M., Fukuhara, N., Saito, K., Sugano, S. & Tsuji, S. (2001). Early-onset ataxia with ocular motor apraxia and hypoalbuminemia is caused by mutations in a new HIT superfamily gene. *Nat Genet*, Vol. 29, No. 2, (Oct), pp. 184-188,

Delia, D., Piane, M., Buscemi, G., Savio, C., Palmeri, S., Lulli, P., Carlessi, L., Fontanella, E. & Chessa, L. (2004). MRE11 mutations and impaired ATM-dependent responses in an Italian family with ataxia-telangiectasia-like disorder. *Hum Mol Genet*, Vol. 13, No. 18, (Sep 15), pp. 2155-2163, 0964-6906

Fernet, M., Gribaa, M., Salih, M.A., Seidahmed, M.Z., Hall, J. & Koenig, M. (2005). Identification and functional consequences of a novel MRE11 mutation affecting 10 Saudi Arabian patients with the ataxia telangiectasia-like disorder. *Hum Mol Genet*, Vol. 14, No. 2, (Jan 15), pp. 307-318, 0964-6906 (Print)

Frischmeyer, P.A., van Hoof, A., O'Donnell, K., Guerrerio, A.L., Parker, R. & Dietz, H.C. (2002). An mRNA surveillance mechanism that eliminates transcripts lacking termination codons. *Science*, Vol. 295, No. 5563, (Mar 22), pp. 2258-2261, 1095-9203

Gilad, S., Chessa, L., Khosravi, R., Russell, P., Galanty, Y., Piane, M., Gatti, R.A., Jorgensen, T.J., Shiloh, Y. & Bar-Shira, A. (1998). Genotype-phenotype relationships in ataxia-telangiectasia and variants. *Am J Hum Genet*, Vol. 62, No. 3, (Mar), pp. 551-561,

Hernandez, D., McConville, C.M., Stacey, M., Woods, C.G., Brown, M.M., Shutt, P., Rysiecki, G. & Taylor, A.M. (1993). A family showing no evidence of linkage between the ataxia telangiectasia gene and chromosome 11q22-23. *J Med Genet*, Vol. 30, No. 2, (Feb), pp. 135-140,

Kawaguchi, Y., Okamoto, T., Taniwaki, M., Aizawa, M., Inoue, M., Katayama, S., Kawakami, H., Nakamura, S., Nishimura, M., Akiguchi, I. & et al. (1994). CAG expansions in a novel gene for Machado-Joseph disease at chromosome 14q32.1. *Nat Genet*, Vol. 8, No. 3, (Nov), pp. 221-228,

Khan, A.O., Oystreck, D.T., Koenig, M. & Salih, M.A. (2008). Ophthalmic features of ataxia telangiectasia-like disorder. *J AAPOS*, Vol. 12, No. 2, (Apr), pp. 186-189, 1528-3933

Klein, C., Wenning, G.K., Quinn, N.P. & Marsden, C.D. (1996). Ataxia without telangiectasia masquerading as benign hereditary chorea. *Mov Disord*, Vol. 11, No. 2, (Mar), pp. 217-220,

Maser, R.S., Monsen, K.J., Nelms, B.E. & Petrini, J.H. (1997). hMre11 and hRad50 nuclear foci are induced during the normal cellular response to Dna double-strand breaks. *Molecular Cell Biology*, Vol. 17, No. 10, pp. 6087-6096,

Matsumoto, Y., Miyamoto, T., Sakamoto, H., Izumi, H., Nakazawa, Y., Ogi, T., Tahara, H., Oku, S., Hiramoto, A., Shiiki, T., Fujisawa, Y., Ohashi, H., Sakemi, Y. & Matsuura, S. (2011). Two unrelated patients with MRE11A mutations and Nijmegen breakage syndrome-like severe microcephaly. *DNA Repair (Amst)*, Vol. 10, No. 3, (Mar 7), pp. 314-321, 1568-7856

Moreira, M.C., Klur, S., Watanabe, M., Nemeth, A.H., Le Ber, I., Moniz, J.C., Tranchant, C., Aubourg, P., Tazir, M., Schols, L., Pandolfo, M., Schulz, J.B., Pouget, J., Calvas, P., Shizuka-Ikeda, M., Shoji, M., Tanaka, M., Izatt, L., Shaw, C.E., M'Zahem, A., Dunne, E., Bomont, P., Benhassine, T., Bouslam, N., Stevanin, G., Brice, A., Guimaraes, J., Mendonca, P., Barbot, C., Coutinho, P., Sequeiros, J., Durr, A., Warter, J.M. & Koenig, M. (2004). Senataxin, the ortholog of a yeast RNA helicase, is mutant in ataxia-ocular apraxia 2. *Nat Genet*, Vol. 36, No. 3, (Mar), pp. 225-227

Nelms, B.E., Maser, R.S., MacKay, J.F., Lagally, M.G. & Petrini, J.H. (1998). In situ visualization of DNA double-strand break repair in human fibroblasts. *Science*, Vol. 280, No. 5363, pp. 590-592

Nicholson, P., Yepiskoposyan, H., Metze, S., Zamudio Orozco, R., Kleinschmidt, N. & Muhlemann, O. (2010). Nonsense-mediated mRNA decay in human cells: mechanistic insights, functions beyond quality control and the double-life of NMD factors. *Cell Mol Life Sci*, Vol. 67, No. 5, (Mar), pp. 677-700, 1420-9071

Petrini, J.H. (2000). The Mre11 complex and ATM: collaborating to navigate S phase. *Curr Opin Cell Biol*, Vol. 12, No. 3, (Jun), pp. 293-296

Pitts, S.A., Kullar, H.S., Stankovic, T., Stewart, G.S., Last, J.I., Bedenham, T., Armstrong, S.J., Piane, M., Chessa, L., Taylor, A.M. & Byrd, P.J. (2001). hMRE11: genomic structure and a null mutation identified in a transcript protected from nonsense-mediated mRNA decay. *Hum Mol Genet*, Vol. 10, No. 11, (May 15), pp. 1155-1162

Savitsky, K., Bar-Shira, A., Gilad, S., Rotman, G., Ziv, Y., Vanagaite, L., Tagle, D.A., Smith, S., Uziel, T., Sfez, S. & et al. (1995). A single ataxia telangiectasia gene with a product similar to PI-3 kinase. *Science*, Vol. 268, No. 5218, pp. 1749-1753

Stewart, G.S., Maser, R.S., Stankovic, T., Bressan, D.A., Kaplan, M.I., Jaspers, N.G., Raams, A., Byrd, P.J., Petrini, J.H. & Taylor, A.M. (1999). The DNA double-strand break repair gene hMRE11 is mutated in individuals with an ataxia-telangiectasia-like disorder. *Cell*, Vol. 99, No. 6, pp. 577-587

Tauchi, H., Matsuura, S., Kobayashi, J., Sakamoto, S. & Komatsu, K. (2002). Nijmegen breakage syndrome gene, NBS1, and molecular links to factors for genome stability. *Oncogene*, Vol. 21, No. 58, (Dec 16), pp. 8967-8980,

Taylor, A.M. (2001). Chromosome instability syndromes. *Best Pract Res Clin Haematol*, Vol. 14, No. 3, (Sep), pp. 631-644,

Taylor, A.M., Groom, A. & Byrd, P.J. (2004). Ataxia-telangiectasia-like disorder (ATLD)-its clinical presentation and molecular basis. *DNA Repair (Amst)*, Vol. 3, No. 8-9, (Aug-Sep), pp. 1219-1225

Taylor, A.M.R., Harnden, D.G., Arlett, C.F., Harcourt, S.A., Lehmann, A.R., Stevens, S. & Bridges, B.A. (1975). Ataxia-telangiectasia, a human mutation with abnormal radiation sensitivity. *Nature*, Vol. 258, No. pp. 427-429,

Uchisaka, N., Takahashi, N., Sato, M., Kikuchi, A., Mochizuki, S., Imai, K., Nonoyama, S., Ohara, O., Watanabe, F., Mizutani, S., Hanada, R. & Morio, T. (2009). Two brothers with ataxia-telangiectasia-like disorder with lung adenocarcinoma. *J Pediatr*, Vol. 155, No. 3, (Sep), pp. 435-438, 1097-6833

Varon, R., Vissinga, C., Platzer, M., Cerosaletti, K.M., Chrzanowska, K.H., Saar, K., Beckmann, G., Seemanova, E., Cooper, P.R., Nowak, N.J., Stumm, M., Weemaes,

C.M., Gatti, R.A., Wilson, R.K., Digweed, M., Rosenthal, A., Sperling, K., Concannon, P. & Reis, A. (1998). Nibrin, a novel DNA double-strand break repair protein, is mutated in Nijmegen breakage syndrome. *Cell*, Vol. 93, No. 3, pp. 467-476

Williams, R.S., Williams, J.S. & Tainer, J.A. (2007). Mre11-Rad50-Nbs1 is a keystone complex connecting DNA repair machinery, double-strand break signaling, and the chromatin template. *Biochem Cell Biol*, Vol. 85, No. 4, (Aug), pp. 509-520, 0829-8211

5

Neuronopathic Forms in Subjects with Mutations in *GBA* Gene

Pilar Giraldo, Jose-Luis Capablo and Miguel Pocovi
Instituto de Investigación Sanitaria de Aragón (IIS), CIBER de Investigación Biomedica en Red de Enfermedades Raras (CIBERER), University of Zaragoza, Zaragoza Spain

1. Introduction

Gaucher disease (GD) (GD, OMIM 230800), is the most common glycosphingolipid storage disorder, with an estimated global prevalence of 1:200,000 of the population (Cox & Schofield, 1997). Impaired activity of the lysosomal enzyme, β-glucocerebrosidase, leads to build-up of glucosylceramide in macrophages, forming dysfunctional, lipid-engorged 'Gaucher cells' that accumulate primarily in the liver, spleen, bone, lungs and nervous system (Grabowski & Horowitz, 1997; Beutler, 1997). Figure 1 Sometimes, bone disease or cellular infiltration in bone marrow, could be lead to fractures or hematomas that cause neurological complications from compression of the spinal cord or peripheral nervous system. In addition, severe deficiency of β-glucocerebrosidase increases the accumulation in the central nervous system of glucosylceramide and other toxic metabolites in the neuronopathic involvement. However the precise mechanisms by which glucosylceramide storage originate them is still unclear. The frequency of neurological GD cases is ranging between 7% and 17%, according to different series (Biegstraaten et al., 2008; Chérin et al., 2010).

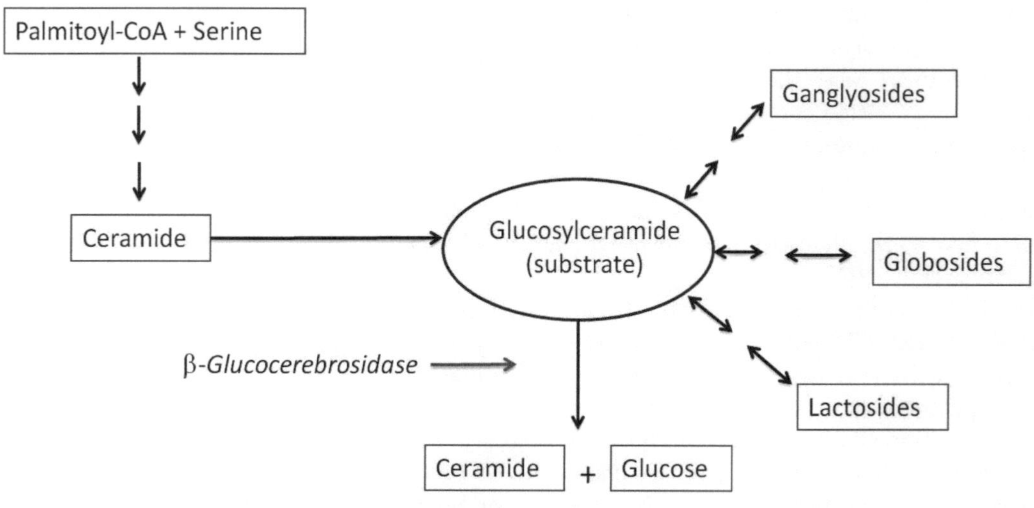

Fig. 1. Biosynthesis and degradation of sphingolipid

2. Clinical characteristics of neurological forms

The neuronopathic forms of GD can be either acute type 2 (GD2) (MIM 230900), or chronic type 3 (GD3) (MIM 231000), the presence of neurological symptoms is the main characteristics for a diagnosis, nevertheless in a low percentage of type 1 GD (GD1) some neurological manifestations could be considered part of the GD1 phenotype.
These forms are considered as ultrarare and estimated at about 5% for GD3 and 1% for GD2 (Charrow et al., 2000).

2.1 Type 2 Gaucher disease

There are many descriptions of type 2 Gaucher disease presenting with hydrops fetalis and joint contractures. In the majority of cases with this severe phenotype, glucocerebrosidase activity is absent or severely deficient. In general, most patients with Gaucher disease do have some residual glucocerebrosidase activity, with no correlation between severity and the level of residual enzyme activity.
The patients with the acute form, usually die within two years. The initial neurological symptoms as paralysis of horizontal gaze supranuclear are followed later, with strabismus, impaired vertical gaze, dysarthria, difficulty in swallowing, chewing, laryngeal stridor and a pyramidal syndrome with opisthotonos. Some of these patients develop a progressive encephalopathy that is neocortical in origin. The molecular and cellular bases for the phenotypic variation and the progression of the neuronopathic features in Gaucher disease are poorly understood. Few studies are available from human tissues that correlate neuronopathic progression, pathologic involvement, and the clinical manifestations. To fill this void, several mouse models with GCase null or point mutations or chemical inhibition were developed. The GCase-null mutations exhibited a defective skin permeability barrier, similar to that in collodion babies. Skin permeability barrier defects lead to death shortly after birth and have limited their utility in understanding the pathogenesis in CNS of type 2 and 3 Gaucher disease (Xu et al, 2008)

2.2 Type 3 Gaucher disease

The patients with chronic form, GD3, the first neurological symptoms usually appear at a mean age of 8 years, and the patients with myoclonic epilepsy variant by age 15 (Park et al., 2003) in these cases the life expectancy can reaches the third decade. Nevertheless, there have been reported some cases of apraxia of gaze without progression to other neurological symptoms (Kraoua et al., 2011). There are other GD3 subtypes, GD3b, the neurological involvement is limited to apraxia of the eyes, but is associated with visceral enlargement and bone disease. (Patterson et al., 1993). Other less common GD3 subtype, have been classified as 3c characterized by heart valves calcification and eye movement disorders (Chabas et al., 1995).
The GD3 has heterogeneous clinical manifestations, and therefore different subtypes have been referred. GD3 subtype a, is characterized by apraxia of gaze and dementia associated with myoclonic epilepsy, ataxia and extrapyramidal signs or spasticity. In addition in this subtype there are several specific forms including the myoclonus epilepsy as the main manifestation (Park et al., 2003). These neurological forms have slight or moderate visceral involvement and bone changes are characterized by chest deformities and kyphoscoliosis, which may have a neurological basis, however bone crises normally are absent (Tylki-Szymańska et al., 2010).

2.2.1 Myoclonic epilepsy

Different lysosomal storage diseases: late-onset GM2 gangliosidosis, type 2 GM1 gangliosidosis, Niemann-Pick disease, sialidosis, galactosialidosis, pseudodeficiencia of arylsulfatase A, Gaucher disease and some forms of ceroid lipofuscinosis have been associated with myoclonic epilepsy (Tinuper et al., 1994; Kowarz et al., 2005).

The main form is an association between Gaucher disease and myoclonic epilepsy in a rare subgroup of patients with GD type 3 who developed a progressive myoclonus epilepsy. All had horizontal saccadic eye movements. The lack of a shared genotype for patients and the variability in clinical presentations suggesting the existence of other modifying factors contributing to this rare phenotype (Park et al., 2003). Have also been documented cases in Spanish population with symptoms of myoclonic epilepsy (Giraldo et al., 2011). In a study of a Spanish patient with neuronopathic type 3 GD and myoclonic epilepsy symptomatic improvement was observed using a combination of substrate reduction therapy with enzyme replacement therapy (Capablo et al., 2007).

Although the mutation N188S in the GBA gene in Gaucher disease was initially considered a mild mutation or a variant modifier has been reported the association of this mutation with the development of myoclonic epilepsy, suggesting that the enzyme could lead to abnormal death of neuronal cells or modify the role of other proteins involved in epilepsy (Kowarz et al., 2005). In recent years, understanding the genetic basis of myoclonic epilepsy has progressed rapidly and several defects have been identified, specific genes and mutations (Scheffer & Berkovic, 2000, Stafstrom et al., 2000, Delgado-Escueta et al. 2001).

Recently genes have been identified for other forms of progressive myoclonus epilepsy:

a. The CLN3 gene has been associated with a type of neuronal ceroid lipofuscinosis, Batten disease, contains 15 exons and spans over 15 Kb. The International Batten Disease Consortium isolated the gene CLN3 between microsatellite markers D16S288 and D16S383 on chromosome 16p12.2.1-16p11 (International Batten Disease Consortium, 1995). It is speculated that the gene product functions as a chaperone involved in folding / unfolding or assembly / disassembly of other proteins, specifically the subunit c of ATP synthase complex (Janes et al., 1996). Biochemically mutation causes multiple deficiencies in the enzyme complexes of the respiratory chain involving NADH-CoQ reductase (complex I) in the cytochrome C oxidase (COX).
b. A mutation at nucleotide 8344 of human mitochondrial DNA causes MERRF (Myoclonus Epilepsy Associated with Ragged-Red Fibers) (Shoffner et al., 1990).
c. The gene for cystatin B (CSTB) is located on chromosome 21 in a segment of about 175KB, between D21S2040 and D21S1259. Expands into three exons over 2500bp, encoding a small protein of 98 amino acids. Mutations in the gene encoding cystatin B are responsible for primary defect in patients with progressive myoclonus epilepsy type Unverricht-Lundborg (EPM1) autosomal recessive (Pennacchio et al., 1996). The encoded protein is a member of the superfamily of cysteine protease inhibitors (Jarvinen & Rinne, 1982, Turk & Bode, 1991).
d. EPM2A gene is located on chromosome 6q24 and contains 5 exons that encode two laforin isoforms, isoform A is located in the rough endoplasmic reticulum and isoform B in the nucleus. Laforin is a dual specificity phosphatase and functions are involved in protein degradation by the proteasome (Lohi et al., 2005) and glycogen metabolism (Worby et al., 2006). Mutations in the gene EPM2A cause deleterious effects on protein encoding the laforin, causing Lafora disease, which is an autosomal recessive progressive myoclonic epilepsy (Minassian et al., 1998).

3. Histological changes in neurological forms

The neuropathological studies (Wong et al., 2004) in patients with different types of GD have found clear pathologic changes in several areas of the brain, mainly in the form of perivascular Gaucher cells, astrogliosis and neuronal loss. Immunohistochemical findings in the same study suggest that, in certain areas, elevated intracellular levels of glucocerebroside would further reduce glucocerebrosidase levels and contribute to citoxicity as well as to abnormalities in calcium homeostasis and increased sensitivity of neurons, thus facilitating spontaneous neuronal discharges. More recent data reinforces the role of citotoxic molecules, but possibly related to the intraneuronal accumulation of the defective enzyme (Futerman; 2006). It has also been proposed that the accumulation of glucosylsphingosine, is responsible for the neurological symptoms (Pelled et al., 2005). On the other hand, the finding that mutation N188S may be associated with the development of myoclonic epilepsy, suggests that the abnormal enzyme might lead to neuronal cell death, or modify the role on other proteins involved in epilepsy (Kowarz et al., 2005). Neuropathological exam in a GD3 patient suggests that cerebellum-dentate degeneration would play a major role in these patients' myoclonus (Verghese et al., 2000). How this relates to in vivo cortical dysfunction is unclear. Probably, other factors in addition to point mutations, environmental, epigenetic and genetic, will ultimately be involved in the development of myoclonic epilepsy in GD patients.

In some cases of myoclonic epilepsy an improvement in neurological symptoms have been observed with substrate reduction therapy (SRT), the biochemical basis of this improvement could be related with small molecules that have been shown to enter the CNS both in animal models and in patients and this was an important argument maybe related to the reduction of glucocerebroside accumulation by the substrate reduction activity. It could also be related to the described chaperoning effect on the defective glucocerebrosidase or a functional improvement, through a yet unknown mechanism, in the defective calcium homeostasis described above (Pelled et al., 2005).

4. Clinical characteristics of type 1 Gaucher Disease

Classically, GD1 is characterized by organomegaly, cytopenias, bone disease and absence of neurological manifestations. However, there are several reports of the co-occurrence of neurological problems, as a consequence of spinal cord or nerve compression following vertebral body collapse or bleeding within confined compartments (Grewel et al., 1991). There is accumulating evidence that in a few GD patients, prominent neurological abnormalities may become evident during adult life (McKeran et al., 1985). Several new lines of evidence have implicated an association between GD and the development of parkinsonism. The first hints of a relationship between the two disorders were suggested by scattered case reports of patients with Gaucher disease who developed early-onset, treatment-refractory parkinsonism (Neudorfer et al., 1996; Machaczka et al., 1999; Tayebi et al., 2001). In a clinic-based series of Parkinson disease patients from Israel, (Aharon-Peretz et al., 2004) screened for the most frequent mutations in glucocerebrosidase gene, they identified 31% with glucocerebrosidase mutations including three N370S homozygotes. This frequency was at least fivefold higher than the observed in their two control groups used.

In an international collaborative study conducted in sixteen countries with 5961 patients with Parkinson disease in all ethnic groups, compared with 4898 controls, the odds ratio estimated for any type of *GBA* mutation has been of 5.43 (Sidransky et al., 2009).

We have studied the characteristics of Gaucher disease in Iberian Peninsula. The Iberian Peninsula (IP) is located in the extreme Southwest of Europe and includes the states of Portugal and Spain. It is the second-largest peninsula in Europe, with an area of 580,000 square kilometers and with a total 55 million of inhabitants. The actual IP genetic pool has been influenced by many major populations and immigrations, including the Paleolithic Iberian population, which already existed by 50,000 B.C. Later, by North Africans who entered the Iberian region between 20,000 and 8,000 B.C. and by the Saharans, who arrived between 8,000 and 4,000 B.C. In addition, there were also people coming from central Europe (also generically called Celt invasions), during the first millennium B.C. At the beginning of the 8th century Islamic peoples (generically called Arabs) entered Spain (Arnaiz Villena et al 1999, Côrte-Real HB et al 1996). Taking into account all these data, nowadays it is believed that, the timing of divergence of populations within Iberia points to a shared ancestry of all populations in the Upper Palaeolithic. Further genetic subdivision is apparent in Catalonia and Andalusia, with increased genetic diversity in the latter. Lineage diversity comparisons of IP populations with European (Tuscan) and North African (Algerian) populations shows the Iberian Peninsula to be more similar to other European populations, although a small number of Iberian lineages can be traced to North Africa.

Since the early 70s, the group of Dr. Chabas in Barcelona (Spain) and the Dr. Sa Miranda in Porto (Portugal) has been dedicated to the identification and study of lysosomal storage diseases including GD (Cormand et al. 1995, 1998; Amaral et al 1993). Moreover since 1993, the Spanish Foundation for the Study and Treatment of Gaucher Disease (FEETEG) keeps the Spanish Registry of GD (SRGD) and also coordinates the screening, diagnosis, characterization, treatment, and follow-up of GD patients in Spain (Giraldo et al. 2000, Alfonso et al 2007).

Of the 436 subjects included in this series, the 96.1% were born in Iberian Peninsula, Balearic and Canary Islands, 92 patient were from Portugal (21.1%) and 327 (75.0%) Spanish origin and 17 were immigrants (3.9%), Patients born at IP were classified at diagnosis: 370 as GD type 1 (88.3%) (age mean: 40.6 ± 20.30 years, range 0.3-87); 28 as GD type 2 (6.7%) (Age: mean 0.4 years, range 0-1) and 21 as GD type 3 (5.0%) (Age: mean 5.9 years, range 2-17). Mean age at diagnosis in the total GD patients was 26.3±19.88 years (range 0-87) and 28.7 years in patients type 1. To date, 63 patients from IP in this series are death (15%) and 373 are alive (85%). According the type distribution 7.6% of type 1; 52.4% of type 3 and 100% of type 2 are death.

4.1 Association of Parkinsonism with Gaucher disease

Parkinson disease (PD), the second most common neurodegenerative disorder after Alzheimer's disease, has a complex and multifactorial etiology, with different contributions: genetic, epigenetic and environmental. It can be classified by age of onset as early PD or late PD and in the form of presentation as family or sporadic PD.

The main clinical phenotype of Parkinson's disease is characterized by motor dysfunction such as bradykinesia, tremor at rest, rigidity and postural instability, but can also affect autonomic functions and knowledge (Poewe, 2008).

The prevalence of the disease is associated with age, and is approximately 1 in 100 individuals at 65 years and increasing to 4-5% at the age of 85 years (Van den Eeden et al., 2003).

Parkinson's disease is mainly due to a progressive degeneration of dopaminergic neurons in the substantia nigra and other monoaminergic cell groups of the brain (Braak et al., 2003), resulting in increased microglial activation and accumulation of proteins in the surviving dopaminergic neurons, known as Lewy bodies and Lewy neurites (Forno, 1996). Symptoms appear when between 50-70% of nigrostriatal dopaminergic neurons are lost.

Although Parkinson's disease has been considered a genetic disorder of not sporadic origin, only 5 to 10% of patients show monogenic forms of the disease. Some genes are associated with Parkinson's disease, and several of them are presented in an autosomal dominant or autosomal recessive.

Autosomal dominant: PARK1/α-sinucleín, PARK4/α-sinucleín, PARK8/Leucine-rich repeat kinase 2 (LRRK2) and microtubule associated protein tau (MAPT).

Autosomal recessive: The PARK2 gene is located on chromosome 6q25.2-q27 and comprises 12 exons with intron structure superexpanded of 1.3 Mb of genomic DNA, which encodes a protein of 465 amino acid N-terminal domain similar to ubiquitin. Mutations in the parkin gene (PARK2) were identified for the first time in several Japanese families with autosomal recessive juvenile parkinsonism (Kitada et al., 1998).

PTEN-induced PARK6/Quinasa 1 (PINK1). Homozygous mutations in this gene were found originally in patients with early-onset Parkinson's, and account for between 1 to 2% of cases of early onset of Parkinson's disease (Hatano et al., 2004).

The PINK1 gene, located on 1p35-36, contains 8 exons spread over 1.8 kb and encodes a protein of 581 amino acids. The transcript is expressed ubiquitously and encodes a protein kinase domain of a highly conserved, which is also in the family of Ca2 + / calmodulin serine-threonine kinases (Valente et al., 2004).

DJ1 PARK7/Oncogen, DJ1 gene, located on chromosome region 1p36, contains 8 exons that span 24 Kb and is located 25 cM from the telomere of the PINK1 gene (Bonifati et al., 2003). Deletions have been identified and mutations that cause amino acid change <1% of early-onset parkinsonism (Lockhart et al., 2004).

Monogenic forms represent less than 10% of Parkinson disease in most populations and are the result of complex interactions between genes and environmental factors. Genetic variations could be susceptibility factors or disease modifiers, affecting the penetrance, age of onset, severity and progression.

The results of different studies show an association between Gaucher and Parkinson's disease by the occurrence of Gaucher disease and atypical parkinsonism in patients, appearing between the fourth and sixth decades of life, and the identification of mutations in the gene the *GBA* in probands with sporadic Parkinson's disease.

There are different hypotheses about how to explain the association of Parkinson disease and Gaucher Disease. One of them claims that glucocerebrosidase gene *(GBA)* mutations can produce an aberrant protein with function gain either hetero or homozygous and facilitate the alpha-synuclein aggregation this effect could induces neuronal toxicity. Wild-type alpha-synuclein could be selectively translocated into lysosomes for degradation by the chaperone-mediated autophagy pathway (Cuervo et al., 2004).

Under these conditions the receptor LAMP2 would saturate their transport capacity, resulting in a jam intracellular alpha-synuclein. Another scenario would involve directly the accumulation of misfolded mutated glucocerebrosidase protein in the endoplasmic reticulum leading to a situation of stress, and decreased activity of parkin, an ubiquitin ligase associated with the occurrence of early onset of Parkinson disease. This stress could trigger the start of the mechanisms of neuronal apoptosis in the substantia nigra, and therefore the onset of disease (Ron et al., 2010).

Moreover, only in patients with the two GBA mutant alleles the functional deficit of glucocerebrosidase, may cause accumulation of glucocerebroside and glucoesphyngosine that interfere with the determination of alpha-synuclein to lipid membranes, facilitating the aggregation of alpha-synuclein and the formation of Lewy bodies (Schlossmacher et al., 2005).

4.2 Other neurological manifestations in type 1 Gaucher Disease

Pastores et al conducted an epidemiological survey in order to ascertain the incidence of neurological symptoms in patients with GD1 (Pastores et al., 2003). This survey revealed that a significant proportion of patients with GD I experience neurological symptoms. In addition, we found that GD1 patients have a greater risk of suffering other common unrelated diseases than carriers or their healthy relatives (Giraldo et al., 2011).

The wide spectrum phenotypic variation and neurological involvement within all types, and the recognition of an increasing number of subgroups of patients, support the view that GD is a disorder with a phenotypic continuum ranging from prenatal lethality to asymptomatic adults (Sidransky, 2004). Figure 2

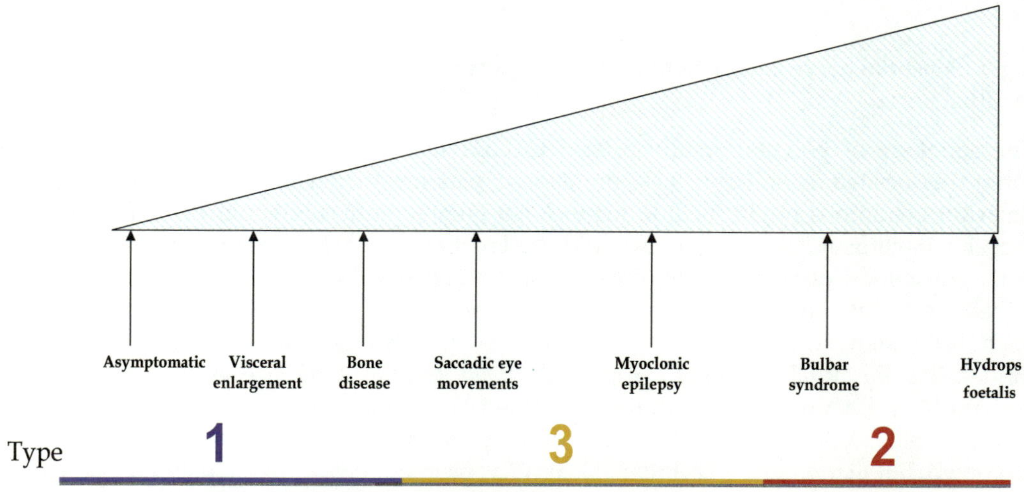

Fig. 2. Phenotype continuum in Gaucher disease

A recent systematic review of published literature identified 86 studies in which patients with GD1, or carriers of a glucocerebrosidase gene mutation, had some form of neurological manifestation (Biegstraaten et al., 2008; Cherin et al., 2010) contrary to the classical neuronopathic phenotypical description. Peripheral nervous system manifestations appear to be of particular relevance in GD1. An epidemiological survey of GD1 patients undergoing long-term enzyme replacement therapy (ERT) revealed that 73% of patients had at least one neurological symptom, including paraesthesia, tremor, muscular weakness, muscle cramps and sciatica, most of which were thought to be due to peripheral nervous system disease (Pastores et al., 2003). A case-control survey in 107 GD1 patients (untreated or receiving ERT) corroborated these findings, reporting a significantly higher frequency of symptoms related to peripheral neuropathy (Halperin et al., 2007). However, the above studies were limited by the absence of a neurological examination and standardised nerve conduction studies, and as yet there are no reliable estimates of the prevalence of peripheral neuropathy in GD1 (Biegstraaten et al., 2010), the vast majority of these cases have subclinical peripheral neuropathy only detected by electroneurophysiological exams. Figure 3

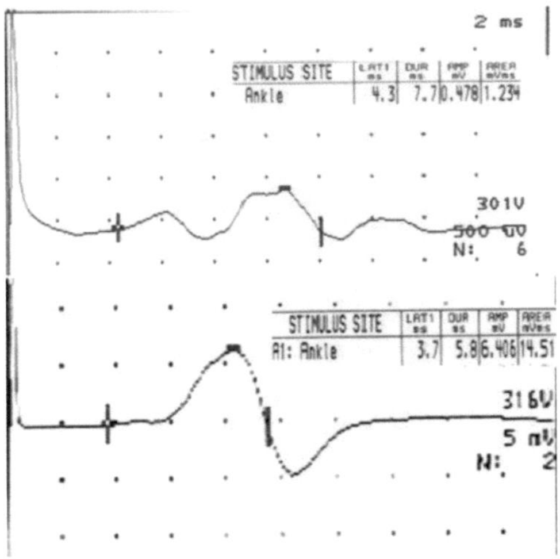

Fig. 3. Sensorial nerve conduction in type 1 Gaucher Disease patient. Abnormal wave forms in radial nerve.

The aetiology of polyneuropathy related to GD1 has not yet been elucidated, although certain associated conditions may predispose patients to develop neurological disease. Relevant conditions might include monoclonal gammopathies, vitamin B_{12} deficiency and diabetes mellitus (Gielchinsky et al., 2001; de Frost et al., 2008; Silverman et al., 2008). The pathophysiology of nerve injury in GD remains speculative, but may be related to an imbalance in calcium homeostasis. Elevated intraneuronal glucocerebroside concentrations have been shown to induce a 300% increase in calcium-induced calcium release by influencing the RyaR channel, which has been proposed as one of the mechanisms responsible for neuronal injury in the central nervous system of neuronopathic GD (Lloyd-Evans et al., 2003). Whether this mechanism plays a role in peripheral nerve injury is unknown, but increased intracellular calcium has been implicated in the pathophysiology of diabetic neuropathy and neuropathic pain (Hall et al., 2001; Yaksh,2006; Finnerup et al., 2007).

In conclusion, polyneuropathy and other peripheral nerve involvement appear to be part of the natural course of disease in patients with GD1, highlighting the need for increased vigilance for peripheral neurological abnormalities

5. Mutations in *GBA* and neuronopatic forms of Gaucher Disease

The gene for human GCase, *GBA*, consists of 11 exon, have 7.2–7.4 kb in size, and maps to chromosome 1q21 (Barneveld et al., 1983). A pseudogene that shares 96% exonic sequence homology with *GBA* is located at 16 kb downstream from the functional gene (Horowitz et al., 1989). Figure 4. The pseudogene is transcribed, but does not produce a functional protein (Sorge et al., 1990). A significant number of mutations are present in the *GBA* pseudogene, and there are mutant alleles caused by gene conversion events with the pseudogene named recombinant alleles, Rec or pseudogene like mutations. Over 300 mutations have been identified worldwide in *GBA* and over 50 different mutations have been described in patients with neuronopatic involvement (Hruska et al., 2008) and also see *http://www.hgmd.org*. They represent a spectrum of non-sense, missense and splice mutations as well as gene rearrangements. Most of these mutations are rare or private mutations, but two missense mutations, N370S and L444P, have significant frequencies in the majority of populations. It has been suggested that the genotype plays an important role in determining the degree of neurological involvement; however genotype-phenotype correlations are not straightforward in GD (Beutler & Grabowski., 2001; Koprivica et al., 2000). The most consistent finding is that the presence of the N370S mutation, either in homozygosity or in heterozygosity, always precludes development of neurological manifestation (Grabowski, 1997).

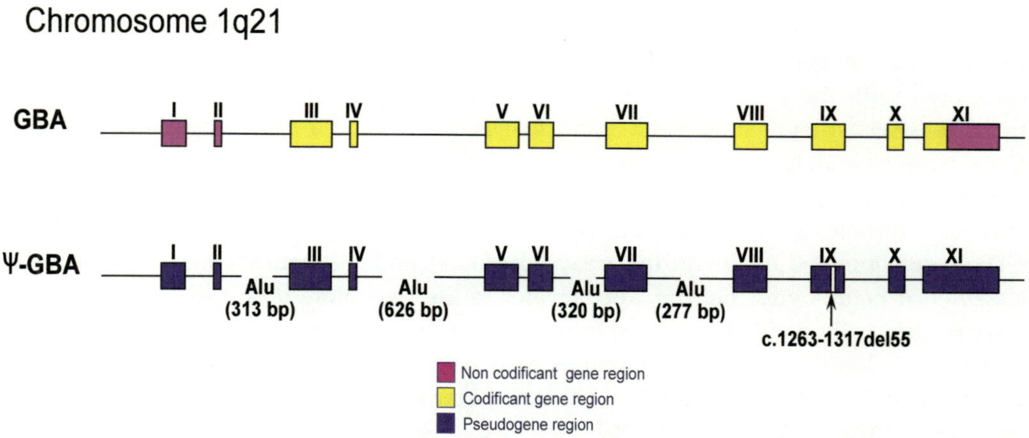

Fig. 4. Structure of glucocerebrosidase gene GBA and Seudogene Ψ-GBA

However, L444 P homozygosity has been shown to be associated with a neuronopathic phenotype in various populations, including Spanish, Swedish, Pole, Ashkenazi Jewish, and other Caucasian populations, while it was clearly associated with non-neuronopathic Gaucher disease in Taiwanese-Chinese (Wan et al., 2006; Goker-Alpan et al., 2005; Koprivica et al., 2000; Stone, 2000). These observations strongly suggest that other factors, such as modifier loci, promoter mutations, environmental factors, and other non-genetic causes, must play roles in the observed genotype-phenotype variability and also that modifying genes could be associated with the ethnic-related genetic diversity (Montfort et al., 2004; Alfonso et al., 2010).

To try to identify relationships genotype-phenotype, two approaches may be useful. First, the use of homogenous populations would tend to diminish genetic variation, as a consequence, the observed phenotype can be attributed to the identified mutants with greater assurance. However, this approach is limited by the need of large sample size to identify sufficient numbers of homozygotes for study, and to guarantee the homogeneity. The second approach is to study patients with most severe disease, and the least amount of residual activity. It is assumed that both mutant alleles have to be highly disruptive in these cases.

An additional problem arises from the analysis method used; most laboratories relied solely on Polymerase Chain Reaction (PCR) based mutation-detection techniques to screen for the presence or absence of specific mutations. PCR amplification of a specific fragment has inherent problems, because a complex allele with more than one mutation, a mutation located at a primer site or a deleted allele could not be detected and therefore the published studies on genotype-phenotype relationship may be biased. Moreover, recombinant alleles would not be identified because using this approach alleles carrying a portion of the pseudogene sequence will not be amplified by primers designed to be specific for the glucocerebrosidase gene, and the patient may mistakenly be designated as a homozygote for the second allele (Torralba et al., 2002; Tayebi et al.,1999)

Given these limitations, we note that some generalizations were observed that suggested genotype–phenotype correlations: 1) homozygosis for the L444P mutation is usually, if not always, associated with neuronopatic forms 2). L444P is the most common mutation identified in patients with the intermediate phenotype. 3) the combination of one allele with L444P mutation and another mutation with a null or very severe allele seemed to be associated with the most severe neurological form, type 2. 4) perinatal lethality due to hydrops fetalis often resulted from homozygosis for a null or a recombinant allele. 5) None of the patients with type 2 are carriers of the N370S mutation, commonly found in GD1.

It is important to point out that there is an overlap between the GD2 and GD3 phenotypes making it difficult to categorize, on the other hand, the differentiation between GD1 and GD3 is sometimes difficult during early adulthood and the patients may have to be re-classified if neurological deficits, appear later in life. Therefore it is possible that Gaucher disease, classically divided into three types have a continuum of phenotypes.

There are a large number of genotypes associated with neuronopatic forms of GD. In Western countries, an association can be drawn between the presence of the N370S allele in combination with other mutation and GD1. Conversely, the L444P allele is most frequently associated to the neuronopathic variants. Data from 47 neurological cases included in the Spanish Gaucher Disease Registry, SGDR, (Alfonso et al., 2007; Giraldo et al., 2000) indicate that the most frequent allele is L444P accounting for 38.3% of the total alleles, followed by D409H 18.1% and the double mutant allele [E326K; L444P] 12.8%. Table 1.

Seventeen per cent of the total neurological GD cases included in the SGDR were homozygous for L444P mutation. It is interesting to note that this genotype was found in two patients classified as GD2 and in 6 GD3 and the homozygous for [E326K; L444P] as GD2. Surprisingly one patient with myoclonic epilepsy was carrier of N370S mutation, genotype N370S/G195W, no other mutations were identified in this patient in spite that the entire *GBA* was sequenced and analysed large rearrangements. It is important to point out that we do not know if in this case the cause of neurological impairment was due to the *GBA* gene or to other gene, gene-gene interaction or gene-environment interaction and therefore we dared not classify them as GD2 or GD3.

As we mentioned before the N370S mutation has been traditionally associated with the absence of neurological disease; however, several studies reported a high proportion of patients with the N370S mutation were diagnosed with GD 1 and showed mild neurological symptoms such tremor, peripheral neuropathy, uncoordinated movements, and hearing loss (as well as Parkinson disease. (Capablo et al., 2008; Giraldo et al., 2011; Pastores et al., 2003). These findings are consistent with the recently established contention that the mutation could not fully protect the patient from the appearance of neurological symptoms (Halperin et al., 2007). These observations reinforce the hypothesis that phenotypes reflect the continuum of the GD (Sidransky et al., 2004).

Genotype	Type2	Type3	Percent
L444P/L444P	2	6	17.0
D409H/D409H		6	12.8
[E326K;L444P]/R463H	3		6.3
G195E/L444P	3		6.3
c.1263_1317del55/L444P	3		6.3
D409H/R120W	2		4.2
D409H/L444P		2	4.2
[E326K;L444P]/[E326K;L444P]	2		4.2
[N188S;E326K]/L444P		2	4.2
R120W/L444P	2		4.2
[E326K;L444P]/D409H		1	2.1
[E326K;L444P]/P182L		1	2.1
[E326K;L444P]/G202R	1		2.1
[E326K;L444P]/W312R	1		2.1
[E326K;L444P]/L444P	1		2.1
G202R/L444P	1		2.1
I270P/L444P	1		2.1
RecNciI/L444P	1		2.1
S364R/L444P	1		2.1
c.203_204insC/L444P	1		2.1
G377S/G195W		1	2.1
R463C/G377S		1	2.1
N392I/L444P	1		2.1
V15M/G195W	1		2.1
Total	**27**	**20**	**100**

Table 1. GBA genotype distribution in 47 neuronopatic forms of GD from Spanish Gaucher Disease Registry

In a recent study, aimed to determine the presence of neurological symptoms and Parkinson's disease in Spanish GD patients and their relatives, we have found that relatives with PD exhibited a wide spectrum of *GBA* mutations L444P, N370S, V398I, R257Q, G202R, c.1439- 1445del7, [E326K; N188S], and c.953delT in the other hand PD was more frequent in carriers of L444P mutation and other rare *GBA* mutations than carriers of N370S (Giraldo et al., 2011).

6. Treatment of neurological forms of Gaucher Disease

The standard care for GD patients is the enzymatic replacement therapy (ERT), unfortunately neurological manifestations of GD are not corrected by ERT. This failure should be attributed to the blood-brain barrier which is largely impermeable to proteins. It is noteworthy that children without neurological symptoms at diagnosis that receive early infusions of ERT, are bound to develop neurological symptoms in type 3 of disease.

The other therapy approach used in glycosphingolipid disease, is the inhibition of the enzyme glusylceramide synthase and is called substrate reduction therapy (SRT), these inhibitors decrease the biosynthesis of the substrate (glucosylceramide). The only licensed

SRT is a small iminosugar molecule (Miglustat) that penetrates the blood–brain barrier. In spite of the trial conducted in children with chronic neuronopathic GD form, Miglustat do not meet its clinical end points and the drug currently is not recommended for neurological manifestations in GD. Nevertheless, there are some reports with specific neurological cases treated with miglustat that showed improvement in neurological manifestations (Capablo et al. 2007). It is interesting that miglustat used by compassionate therapy, in some type3 Gaucher disease gets to slow the progression of neurological manifestations, in similar manner that occurs in the licensed therapy with Miglustat in Niemann–Pick disease type C, another lysosomal disease that affects the brain in which there is disturbed cholesterol trafficking to lysosomes and causes secondary accumulation of glycosphingolipids in neurons (Wraith et al. 2010).

Bone marrow hematopoietic stem-cell transplantation, is not in current general use for GD, partly because of the difficulty to found ideal donors and procedural risks. The introduction of successful ERT has superseded this treatment in many countries. Only neurological forms in early stages could be rescued by this procedure.

The gene therapy is an interesting future option. The use of lentivirus-transduced autologous hematopoietic stem cells has been applied in other neurodegenerative disease as adrenoleukodystrophy (Cartier et al 2009) and currently in clinical trials for metachromatic leukodystrophy. Gene therapy has the advantage of being one procedure that requires less powerful myeloablative conditioning and thus is applicable for patients predicted to be at risk of severe neurological disease (Cox 2010).

7. Conclusions

Gaucher Disease is divided classically in three types based on the presence and rate of progression of the neurologic manifestations: type 1 non-neuronopathic, type 2 acute neuronopathic , and type 3 subacute neuronopathic. However there is an overlap between the different types suggesting that the disease have a continuum of phenotypes. There is accumulating evidence that in some Gaucher Disease patients classified as type 1, will develop neurological abnormalities during adult life such as peripheral neuropathy or early onset Parkinson Disease.

In spite of that, there are some glucocerebrosidase gene mutations associated more frequently to neurological forms, nevertheless genotype-phenotype correlations are not straightforward in Gaucher Disease.

The origin of neurological changes has not been clearly established, the neuropathological studies have demonstrated damage in several areas of the brain with perivascular Gaucher cells, astrogliosis and neuronal loss that could be attributed to intracellular deposits of glucocerebroside, and to abnormalities in calcium homeostasis.

8. Ackowledgements

Research into Gaucher disease from the author's group is supported in part by the grant PS09/2556, and by the CIBERER U-752, Fundación Ramón Areces and Spanish Gaucher Disease Foundation (FEETEG). The team of researchers: Pilar Alfonso, Alicia Saénz de Cabezón, Pilar Irún, Javier Gervas, Beatriz García-Rodríguez and all components of FEETEG.

9. References

Aharon-Peretz, J.; Rosenbaum. H. & Gershoni-Baruch, R. (2004) Mutations in the glucocerebrosidase gene and Parkinson´s disease in ashkenazi Jews. N. Engl. J. Med; 351: 1972–1977.

Alfonso, P.; Aznarez, S.; Giralt, M.; Pocovi, M. & Giraldo, P.(2007) Spanish Gaucher's Disease Registry. Mutation analysis and gassoenotype/phenotype relationships of Gaucher disease patients in Spain. J Hum Genet; 52:391-6.

Alfonso, P.; Pampín, S.; García-Rodríguez, B.; Tejedor, T.; Domínguez, C. et al (2011). Characterization of the c.(-203)A>G variant in the glucocerebrosidase gene and its ciation with phenotype in Gaucher disease.Clin Chim Acta;412:365-369

Amaral, O,; Lacerda, L;, Santos, R.; Pinto, RA.; Aerts, H. et al (1993). Type 1 Gaucher disease: molecular, biochemical, and clinical characterization of patients from northern Portugal. Biochem Med Metab Biol.;49:97-107

Arnaiz-Villena, A.; Martínez-Laso, J.& Alonso-García, J. (1999) Iberia: population genetics, anthropology, and linguistics. Hum Biol.;71:725-43

Barneveld, R.; Keijzer.; Tegelaers, FP.; Ginns, EI.; Geurts van Kessel, A. et al. (1983) Assignment of the gene coding for human beta-glucocerebrosidase to the region q21-q31 of chromosome 1 using monoclonal antibodies. Hum Genet: 64: 227–231.

Beutler, E.(1997) Gaucher disease. Curr Opin Hematol;4:19-23.

Beutler, E. & Grabowski, GA. Gaucher disease. In: Scriver CR, Beaudet AL, Sly WS, Valle D, eds. The metabolic and molecular basis of inherited disease, 8th ed. New York, NY: McGraw-Hill, 2001:3635–6

Biegstraaten, M.; van Schaik, IN.; Aerts, JM. & Hollak, CE. (2008). 'Non-neuronopathic' Gaucher disease reconsidered. Prevalence of neurological manifestations in a Dutch cohort of type I Gaucher disease patients and a systematic review of the literature. J Inherit Metab Dis;31:337-349.

Biegstraaten, M.; Mengel, E.; Maródi, L.; Petakov, M.; Niederau, C. et al (2010). Peripheral neuropathy in adult type 1 Gaucher disease: a 2-year prospective observational study. Brain,.133:2909-19.

Bonifati, V.; Rizzu, P.; van Baren, MJ.; Schaap, O.; Breedveld, GJ et al. (2003) Mutations in the DJ-1 gene associated with autosomal recessive early-onset parkinsonism. Science; 299: 256-259.

Braak, H.; Rüb, U.; Gai, W. & Del Tredici, K.(2003) Idiopathic Parkinson's disease: possible routes by which vulnerable neuronal types may be subject to neuroinvasion by an unknown pathogen. J Neural Transm; 110: 517-536.

Capablo, JL.; Franco, R.; de Cabezón, AS.; Alfonso, P.; Giraldo, P.(2007) Neurologic improvement in a type 3 Gaucher disease patient treated with imiglucerase/miglustat combination. Epilepsia;48:1406-8.

Capablo, JL.; Saenz de Cabezón, A.; Fraile, J.; Alfonso, P.; Giraldo, P. (2008) Neurological evaluation of patients with Gaucher disease diagnosed as type 1. J Neurol Neurosurg Psychiatry ;79:219-22.

Cartier, N.; Hacein-Bey-Abina, S.; Bartholomae, CC.; Bougnères, P.; Fischer, A. et al. (2009) Hematopoietic stem cell gene therapy with a lentiviral vector in X-linked adrenoleukodystrophy. Science.;326:818–823.

Chabás, A.; Cormand, B.; Grinberg, D.; Burguera, JM.; Balcells, S.; Merino, JL. et al (1995) Unusual expression of Gaucher's disease: cardiovascular calcifications in three sibs homozygous for the D409H mutation. J Med Genet;32:740-2.

Charrow, J.; Andersson, H.; Kaplan, P.; Kolodny, EH.; Mistry, P. et al.(2000) The Gaucher registry: demographics and disease characteristics of 1698 patients with Gaucher disease. Arch Intern Med;160:2835–2843.

Chérin, P. ; Rose, C. ; de Roux-Serratrice, C. ; Tardy, D. ; Dobbelaere, D. et al. (2010) The neurological manifestations of Gaucher disease type 1: the French Observatoire on Gaucher disease (FROG). J Inherit Metab Dis; 33:331–338

Cormand, B.;, Vilageliu, L.;, Burguera, JM,; Balcells, S.; Gonzàlez-Duarte, R. et al (1995). Gaucher disease in Spanish patients: analysis of eight mutations. Hum Mutat;5:303-9.

Cormand, B.; Grinberg, D.; Gort, L.; Chabas, A.; Vilageliu, L (1998). Molecular analysis and clinical findings in the Spanish Gaucher Disease population: putative haplotype of the N370S ancestral chromosome. Hum Mutat 11:295–305.

Côrte-Real, HB.; Macaulay, VA.; Richards, MB.; Hariti, G.; Issad, MS. Et al (1996). Genetic diversity in the Iberian Peninsula determined from mitochondrial sequence analysis. Ann Hum Genet.;60:331-50

Cox, TM, & Schofield, JP.(1997). Gaucher's disease: clinical features and natural history. Baillieres Clin Haematol;10:657-689.

Cox TM. (2010). Gaucher disease: clinical profile and therapeutic developments. Biologics. ;4:299-313.

Cuervo, AM.; Stefanis, L.; Fredenburg, R.;Lansbury, PT. & Sulzer, D.(2004). Impaired degradation of mutant alpha-synuclein by chaperone-mediated autophagy. Science;305:1292-5.

de Fost, M.; Out, TA.; de Wilde, FA.; Tjin, EP. Pals, ST. et al. (2008). Immunoglobulin and free light chain abnormalities in Gaucher disease type I: data from an adult cohort of 63 patients and review of the literature. Ann Hematol;87:439-449.

Delgado-Escueta, AV.; Ganesh, S. & Yamakawa, K. (2001). Advances in the genetics of progressive myoclonus epilepsy. Am J Med Gent; 106: 129-138.

Finnerup, NB.; Sindrup, SH. & Jensen, TS.(2007). Chronic neuropathic pain: mechanisms, drug targets and measurement. Fundam Clin Pharmacol;21:129-136.

Forno, LS. (1996). Neuropathology of Parkinson's disease. J Neuropathol Exp Neurol; 55: 259-272.

Futerman, AH.(2006). Intracellular trafficking of sphingolipids: Relationship to biosynthesis Biochim Biophys Acta. 1758:1885-92.

Gielchinsky, Y.; Elstein, D.; Green, R. Miller, JW.; Elstein, Y. et al. (2001). High prevalence of low serum vitamin B12 in a multi-ethnic Israeli population. Br J Haematol;115:707-709.

Giraldo, P.; Pocoví, M.; Pérez-Calvo, J.; Rubio-Félix, D. & Giralt M.(2000). Report of the Spanish Gaucher's disease registry: clinical and genetic characteristics. Haematologica;85:792-799

Giraldo, P.; Capablo, JL.; Alfonso, P.; Garcia-Rodriguez, B.; Latre, P, et al (2011). Neurological manifestations in patients with Gaucher disease and their relatives, it is just a coincidence?. J Inherit Metab Dis;34:781-787

Goker-Alpan, O.; Hruska, K.S.; Orvisky, E.; Kishnani, P.S.; Stubblefield, B.K. et al (2005), Divergent phenotypes in Gaucher disease implicate the role of modifiers, J. Med. Genet; 42; e37.

Grabowski, GA. & Horowitz, M. (1997). Gaucher's disease: molecular, genetic and enzymological aspects. Baillieres Clin Haematol;10:635-656.

Grabowski, GA. (1997). Gaucher disease: gene frequencies and genotype/phenotype correlations. Genet Test; 1:5-12.

Grewel, RP.; Doppelt, SH.; Thompson, MA.; Katz, D.; Brady, RO, et al (1991). Neurological complications of no n-neuronopathic Gauchers' disease. Arch Neurol; 48:1271-1272.

Hall, KE,; Liu, J.; Sima, AA. & Wiley, JW. (2001). Impaired inhibitory G-protein function contributes to increased calcium currents in rats with diabetic neuropathy. J Neurophysiol;86:760-770.

Halperin, A.; Elstein, D, & Zimran, A. (2007). Are symptoms of peripheral neuropathy more prevalent in patients with Gaucher disease? Acta Neurol Scand;115:275-8.

Hatano, Y.; Li, Y.; Sato, K.; Asakawa, S.; Yamamura, Y. et al (2004). Novel PINK1 mutations in early-onset parkinsonism. Ann Neurol;56:424-427.

Horowitz, M.; Wilder, S.; Horowitz, Z.; Reiner, O.; Gelbart, T. et al (1989). The human glucocerebrosidase gene and pseudogene. Structure Evol Genomics: 4: 87–96.

Hruska, KS.; LaMarca, ME.; Scott, CR. & Sidransky ,E. (2008). Gaucher disease: mutation polymorphism spectrum in the glucorebrosidase gene (GBA). Hum Mutat;29:567-83

International Batten Disease Consortium.(1995). Isolation of a novel gene underlying Batten disease, CLN3. Cell.; 82: 949-957

Janes, RW.; Munroe, PB.; Mitchison, HM.; Gardiner, RM.; Mole, SE. et al (1996). A model for Batten disease protein CLN3: functional implications from homology and mutations. FEBS Lett.; 399: 75-77.

Järvinen, M .& Rinne, A. (1982). Human spleen cysteineproteinase inhibitor. Purification, fractionation into isoelectric variants and some properties of the variants. Biochim Biophys Acta; 708: 210-207.

Kitada, T.; Asakawa, S.; Hattori, N.; Matsumine, H.; Yamamura, Y.et al. (1998). Mutations in the parkin gene cause autosomal recessive juvenile parkinsonism. Nature; 392: 544-545.

Koprivica, V.; Stone, D.; Park, JK.; Callahan, M.; Frisch, A. et al (2000). Analysis and classification of 304 mutant alleles in patients with type 1 and type 3 Gaucher disease. Am J Hum Genet; 66:1777-86

Kowarz, L.; Goker-Alpan, O.; Banerjee-Basu, S.; LaMarca, ME,; Kinlaw, L. et al (2005). Gaucher Mutation N188S Is Associated With Myoclonic Epilepsy. Human Mutation; 26: 271-273.

Kraoua, I.; Sedel, F.; Caillaud, C.; Froissart, R.; Stirnemann, J, et al (2011). A French experience of type 3 Gaucher disease: Phenotypic diversity and neurological outcome of 10 patients. Brain Dev;33:131-9.

Lockhart, PJ.; Lincoln, S.; Hulihan, M.; Kachergus, J.; Wilkes, K. et al. (2004). DJ-1 mutations are a rare cause of recessively inherited early onset parkinsonism mediated by loss of protein function. J Med Genet.; 41: e22.

Lohi, H.; Ianzano, L.; Zhao, XC.; Chan, EM.;Turnbull, J. et al.(2005). Novel glycogen synthase kinase 3 and ubiquitination pathways in progressive myoclonus epilepsy. Hum Mol Genet.; 14: 2727-2736.

Lloyd-Evans, E.; Pelled, D.; Riebeling, C.; Bodennec, J.; de-Morgan, A. et al.(2003). Glucosylceramide and glucosylsphingosine modulate calcium mobilization from brain microsomes via different mechanisms. J Biol Chem;278:23594-23599.

Machaczka, M.; Rucinska, M.; Skotnicki, AB, & Jurczak, W. (1999). Parkinson´s syndrome preceding clinical manifestation of Gaucher´s disease. Am J Hematol;. 61: 216–217.

McKeran, R.; Bradbury, P.; Taylor, D. & Stern, G. (1985)Neurological involvement in type 1 (adult) Gaucher´s disease. J Neurol Neurosurg Psychiatry; 48: 172-175

Minassian, BA.; Lee, J.;, Herbrick, JA.; Huizenga, J.; Soder, S. et al.. (1998). Mutations in a gene encoding a novel protein tyrosine phosphatase cause progressive myoclonus epilepsy. Nat Genet; 20: 171-174.

Montfort, M.; Chabás, A.; Vilageliu, L, & Grinberg, D. (2004). Functional analysis of 13 GBA mutant alleles identified in Gaucher disease patients: pathogenic changes and "modifier" polymorphisms. Hum Mutat;23:567–75

Neudorfer, O.; Giladi, N.; Elstein, D.; Abrahamov, A.; Turezkite, T. et al (1996). Occurrence of Parkinson´s syndrome in type I Gaucher disease. QJM; 89: 691–694.

Park, JK.; Orvisky, E.; Tayebi, N.; Kaneski, C.; Lamarca, ME. et al (2003). Myoclonic epilepsy in Gaucher disease: genotype-phenotype insights from a rare patient subgroup. Pediatr Res;53:387-95.

Pastores, GM.; Barnett, NL.; Bathan, P. & Kolodny, EH. (2003). A neurological symptom survey of patients with type I Gaucher disease. J Inherit Metab Dis;26:641-645.

Patterson, MC.; Horowitz, M.; Abel, RB.; Currie, JN.; Yu, KT. et al.(1993) Isolated horizontal supranuclear gaze palsy as a marker of severe systemic involvement in Gaucher's disease. Neurology;43:1993-7.

Pelled, D.; Trajkovic-Bodennec, S.; Lloyd-Evans, E.; Sidransky, E.; Schiffmann, R, et al (2005). Enhanced calcium release in the acute neuronopathic form of Gaucher disease. Neurobiol Dis;18:83-8.

Pennacchio, LA.; Lehesjoki, AE.; Stone, NE.; Willour, VL.; Virtaneva, K. et al. (1996). Mutations in the gene encoding cystatin B in progressive myoclonus epilepsy (EPM1). Science; 271: 1731-1734.

Poewe, W (2008). Non-motor symptoms in Parkinson's disease. Eur J Neurol; 15 Supl: 14-20.

Ron, I.; Rapaport, D. & Horowitz, M. (2010). Interaction between parkin and mutant glucocerebrosidase variants: a possible link between Parkinson disease and Gaucher disease. Hum Mol Genet; 19:3771-81.

Scheffer, IE. & Berkovic, SF.(2000). Genetics of the epilepsies. Curr Opin Pediatr; 12: 536-542.

Schlossmacher, MG. & Shimura, H. (2005). Parkinson's disease: assays for the ubiquitin ligase activity of neural Parkin. Methods Mol Biol;301:351-69.

Shoffner, JM.; Lott, MT.; Lezza, AM.; Seibel, P.; Ballinger, SW. et al (1990). Myoclonic epilepsy and ragged-red fiber disease (MERFF) is associated with a mitocondrial DNA tRNA (Lys) mutation. Cell; 61: 931-937.

Sidransky, E. (2004). Gaucher disease: complexity in a "simple" disorder. Mol Genet Metab; 83: 6-15

Sidransky, E.; Nalls, MA.; Aasly, JO.; Aharon-Peretz, J.; Annesi, G. et al (2009). Multicenter analysis of glucocerebrosidase mutations in Parkinson's disease. N Engl J Med;361:1651-61.

Silberman, J, & Lonial S (2008). Review of peripheral neuropathy in plasma cell disorders. Hematol Oncol;26:55-65.

Sorge, J.; Gross, E.; West, C. & Beutler, E. (1990). High level transcription of the glucocerebrosidase pseudogene in normal subjects and patients with Gaucher disease. J Clin Invest: 86: 1137–1141.

Stafstrom, CE. & Temperl, BL.(2000). Epilepsy genes: the link between molecular dysfunction and pathophysiology. Ment Retard Dev Disabil Res Rev; 6: 281-292.

Stone, DL.; Tayebi, N.; Orvisky, E.; Stubblefield, B.; Madike, V. et al (2000), Glucocerebrosidase gene mutations in patients with type 2 Gaucher disease, Hum. Mutat; 15: 181–188.

Tayebi, N.; Stubblefield, B.; Stone, D.; Callahan, M.; Madike, V. et al (1999). Homologous and non-homologous recombinations at the glucocerebrosidase locus: Implications for Gaucher disease. Am J Hum Genet Suppl; 65:A493

Tayebi, N.; Callahan, M.; Madike, V.; Stubblefield, BK.; Orvisky, E. et al (2001). Gaucher disease and parkinsonism: a phenotypic and genotypic characterization. Mol Genet Metab;73: 313–321.

Tinuper, P.; Plazzi, G.; Monari, L.; Sangiorgi, S.; Pellissier, JF. et al. (1994). Arylsulfataser A pseudodeficiency and Lafora bodies in a patient with progressive myoclonic epilepsy. Epilepsia; 35: 332-335

Torralba, MA.; Alfonso, P.; Pérez-Calvo JI. Cenarro, A.; Pastores, GM.; Giraldo, P. et al (2002). High prevalence of the 55-bp deletion (c.1263del55) in exon 9 of the glucocerebrosidase gene causing misdiagnosis (for homozygous N370S (c.1226A > G) mutation) in Spanish Gaucher disease patients. Blood Cells Mol Dis;29:35-40.

Turk, V. & Bode, W. (1991). The cystatins: protein inhibitors of cysteine proteinases. FEBS Lett;285(2):213-219.

Tylki-Szymańska, A.; Vellodi, A.; El-Beshlawy, A.; Cole, JA. & Kolodny, E. (2010). Neuronopathic Gaucher disease: demographic and clinical features of 131 patients enrolled in the International Collaborative Gaucher Group Neurological Outcomes Subregistry. J Inherit Metab Dis;33:339-46.

Valente, EM.; Abou-Sleiman, PM,; Caputo, V.;, Muqit, MM.; Harvey, K. ,et al. (2004). Hereditary early-onset Parkinson´s disease caused by mutations in PINK1. Science; 304: 1158-1160.

Verghese, J.; Goldberg, RF.; Desnick, RJ.; Grace, ME.; Goldman, JE. et al. (2000). Myoclonus from selective dentate nucleus degeneration in type 3 Gaucher disease Arch Neurol;57:389-395.

Van Den Eeden, SK.; Tanner, CM.; Bernstein, AL.; Fross, RD.; Leimpeter, A. et al. (2003). Incidence of Parkinson's disease: variation by age, gender, and race/ethnicity. Am J Epidemiol; 157: 1015-1022.

Wan, L.; Hsu, CM,;Tsai ,CH.; Lee, CC.; Hwu, WL. et al.(2006), Mutation analysis of Gaucher disease patients in Taiwan: high prevalence of the RecNciI and L444P mutations, Blood Cells Mol. Diseases;36:422–425.

Wong, K.; Sidransky, E.; Verma, A.; Mixon, T.; Sandberg, GD. et al (2004). Neuropathology provides clues to the pathophysiology of Gaucher disease. Molecular genetics and metabolism ; 82: 192-207

Wraith, JE.; Vecchio, D.; Jacklin, E. ; Abel, L.; Chadha-Boreham, H. et al. (2010) Miglustat in adult and juvenile patients with Niemann-Pick disease type C: long-term data from a clinical trial. Mol Genet Metab.;99:351–357.

Xu, YH.; Reboulet, R.; Quinn, B.; Huelsken, J.; Witte, D. et al (2008) Dependence of reversibility and progression of mouse neuronopathic Gaucher disease on acid beta-glucosidase residual activity levels. Mol Genet Metab;94:190-203.

Yaksh, TL. (2006). Calcium channels as therapeutic targets in neuropathic pain. J Pain;7:S13-S30.

6

The Role of Gene Mutations Detection in Defining the Spectrum of ß – Thalassemia in Various Ethnic Regions

Fakher Rahim[1], Najmaldin Saki[2,3] and Mohammad Ali Jalalai far[2,3]
[1]*Endocrinology and Metabolism Research Center (EMRC), Tehran University of Medical Sciences, Tehran*
[2]*Department of Medical Laboratory Science, Ahvaz Jundishapur University of Medical Sciences, Ahvaz*
[3]*Thalassemia and Hemoglobinopathies Research Center, Ahvaz Jundishapur University of Medical Sciences, Ahvaz*
Iran

1. Introduction

The thalassemia is a widespread with about 5% of the world population affected by it and is found in some 60 countries, with the highest prevalence in the Mediterranean region, parts of North and West Africa, the Middle East, the Indian subcontinent, southern Far East and south-eastern Asia, together comprising the so-called thalassemia belt. In western countries, thalassemia affects mostly individuals whose ancestry is traceable to high prevalence areas. As an example, there are around 1,000 cases of β-thalassemia major in the United States, most of whom are descendants of Mediterranean, Asian Indian, South Asian or Chinese ancestors. This figure is even less than half of the number of β-thalassemic patients in Fars Province, a region only 120,000 km 2 large in southern Iran (Haghshenas and Zamani, 1997; Rahim et al., 2007). The gene frequency of ß-thalassemia, however, is varies from area to area, having its highest rate of more than 10% around the Caspian Sea and Persian Gulf. The prevalence of the disorder in other areas is between 4-8% (Rahim and Abromand, 2008). There are many genes coding for the globins. They are found on chromosome 11 (β-globin cluster) or chromosome 16 (α-globin cluster) figure1.

1.1 Beta-Thalassemia

Beta-Thalassemia, one of the most widespread genetic diseases in the world, is a common autosomal recessive disorder caused by point mutations in the ß- globin gene that is located as a cluster on the short arm of chromosome 11 (Weatherall et al., 1989; Sack, 1999; Oliveri, 1999). More than 200 different mutations affecting diverse levels of beta-globin genes expression have so far been identified (Trent, 1997; Ho and Thein, 2000). South-western region of Iran also represented various ß-thalassemia mutations (Figure 2). Different strategies of classification individuals genotypes by ß-globin gene cluster and cloning nucleotides sequencing lead to identification of several mutations in Mediterranean (Orkin et al., 1982), Asian Indians (Kazazian et al., 1984, Ohba et al., 1997), American Blacks

(Antonarakis et al., 1984) and Chinese (Cheng et al., 1984). The global distribution indicates a high prevalence in a belt around the earth, which is around the 40th parallel in the Mediterranean area but eastwards moves further south, reaching the equator in Indonesia. More than two million carriers of ß-thalassemia live in Iran. The Iranian populations are mixture of different ethnic groups.

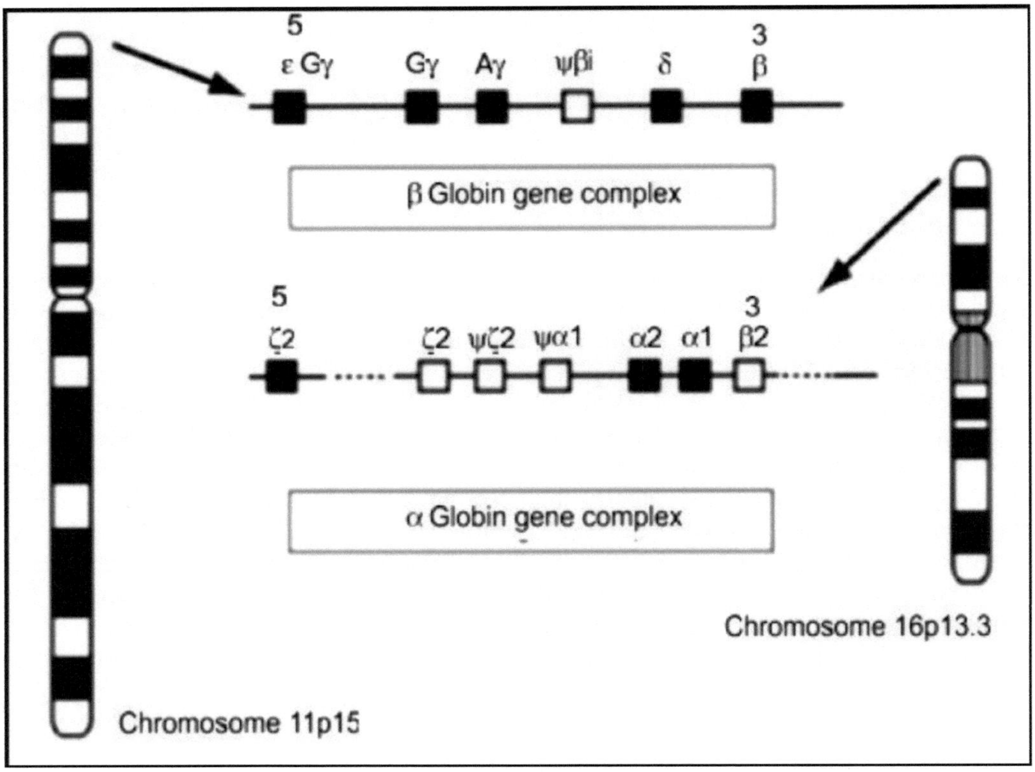

Fig. 1. Two globin gene clusters including α- and β- represented here.

1.2 Alpha thalassemia

Alpha thalassemia disorders are a group of hereditary anemias caused by absent or decreased production of the alpha chain of hemoglobin (Hb) (Vichinsky, 2009). freeAll affected individuals have a variable degree of anaemia (low Hb), reduced mean corpuscular hemoglobin (MCH/pg), reduced mean corpuscular volume (MCV/fl) and a normal/slightly reduced level of HbA2. Molecular analysis is usually required to confirm the hematological observations (especially in silent alpha thalassemia and α-thalassemia trait). A single gene, two-gene, three-gene or four-gene deletions result in alpha thalassemia silent carrier status, thalassemia trait (minor), HbH, and hemoglobin Bart's (Hb Bart's), respectively (Figure 3).

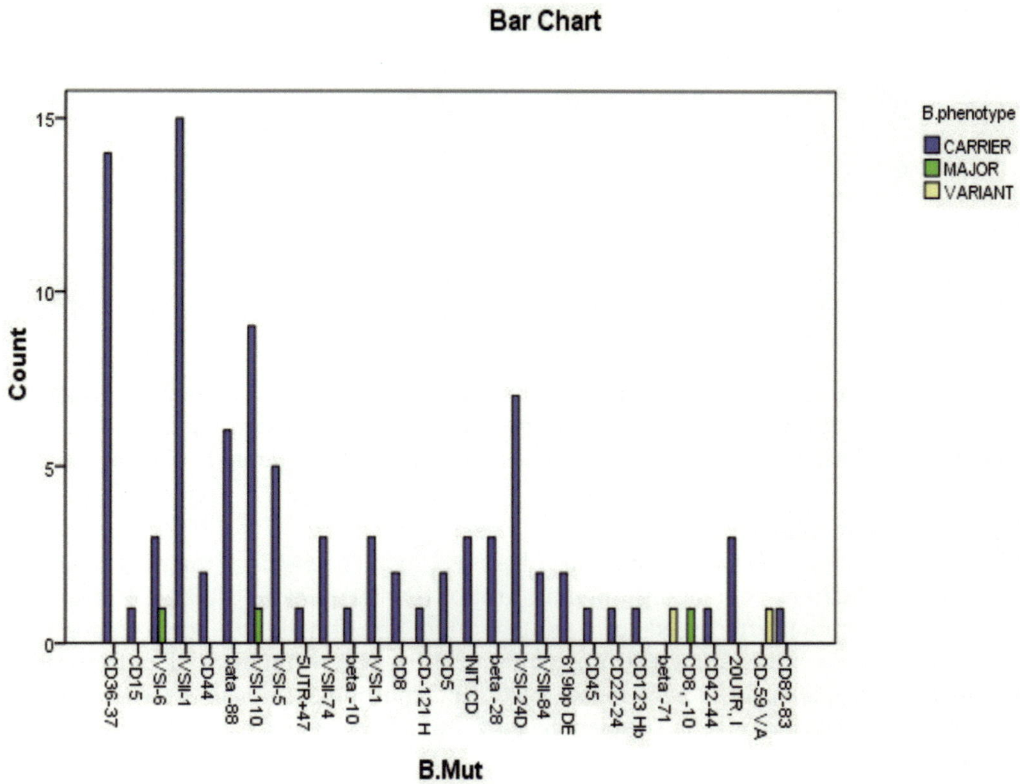

Fig. 2. Different ß-thalassemia mutations detected in our region of study (South-western region of Iran), different explained groups are carrier, which represents the heterozygous type; Major, which represents the homozygous type; Variants, which represents the hemoglobin variants

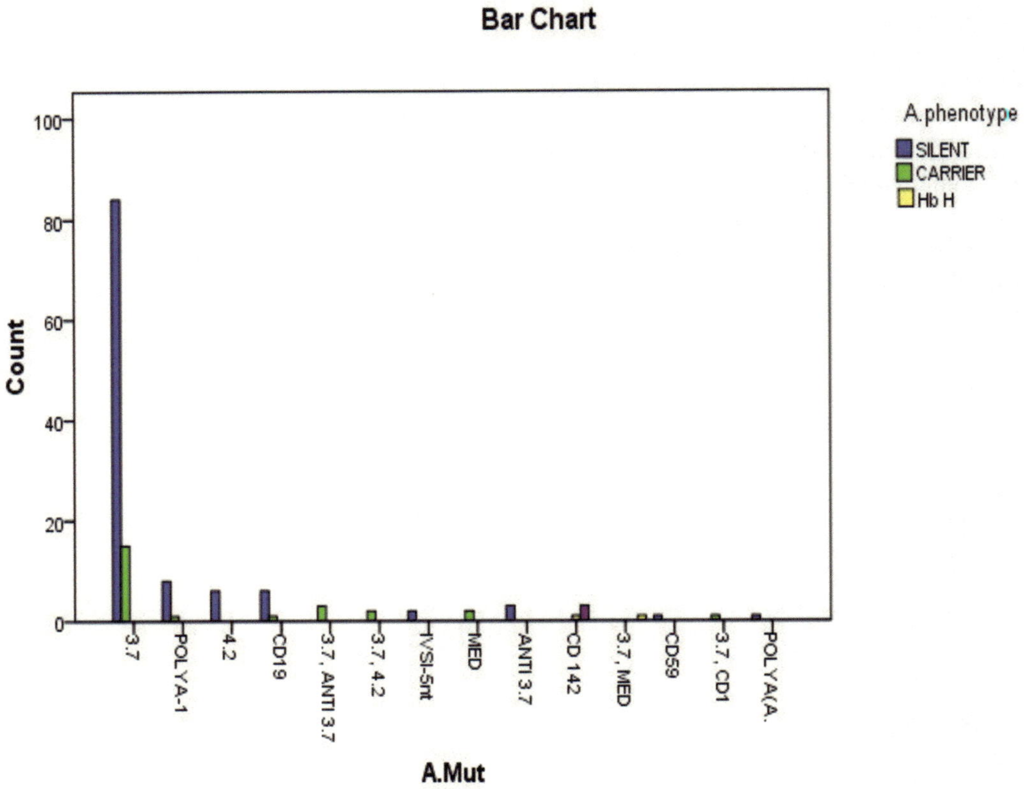

Fig. 3. Different α -thalassemia mutations detected in our region of study (South-western-region of Iran), different explained groups are carrier, which represents the heterozygous type; Major, which represents the homozygous type; HbH, Hemoglobin H disease

1.3 Thalassemia intermedia

Thalassemia intermedia are a clinical phenotype which displays marked genotypic variability in different populations or ethnic groups (Panigrahi et al., 2009). This disorder is a clinical designation often used to characterize individuals who are homozygous for b-thalassemia genes but maintain hemoglobins of 6–9 g/dL without regular transfusions (Galanello et al., 2001). They have more severe RBC morphological abnormalities than the trait, as well as varying degrees of splenomegaly, thrombosis and skeletal changes (Taher et al., 2008).

1.4 Hemoglobin H (Hb H)

Hemoglobin H (Hb H) disease is the most common form of thalassemia intermedia. Hb H (beta4) disease results from double heterozygosity for alpha(0)-thalassemia due to deletions that remove both linked alpha-globin genes on chromosome 16, and deletional alpha(+)-thalassemia from single alpha-globin gene deletions (--/-alpha). However, Hb H disease may occur from interactions between alpha (0)-thalassemia with nondeletional mutations or with abnormal hemoglobins such as Hb Constant Spring, Hb Paksé, Hb Quong Sze, and Hb Pak Num Po (Fucharoen and Viprakasit, 2009).

1.5 Hemoglobin (Hb) Bart's

Hemoglobin (Hb) Bart's hydrops fetalis is a generally fatal intrauterine condition associated with homozygous alpha (0)-thalassemia. It is moderately insoluble, and therefore accumulates in the red blood cells (Karnpean et al., 2009; Singer, 2009).

1.6 Simultaneous α-and β-thalassemia

Some case of complex beta- and alpha-thalassemia coinheritance is described. The chance of finding an individual with co-inheritance of α^0- and β-thalassemia is theoretically 1: 1000. In other words, one in every 25 b-thalassemia carriers co-inherits a^0- thalassemia (Rahim, 2010; Rahim et al., 2008). Routine screening testing, such as mean cell volume (MCV) and Hb A2 level, cannot distinguish double heterozygotes for α and β-thalassemia from the pure β-thalassemia heterozygotes. The α^0-thalassemia can be distinguished simply from double α^0- and β-thalassemia by a normal Hb A2 level (Table 1).

Case	Sex	Age (Y)	Hb (g/dl)	MCV(fl)	MCH(pg)	HbF(%)	HbA2(%)	α-genotype	β-genotype	HbH
1	M	24	13.9	72.1	23.4	1.1	5.3	$-\alpha^{3.7}/\alpha\alpha$	A	-
2	M	32	11.7	70.7	22.6	0.4	5.1	$-\alpha^{3.7}/\alpha\alpha$	B	-
3	M	29	11.4	73.0	22	0.5	5.1	$-\alpha^{3.7}/-\alpha^{3.7}$	C	-
4	F	27	11.9	71.5	22.6	1.5	4.2	$\alpha\alpha/-\alpha^{4.2}$	D	-
5	F	30	10.4	65.0	21	1.4	4.5	$-\alpha^{3.7}/\alpha\alpha$	E	-
6	F	25	11.7	61.4	19.8	0.9	4.3	$-\alpha^{3.7}/\alpha\alpha$	F	-
7	F	23	13.2	69.7	23.2	1.3	5.3	$\alpha\alpha/--_{MED}$	G	-
8	M	29	11.5	75.5	23.2	1.9	4.9	$\alpha\alpha/-\alpha^{4.2}$	H	-
9	M	27	13.3	67.3	22.6	1.4	5.5	$\alpha\alpha/--_{MED}$	I	+
10	M	29	11.1	69.5	23.8	0.9	5.4	$\alpha\alpha/--_{MED}$	J	+

A, $\beta^{IVS\ 1\text{-}5}/\beta^N$; B, $\beta^{IVS\ 1\text{-}25}/\beta^N$; C, $\beta^{IVS\ 2\text{-}1}/\beta^N$; D, $\beta^{CD8(-AA)}/\beta^N$; E, $\beta^{CD121(G\text{-}C)}/\beta^N$; F, $\beta^{CD6(CTC\text{-}GAG)}/\beta^N$;G, $\beta^{IVS\ 2\text{-}1}/\beta^N$; H, $\beta^{CD121(G\text{-}C)}/\beta^N$;I, $\beta^{CD41/42)}/\beta^N$; J, $\beta^{CD8(-AA)}/\beta^N$

Table 1. Hematologic and genotypic findings in the 10 double heterozygotes for α- and β-thalassemia

1.7 Co-inheritance of α-and hemoglobin variants

The chance of finding an individual with co-inheritance of α^0- thalassemia with different hemoglobin variants is also presented. In other words, this chance and presentation is rare (Rahim, 2009).

2. Diagnosis

The key to successful detection and characterization of the hemoglobinopathies, particularly the thalassemias, is the initial hematological data. The clue for a thalassemia comes with a low mean corpuscular volume (MCV) or mean corpuscular hemoglobin (MCH). Although iron deficiency is the other explanation for a low MCV or MCH, it is likely that this finding will point to thalassemia in regions of countries with at-risk ethnic populations (Table 2).

Group(number of cases)	*Hb mean ± SD (Range)*	*MCV mean ± SD (Range)*	*MCH mean ± SD (Range)*
Beta-thalassemia Trait(171)	9.53 ± 1.43 (5.60 - 12.10)	62.9 ± 5.3 (49 - 78.90)	20.03 ± 1.80 (15 - 26)
Beta-thalassemia Major(13)	7.5 ± 1.34 (5.20 - 9.28)	71.6 ± 5.20 (63 - 79)	22.9 ± 2.1 (20.9 - 25.6)
Iron deficiency(42)	7.75 ± 2.05 (4.3 - 12.95)	69.35 ± 6.95 (52.0 - 77.8)	17.52 ± 2.84 (12.10 - 23.12)
Alpha-thalassemia Trait(88)	11.1 ± 1.25 (9.20 - 12.25)	73.6 ± 4.67 (60 - 79)	23.9 ± 1.82 (19 - 26.20)
Hb Variants(11) *	12.1 ± 2.63 (7.8 - 15.20)	73.9 ± 4.4 (66 - 79)	23.5 ± 1.65 (21 - 26.5)

*Includes hemoglobin S (HbS), hemoglobin C (HbC) and hemoglobin DPunjab (HbDPunjab)

Table 2. Hematological parameters in different groups with microcytic hypochromic anemia

2.1 Differential diagnosis of beta-thalassemia

We can differentiate β -thalassemia from other disorders such as iron deficiency anemia with the help of discriminate indices including Mentzer Index, England and Fraser Index, Srivastava Index, Green and King Index, Shine and Lal Index, red blood cell (RBC) count, red blood cell distribution width index (RDWI), Mean Density of Hemoglobin per Liter of blood (MDHL) and mean cell hemoglobin density (MCHD) (Rahim and Keikhaei, 2009). If iron deficiency is present, it is essential to correct this and then repeat the full-blood count and all other investigations. The first step after the initial abnormal blood count is to exclude iron deficiency and if present, to treat it. The blood count is then repeated and if the MCV/MCH remains low, a thalassemia is most likely. Therefore, ferritin levels (and if necessary serum iron, iron binding capacity and percentage saturation) are sought. This is recommended because at times, particularly during pregnancy, it is possible that iron stores will be low or, in the presence of iron deficiency, it is possible that the MCV or MCH are influenced by the iron deficiency. It is also occasionally seen that the HbA_2 level can be falsely lowered by iron deficiency. In this context there are special hemoglobin tests which may help in the primary detection scenarios (Table 3).

2.2 Molecular diagnostic methods

Almost all the methods for DNA analysis of the hemoglobinopathies used today are based on the polymerase chain reaction (PCR). Different well-known and applied methods have been described in table 4. Therefore whether a mutation is a deletion, a rearrangement or a point mutation, a similar test will be performed with the variability and specificity coming

Test	What does it measure or detect Y	What does it mean
HbEPG	Electrophoresis of globin proteins. Different techniques possible from gel or membrane-based kits to HPLC. Abnormal bands apart from the usual HbA, HbF and HbA_2 peaks can be detected	(1) Gives some idea of the HbA_2 level but more importantly (2) identifies if there are any variant Hbs - particularly Hbs such as HbE and HbS.
HbA_2	Globin electrophoresis and quantization of the HbA_2 peak. Different techniques used from membrane or column-based kits to the more universally suited HPLC are in use.	A raised HbA_2 is the key parameter indicating the presence of β-thalassemia. It is said that variant Hbs can raise the HbA_2 but this must be a rare event. More of an issue is the borderline normal-raised HbA_2 because this might indicate silent β-thalassemia. A low HbA_2 is also important to note as this might indicate δ thalassemia
HbF	Globin electrophoresis and quantization with different methods available for the latter.	A slightly raised HbF to 2-3% (normal is <1% in an adult) might indicate heterocellular HPFH or may be a subtle pointer to an underlying silent β-thalassemia. HbF levels 5% and above are more likely to be due to δβ thalassemia or HPFH (heterocellular or pancellular). In the case of δβ thalassemia or deletional HPFH one would expect the HbA_2 level to be low.
Kleihauer	Red blood cells are stained to detect HbF. This test is used to distinguish heterocellular from pancellular HPFH.	Not a particularly useful test for distinguishing the types of HPFH because these are very rare and most laboratories are not sure how to interpret the results. The only practical value for a Kleihauer stain might be in fetal blood sampling to confirm that maternal blood has not contaminated a fetal sample (the latter would be homogeneously stained for HbF). Any cells not staining for HbF would represent maternal blood.
HbH inclusions	Red blood cells are stained to detect HbH inclusions (aggregates of β globin protein)	Requires patience and skill to find the HbH inclusions and even with a 2-gene deletion α thalassemia, only 1-2 such inclusions might be found after a search lasting many minutes. There fore, HbH inclusions are easy to miss if the labora tory is inexperienced or the individual looking down the microscope does not spend enough time searching for these inclusions.
Sickle solubility and instability tests	Various tests ranging from biochemical to immunoassay are used to detect HbS and unstable variant Hbs	HbS diseases as well as interactions of HbS with β-thalassemia are increasingly being detected in many Iranian cities. Therefore, efficient and accurate tests for sickling (sickle solubility, HbEPG) are important components of the hemoglobinopathy workup.

Table 3. Special hematologic tests requested once a hemoglobinopathy is suspected based on family history and/or full-blood count.

from the primers used. The sensitivity and specificity of PCR has revolutionized the molecular diagnostic field. It has almost eliminated the use of radioactive isotopes for detecting sequences and has enabled diagnosis to be made on much smaller quantities of DNA. The PCR-based techniques used in hemoglobin diagnostics include allele-specific oligonucleotide (ASO) hybridization or dot-blot analysis, reverse dot-blot analysis, allele-specific priming or amplification refractory mutation system (ARMS), restriction enzyme analysis, amplification created restriction analysis, mutagenically separated PCR and gap-PCR. These PCR-based techniques are useful for identifying a known mutation; PCR-based approaches for scanning or screening for unknown mutations take advantage of altered conformation of single-stranded DNA and include denaturing gradient gel electrophoresis (DGGE), single-strand conformation polymorphism (SSCP) and heteroduplex analysis. The characteristic altered patterns of migration and their position in the scanning methods act as a guide for the location of the mutation, targeting the region for identification by other means. The ultimate method of mutation identification is by direct sequence analysis of specifically amplified DNA. In the last decade, the use of automated sequencers has led to nonradioactive, more robust and more rapid sequencing, making it suitable as a routine diagnostic tool. Direct sequencing analysis is particularly applicable to the globin genes which are compact and relatively small (1.2-1.6kb) with most of the point mutations within the gene or its flanking sequences (Fakher et al., 2006).

Southern blotting is one of the few non-PCR based molecular techniques that still have a significant role to play in the molecular diagnosis of the hemoglobinopathies. It is very useful in the screening for large deletions or rearrangements and is essential in characterizing novel deletions. The more common deletions can be detected by gap-PCR once the deletion break points have been defined and specific primers flanking the deletion designed. Each of these techniques has its own limitations; the particular repertoire chosen by a laboratory for molecular diagnosis of the hemoglobinopathies depends on the spectrum of mutations encountered in their catchment area and the technical expertise available in the diagnostic laboratory. It is good practice for any DNA diagnostic laboratory to have at least two alternative methods for detecting each mutation (Vrettou et al., 2003).

2.3 Prenatal Diagnosis (PND) & Foetal DNA analysis

Although historically, the prevention program, abortion, was considered unacceptable in Iran, intensive consultation led to the clerical approval of induced abortion in cases with β-thalassemia major in 1997, and a nationwide prevention program with screening, counseling and prenatal diagnosis (PND) network has been developed (Najmabadi et al., 2006 ;Rahim et al., 2007) (Table 4). Many laboratories offering DNA diagnostics of the Hb disorders are also involved in analysis of fetal DNA for the prenatal diagnosis of these disorders. Fetal DNA is usually and preferably, obtained through chorionic villus sampling in the first trimester of pregnancy (10-12 weeks). Chorionic villus sampling provides a good yield of DNA which is isolated using conventional methods of phenol chloroform extraction after careful microscopic dissection to remove any contaminating maternal deciduas. Occasionally, if the sample is too small, it may need to be cultured increasing the risk of maternal contamination. Amniocytes obtained in the second trimester can also be used as a source of fetal DNA but the fetal cells are often contaminated with maternal cells and the results have to be interpreted with caution after analysis for maternal contamination.

Every prenatal diagnosis should be accompanied by copies of haematology results of the parents and prior confirmation of the parental phenotypes and genotypes. The PCR-based techniques that best suit the expertise of the laboratory are then used to screen for the presence of the parental mutations in the fetal DNA. Parental, appropriate positive and negative controls must always be included in the investigations. A limited number of PCR cycles (25-28) should be performed to avoid amplification of any minor DNA species and to minimize amplification of any contaminating maternal DNA. As an added precaution, maternal DNA contamination should be checked for by using polymorphic DNA markers including the variable tandem repeats (VNTRs) such as ApoB and the short tandem repeats or micro satellites. This is particularly important when the fetal genotype is the same as the maternal genotype. Fetal DNA analysis should also be performed in duplicate and confirmed by an independent PCR-based technique. To confirm maternal DNA contamination we used polymorphic DNA markers including the variable tandem repeats (VNTRs) in all cases.

Mutation	Type	Ethnic origin	Heterozygous cases	Homozygote cases	No. of chromosomes (%frequency)
Fr 36/37(-T)	*β0*	Kurd, Iranian	16	6	28(14.7)
IVS 2-1(G to C)	*β0*	Iranian	14	7	28(14.7)
CD 6 (Hb S)	*βs*	----------------	4	9	22(13)
IVS 1-110 (G to A)	*β+*	Mediterranean	5	5	15(8.8)
IVS 1 –6 (T→C)	*β+*	Mediterranean	0	5	10(5.89)
CD 44 (-C)	*β0*	Kurdish	4	2	8(4.7)
IVS 1-5 (G to C)	*β0*	Asian Indian, SE Asian, Melanesian	2	2	6(3.5)
CD 39(C to T)	*β0*	Mediterranean	4	0	4(2.35)
Fr 8/9 (+G)	*β0*	Asian Indian, Japanese	2	1	4(2.35)
IVS 2-745 (C to G)	*β+*	Mediterranean	4	0	4(2.35)
IVS 1-1(G to A)	*β0*	Mediterranean	2	1	4(2.35)
IVS 1(3' end)-25bp	*β0*	Asian Indian, UAE	2	1	4(2.35)
CD 8 (-AA)	*β0*	Mediterranean	1	1	3(1.8)
CD 5 (-CT)	*β0*	Mediterranean	2	0	2(1.17)
-88(C to A)	*β+*	Kurds	2	0	2(1.17)
CD 82/83(-G)	*β0*	Czech, Azerbaijan	1	0	1(0.59)
IVS 2-2,3(+11, -2)	*β+*	Iranian	1	0	1(0.59)
IVS 1-130 (G to A)	*β0*	Egyptian	1	0	1(0.59)
Unknown			23	0	23(14.1)
Total			90	40	170(100)

Table 4. Globin mutations identified by reverse- hybridization and DNA sequencing in 254 thalassemia patient and prenatal DNA sample were initially tested for 22 common mutations by reverse – hybridization (Fakher et al., 2006).

3. Discussion

Iran is a country which has a population with a different ethnic identity and different languages. As we saw mutation in ß-globin gene will lead to thalassemia. Although, all this mutations were found in coastline areas but their geographic distribution has special characteristic properties. In most parts of the world, a small number of thalassemia mutations predominant and the most common ones tend to be those that are geographically the most widespread and presumably also the oldest. For instance, in China and Southeast Asia, four alleles account for 91% of the genes (Kazazian et al., 1986), and in the Mediterranean Basin, six mutation account for 92% of the genes (Najmabadi et al., 2002). However, mutation 619 bp deletion is predominant in India or mutations IVS I-110 and IVS II-1 are most predominant in Arab populations (El-Hazmi et al., 1995). Because of Wars and trade off between different countries in the past years there was exchange of genetic materials between different populations. In one study it show that IVS II-1, IVS I-110, IVS I-1, and CD 8/9. These mutations are the most frequent in Iran and IVS II-1(24%) is most predominant in Khuzestan (Rahim and Abromand, 2008). In a similar work on 1217 patients

with ß- thalassemia the most predominant mutation in North part of Iran was IVS II-1(34%) and in South part was IVS I-5(%) (Najmabadi et al., 2002).
Najmabadi et al (2002), have studied ß -globin mutations and claimed the most common ß - globin mutations is IVS I-130 (G-C), which was identified in six subjects from the North of Iran, three subjects from the Southwest, as well as in one DNA of unknown geographical origin. We have found that most predominant in South was IVSII-I (34%) follows by IVS I-110(15.7%) and CD 8/9(13.3%) (Rahim and Abromand, 2008). Previous research work showed most predominant mutation in Pakistan is IVS I-5(37%) therefore this mutation is most predominant in Sistan-Baloochestan (44.8%)(Southeast of Iran) because it is a neighborhood area to Pakistan (Kazazian et al., 1984). In a work done on thalassemia patients in Hormozgan (Southern part of Iran) claimed that most predominant mutation there is IVS I-5(69%) followed by IVS II- 1(9.6%) (Yavarian et al., 2001).
Research work done in 8 Gulf (Arab) Countries showed that most predominant mutations are IVS I-110 and IVS II-1 followed by IVS I-5, CD39, CD6, IVS I(3' end)-25 bp del (Adekile et al., 2005). Our finding was similar to the work done in Kuwait which showed 6 mutations are most predominant involve IVS II-1, IVS I-6, CD39, IVS I-110, CD8, IVS I-1(all give 64%) and followed by another 2 involve CD44, CD 36/37 (Kurd, Iranian types) that give 10% of the population. We detected different ß-thalassemia mutations in the studied chromosomes and 5 different areas from Iran which showed IVS-II-I (G → A) was the predominant mutation found in all ethnic regions. . The presence of such a high frequency of various local mutants alleles confirms support for a role of non-isolating genetically areas. In likelihood, both founder effect and natural selection caused by migration from neighboring areas have complemented each other to produce the high frequency of unique alleles within each region (Figure 4).

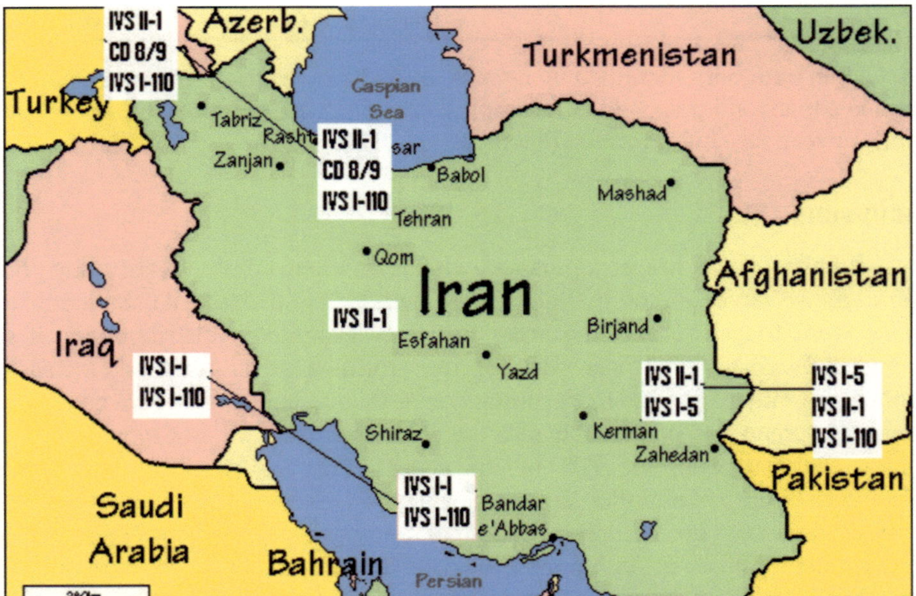

Fig. 5. The origin of mutant alleles with high frequency within different parts of Iran. The most frequent beta-gene mutations in each ethnic region indicated individually.

4. References

Adekile A, Haider M, Kutlar F. Mutations Associated with Beta-Thalassemia intermedia in Kuwait. Medical Principles and Practice 2005;14(Suppl.1):69-72.

Antonarakis SE, Irkin SH, Cheng TC, Scott AF, Sexton JP, Trusko SP, et al. beta - Thalassemia in American Blacks: novel mutations in the "TATA" box and an acceptor splice site. ProcNatlAcadSci USA. 1984;81(4):1154-8.

Cheng TC, Orkin SH, Antonarakis SE, Potter MJ, Sexton JP, Markham AF, et al. beta-Thalassemia in Chinese: use of in vivo RNA analysis and oligonucleotide hybridization in systematic characterization of molecular defects. ProcNatlAcadSci USA 1984;81(9):2821-5.

El-Hazmi MA, Warsy AS, Al-Swailem AR. The frequency of 14 beta- thalassemia mutations in the Arab populations.Hemoglobin 1995;19(6):353-60.

Fakher R, Bijan K, Taghi AM. Application of diagnostic methods and molecular diagnosis of hemoglobin disorders in Khuzestan province of Iran. Indian J Hum Genet 2007;13:5-15

Fucharoen S, Viprakasit V. Hb H disease: clinical course and disease modifiers. Hematology Am Soc Hematol Educ Program. 2009:26-34.

Galanello R, Piras S, Barella S, Leoni GB, Cipollina MD, Perseu L, et al, Cholelithiasis and Gilbert's syndrome in homozygous betathalassemia. Br J Haematol 2001. 115: 926-928.

Haghshenas M, Zamani J. [Thalassemia]. 1st ed. Shiraz University of Medical Sciences Publishing Center: Shiraz; 1997. [Book in Persian]

Ho PJ, Thein SL. Gene regulation and deregulation: a beta globin perspective. Blood Rev 2000;14(2):78 -93.

Jeffreys AJ. Gene evolution. *In*: Genetic engineering, 2nd ed. Robert Williamson, Academic Press: 1981. p. 1-48.

Karnpean R, Fucharoen G, Fucharoen S, Sae-ung N, Sanchaisuriya K, Ratanasiri T. Accurate prenatal diagnosis of Hb Bart's hydrops fetalis in daily practice with a double-check PCR system. Acta Haematol. 2009; 121(4):227-33.

Kazazian HH, Jr, Orkin SH, Antonarakis SE, Sexton JP, Boehm CD, Goff SC, et al. Molecular characterization of seven beta - Thalassemia mutations in Asian Indians. EMBO J 1984;3(3):593-6.

Kazazian HH, Jr., Dowling CH, Waber PG, Hung S, LO, WHY.The spectrum of Beta - thalassemia genes in China and Southeast Asia. Blood 1986;68:964-6.

Kazazian HH. Jr., Orkin SH, Markham AF, Chapman CR, Youssoufian H, Waber PG. On the origin and spread of beta-thalassemia: recurrent observation of four mutations in different ethnic groups. Nature 1984;310:152-4.

Najmabadi H, Ali A. Pourfathollah, Neishabury M, Sahebjam F. Rare and unexpected mutations among Iranian ß -thalassemia patients and prenatal samples discovered by reverse-hybridization and DNA sequencing. Haematologica 2002;87(10).

Najmabadi H, Ghamari A, Sahebjam F, Kariminejad R, Hadavi V et al. Fourteen –Years Experience of Prenatal Diagnosis of Thalassemia in Iran. Com Gen 2006; 9:93-97.

Ohba Y, Hattori Y, Harano K, Fukumaki Y, Ideguchi H. ß-thalassemia mutations in Japanese and Koreans. Hemoglobin 1997;21:191-200.

Oliveri NF. The beta- thalassemias. New Eng J Med 1999;341:99-109.

Orkin SH, Kazazian HH, JrAntonarakis SE, Goff SC, Boehm CD, Sexton JP, et al. Linkage of beta - thalassemia mutations and beta-globin gene polymorphisms with DNA polymorphisms in human beta-globin gene cluster. Nature 1982;296(5858):627-31.

Panigrahi I, Marwaha RK, Kulkarni K. The expanding spectrum of thalassemia intermedia. Hematology. 2009 Dec; 14(6):311-4.

Rahim F, Abromand M. spectrum of ß –thalassemia mutations in various ethnic regions of Iran. Pak J Med Sci 2008 ;24(3):410-15

Rahim F, Kaikhaei B, Zandian K, Hoseini A. Co-inheritance of alpha-and beta-thalassemia in Khuzestan Province, Iran. Hematology. 2008 Feb; 13(1):59-64.

Rahim F, Keikhaei B, Aberumand M. Prenatal Diagnosis (PND) of β-Thalassemia in the Khuzestan Province, Iran. Journal of Clinical and Diagnostic Research. 2007Dec; 1(6):454-459

Rahim F, Keikhaei B. Better differential diagnosis of iron deficiencyanemia from beta-thalassemia trait. Turk J Hematol. 2009; 26(3): 138-145

Rahim F. Correlation of beta-thalassemia mutations with alpha-thalassemia: an experience of the southwestern region of Iran. Hematology. 2010 Dec; 15(6):430-3.

Rahim F. Microcytic hypochromic anemia patients with thalassemia: genotyping approach. Indian J Med Sci. 2009 Mar; 63(3):101-8.

Sack GH. Autosomal recessive disorders.Medical Genetics, McGraw-Hill, New York. 1999;61-3.

Singer ST. Variable clinical phenotypes of alpha-thalassemia syndromes. ScientificWorldJournal. 2009 Jul 13; 9:615-25.

Taher AT, Otrock ZK, Uthman I, Cappellini MD, Thalassemia and hypercoagulability. Blood Rev 2008. 22: 283-292.

Trent RJ. Medical Genetics.Molecular Medicin, Longman Singapore Ltd., Singapore. 1997;37-717.

Vichinsky EP. Alpha thalassemia major--new mutations, intrauterine management, and outcomes. Hematology Am Soc Hematol Educ Program. 2009:35-41.

Vrettou C, Traeger-Synodinos J, Tzetis M, Malamis G, Kanavakis E, Rapid screening of multiple betaglobin gene mutations by real-time PCR on the LightCycler: application to carrier screening and prenatal diagnosis of thalassemia syndromes. Clin Chem 2003. 49: 769-776.

Weatherall DJ, Clegg JB, Higgs DR, Wood WG. The hemoglobinopathies.The Metabolic and Molecular Bases of Inherited Disease.McGraw - Hill, New York. 1989;3417-83.

Yavarian M, Harteveld CL, Batelaan D, Bernini LF, Giordano PC. Molecular spectrum of beta-thalassemia in the Iranian Province of Hormozgan. Hemoglobin. 2001 Feb;25(1):35-43.

7

CCL Chemokines Levels in Tear Fluid of Patients with Cystic Fibrosis

Malgorzata Mrugacz
Medical University of Bialystok
Poland

1. Introduction

Cystic fibrosis (CF) is inherited as an autosomal recessive disorder in white populations, caused by a mutation in a gene that encodes cystic fibrosis transmembrane conductance regulator (CFTR) protein, which is expressed in many epithelial cells and blood cells. Although CFTR functions mainly as a chloride channel, it has many other regulatory roles, including inhibition of sodium transport through the epithelial sodium channel, regulation of the outwardly rectifying chloride channel, regulation of ATP channels, regulation of intracellular vesicle transport, acidification of intracellular organelles, and inhibition of endogenous calcium-activated chloride channels (O'Sullivan & Freedman, 2009; Reisin et al., 1994; Schwiebert et al., 1995; Stutts et al., 1995; Vankeerberghen et al., 2002; Mehta, 2005). CFTR is also involved in bicarbonate-chloride exchange. A deficiency in bicarbonate secretion leads to poor solubility and aggregation of luminal mucins (Quinton, 2008). More than 1500 CFTR mutations have been identified, but only the functional importance of a small number is known. The absence of phenylalanine at position 508 accounts for about two-thirds of mutated alleles in northern European and North American populations (Walters & Mehta, 2007).

The clinical manifestations of the disease vary greatly between affected individuals, which has led to interest in the relation between genotype and phenotype. It is presumed that disease affects all secretory epithelia including the eye (Castagna, 2001; Turner et al., 2002; Mrugacz et al., 2006; Mrugacz et al., 2007; Mrugacz et al., 2007). The pathogenesis of ocular changes in CF is still unknown. CF belongs to the group of ocular surface diseases termed keratoconjunctivitis sicca or dry eye syndrome. The causes of dry eye are multi-factorial and can be connected with deficiencies in any one of the components of the ocular surface and tear fluid. It is known that inflammation plays a key role in the pathogenesis of dry eye (Baudouin, 2001; Brignole et al., 2000; Pflugfelder, 2004; Pisella et al., 2000), especially with the participation of chemokines.

Chemokines are a family of small protein molecules that play an important role in normal leukocyte trafficking as well as in leukocyte recruitment during inflammation. These chemokines are grouped into CXC, CC, C, and CX3C subfamilies on the basis of the arrangement of the conserved cysteine residues. This molecular subvivision generally correlates with their function. Most recently, chemokines have been classified according to their physiological features: inflammatory or inducible chemokines and homeostatic or constitutive chemokines. Chemokines act through both specific and shared receptors that belong tho the superfamily of G-protein-coupled receptors. The chemokine receptors also comprise four groups, including the CC receptors (CCR), which bind CC chemokines; and CXC receptors (CXCR), which bind CXC chemokines. Chemokine and chemokine receptor expression can increase in acute and chronic inflammatory conditions due to inflammatory mediators, such as cytokines. The CC chemokines are involved in the pathogenesis of immune-mediated inflammation through monocytes/macrophages activation and recruitment. CC chemokines, such as CCL3/macrophage inflammatory protein-1α (CCL3/MIP-1α) and CCL4/macrophage inflammatory protein-1ß (CCL4/MIP-1ß) are efficient chemoattractant for Th1 cells and contribute to the inflammatory processes in the eye (Locati & Murphy, 1999; Manczak & Yiang, 2002).

The aim of this study was to assess the potential role of chemokines in the pathogenesis of ocular changes in patients with CF. We assayed CCL3/MIP-1α and CCL4/MIP-1ß levels in tear fluid of CF patients. We also investigated the correlation between the tear levels of these chemokines and clinical severity of CF and ocular surface disease.

2. Materials and methods

2.1 Patients

We studied 28 patients with CF with a mean age 14.75±3.95 years (range 6-23) (14 women, 14 men) who attended 3th Department of Pediatric Diseases, Medical University of Bialystok, Poland. Twenty-seven normal subjects with a mean age of 15.21±4.35 years (range 8-23) (13 women, 14 men) were also included. All the CF patients had a comprehensive assessment every 6-12 months and were receiving vitamin A supplementation. They did not receive any systemic steroid therapy.

The clinical status was scored according to Schwachmann and Kulczycki (Schwachman Score, scale 100-0: 100=excellent, 100-55=without pulmonary insufficiency, below 55=severe of CF) (Schwachmann & Kulczycki, 1958).

2.2 Tear sample collection

Tear samples were collected in graduated 30-µl disposable microcapillaries (ACCU-FILL 90 MICROPET, Becton Dickinson and Company, Franklin Lakes, NJ) unilaterally or bilaterally from the conjunctival cul-de-sac without anesthesia. Care was taken to avoid touching the lid margin or corneal surface. We collected 50 to 100 µl of basal tears from each eye. The CCL3/MIP-1α and CCL4/MIP-1ß levels in tears were determined by ELISA using highly sensitive immunoassay kit (Endogen system, MA, USA). The collected tears were immediately frozen to -80°C; they were thawed just before assaying. All the samples were coded and read blind in the assay. The procedure recommended by the manufacturer was followed without any modification.

2.3 Ophthalmic examination including dry eye tests

The ophthalmologic examination included subjective assessment, visual acuity and biomicroscopy. Subject complaints, such as redness, foreign body sensation, irritation, intense burning, and blurred vision were noted. Both patients and controls were performed tests for keratoconjunctivitis sicca. Tear break-up time (TBUT) was measured to assess tear

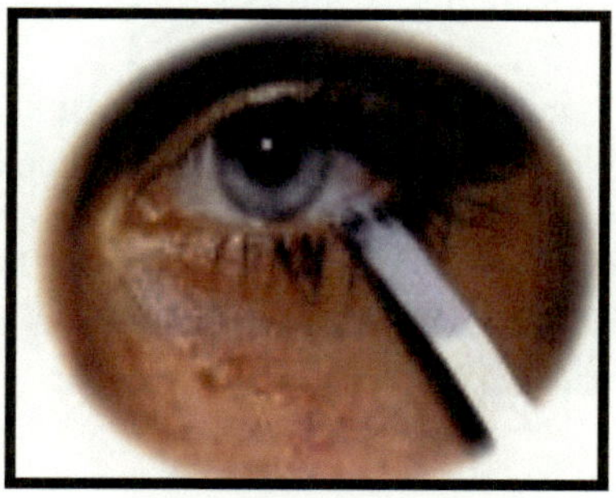

1

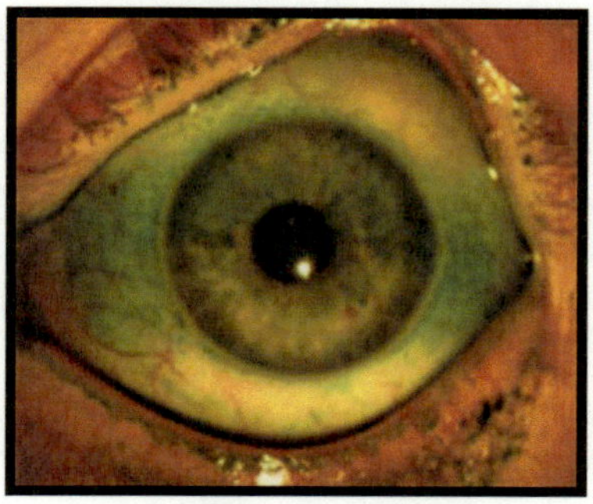

2

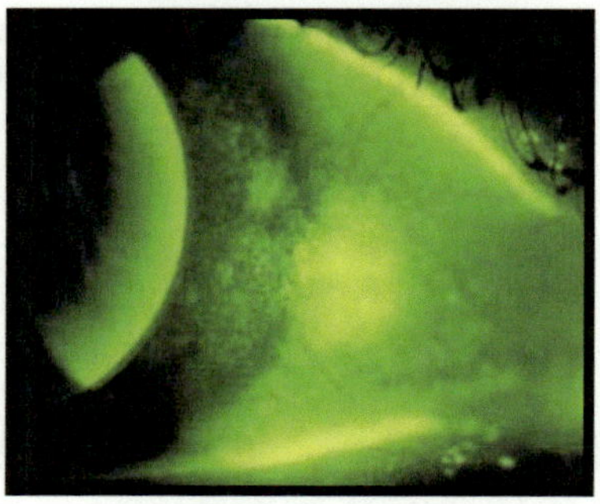

3

Fig. 1. Dry eye tests. 1- Schirmer test, 2- Tear break-up time (TBUT), 3- Lissamine green staining

film stability. A value of <10 seconds was abnormal. Schirmer test was used to estimate tear film quantity; a value of <5 mm after 5 minutes was abnormal. The lissamine green instilled into the inferior fornix was used to assess the amount of dead epithelial cells at the ocular surface. If two of these variables were abnormal then dry eye syndrome was the diagnosis according to the Copenhagen criteria (Manthorpe 1986). All clinical examinations were performed before any topical or systemic treatment was administered to the eye.

2.4 Statistical analysis

Non- parametric analysis was conducted in this study. Wilcoxon's sum rank test was used to identify differences between tear chemokine levels in patients group and controls. Spearman's rank correlation test was used to establish the significance of correlation between tear chemokine levels and severity of CF and the eye disease. A level of $p < 0.05$ was accepted as statistically significant.

3. Results

3.1 Chemokines levels

The tear fluid levels of CCL3/MIP-1α were 144.50±18.51 pg/mL (mean±SD) in CF patients, whereas in normal controls, they were 41.85±11.25 pg/mL (mean±SD). There is significant difference between serum levels of MIP-1α in CF patients and healthy controls (p=0.001)
The tear fluid levels of CCL4/MIP-1ß were 4.25±1.15 pg/mL (mean±SD) in CF patients and 0.52±0.36 pg/mL (mean±SD) in healthy controls. The tear fluid levels of MIP-1beta were significantly raised in CF group compared to controls (p<0.001).

3.2 Assessment of dry eye syndrome

Dry eye syndrome were observed in 10 (36%) CF patients (five girls and five boys). However, the tear fluid levels of CCL3/MIP-1α and CCL4/MIP-1ß were significantly higher in CF patients with dry eye syndrome than in CF patients without dry eye symptoms: 165.50±20.32 pg/mL (mean±SD) and 132.22±17.35 pg/mL (mean±SD) of CCL3/MIP-1α, respectively; and 5.25±1.26 pg/mL (mean±SD) and 3.18±0.80 pg/mL (mean±SD) of CCL4/MIP-1ß, respectively (p<0.05).

3.3 Assessment of pulmonary insufficiency

Symptoms of pulmonary insufficiency (below 55 according to the Schwachman- Kulczycki Score) were found in 45% (13 out of 28) of the CF patients. Spearman correlation coefficient indicated a positive correlation between the tear levels of CCL3/MIP-1α and CCL4/MIP-1ß and severe clinical status of CF patients (R=0.869, p< 0.001). However, negative correlation was found between the tear levels of these chemokines and mild CF (R=–0.817, p< 0.001). Fifteen of our CF patients (55%) with high levels of CCL3/MIP-1α and CCL4/MIP-1ß had clinical evidence of dry eye. Spearman correlation coefficient indicated a positive correlation between the tear levels of these chemokines and dry eye findings in CF patients.

4. Discussion

One of the major problems in understanding the mechanisms of dry eye symptoms in CF patients, is to determine the factors involved in this disease. It is known that inflammation

plays a key role in the pathogenesis of dry eye syndrome, especially with the participation of chemokines. Chemokines are expressed at sites of inflammation to attract and amplify the leukocyte response. It is important to identify chemokines that play a role in mediating response. The recruitment of leukocytes to tissue is essential for inflammation. This process may be controlled by MIP-1α and CCL4/MIP-1beta that contribute to the recruitment of inflammatory cells into the eye and plays an important role in pathogenicity.
In this study, we have documented, for the first time, raised levels of CCL3/MIP-1α and CCL4/MIP-1beta in tear fluid in CF patients. The highest levels of these chemokines were detected in patients with dry eye syndrome and severe CF. The high levels of suggest of CCL3/MIP-1α and CCL4/MIP-1beta suggest that these chemokines may be produced locally and may be a factor for evaluation of the clinical status of this disease. It may confirm the involvement of CCL4/MIP-1beta in the local inflammatory process. Functional consequence of elevated levels of these chemokines has yet to be determined exactly. Moreover, there is evidence that dry eye stimulates the production of inflammatory cytokines from the ocular surface epithelium (Luo et al., 2004). The increased levels of MIP-1α and MIP-1beta observed in this study may be a consequence of increased secretion from the corneal epithelium or from the another noncorneal cell type. The tear film containing numerous specific and nonspecific immune components (Solomon et al., 2001) may act as a vehicle of chemokines produced by the lacrimal gland or other epithelia of the ocular surface.
There is a little information about the role of CCL3/MIP-1α and CCL4/ MIP-1beta in eye inflammation. Despite advances in tissue typing, surgery and immunosuppressive treatment allogenic rejection is the most common cause of corneal graft failure. Allograft rejection is characterized by infiltration of leucocytes into the donor tissue, a response that has been associated with chemokine expression, with CCL2/MCP-1, CCL3/ MIP-1α and CCL4/ MIP-1beta showing ans increased expression in rejected grafts in mice (Yamagami et al., 1999). In recent studies of CCL3/MIP-1α and CCL4/ MIP-1ß, Verma and others have shown that these chemokines were significantly increased in the aqueous humor during the active stages of human autoimmune anterior uveitis (AAU) and correlated with the clinical severity of the disesase (Verma et al., 1997). Anti-MIP-1α and anti-MIP-1ß treatment suppressed clinical signs of recurrent anterior uveitis (RAU) in the Lewis rats, suggesting that these chemokines may also influence the migration of memory T cells across the blood ocular barrier in recurring episode of AAU. In addition, during acute AAU associated with experimental autoimmune encephalomyelitis (EAE), CC chemokines, such as CCL2/MCP-1, CCL5/RANTES, CCL3/MIP-1α and CCL4/MIP-1ß, contributed to the inflammatory processes in the eye and central nervous system (CNS) (Manczak et al., 2002). Treatment with anti-CCL4/ MIP-1ß delayed onset and reduced duration of AAU (Adamus et al., 2001). The retinal ischemia- reperfusion model showed an upregulation of CCL4/MIP-1beta in the retinal vessels and these results confirm that this chemokine may be involved in the inflammatory element of pathogenesis of retinal neovascularization (Jo et al., 2003).

5. Conclusion

In conclusion, the results of this study demonstrate that increased levels of chemokines in the tear fluid may play an important role in the pathogenesis of dry eye in patients with cystic fibrosis. The tear levels of CCL3/MIP-1α and CCL4/MIP-1ß may be a candidate marker to evaluate the clinical status of cystic fibrosis and eye disease. Our findings may contribute to further understanding of local and systemic immune responses and might lead to the development of new clinical approaches to inflammatory disorders. Clarification of the role of chemokines in the pathogenesis of ocular findings in CF patients will be useful in establishing immunotherapeutic strategies for this disease.

6. Acknowledgment

I think Prof. Maciej Kaczmarski (3th Department of Pediatrics, Medical University of Bialystok, Poland) and Beata Żelazowska-Rutkowska (Department of Pediatric Laboratory Diagnostic Medical University of Bialystok, Poland) for their assistance.

7. References

Adamus, G.; Manczak, M. & Machnicki, M. (2001). Expression of CC chemokines and their receptors in the eye in autoimmune anterior uveitis associated with EAE. *Invest Ophthalmol Vis Sci*, 42, pp. 2894-2903, ISSN 1552-5783

Baudouin, C. (2001). The pathology of dry eye. *Surv Ophthalmol*, 45: pp. 211-20, ISSN 0039-6257

Brignole, F.; Pisella P.J.; Goldshild, M.; De Saint Jean, M.; Goguel, A. & Baudouin, C. (2000). Flow cytometric analysis of inflammatory markers in conjunctival epithelial cells of patients with dry eyes. *Invest Ophthalmol Vis Sci*, 41, pp. 1356-1363, ISSN 1552-5783

Castagna, I.; Roszkowska, A.M.; Fama, F.; Sinicropi, S. & Ferreri, G. (2001). The eye in cystic fibrosis. *Eur J Ophthalmol*, 11, pp. 9-14, 1120-6721

Jo, N.; Wu, G.S. & Rao, N.A. (2003). Upregulation of chemokine expression in the retinal vasculature in ischemia-reperfusion injury. *Invest Ophthalmol Vis Sci*, 44, pp. 4054-60, ISSN 1552-5783

Locati, M. & Murphy, P. (1999). Chemokines and chemokine receptors: biology and clinical relevance in inflammation and AIDS. *Annu Rev Medicine*, 50, pp. 425-440, ISSN 0163-7525

Luo, L.; Li, D,Q. & Doshi, A. (2004). Experimental dry eye stimulates production of inflammatory cytokines and MMP-9 and activates MARK signaling pathways on the ocular surface. *Invest Ophthalmol Vis Sci*, 45, pp. 4293-4301, ISSN 1552-5783

Manczak, M.; Jiang, A.; Orzechowska, B. & Adamus, G. (2002). Crucial role of CCL3/MIP-1α in the recurrence of autoimmune anterior uveitis induced with myelin basic protein in Lewis rats. *J Autoimmun*, 18, pp. 259-270, ISSN 0896-8411

Manthorpe, R.; Oxholm, P. & Prause JU. (1986). The Copenhagen criteria for Sjogren's syndrome. *Scand J Rheumatol (suppl)*, 61, pp. 19-21, ISSN 0300-9742

Mehta, A. (2005). CFTR: more than just a chloride channel. *Pediatr Pulmonol*, 39, pp. 292–98, ISSN 1054-187X

Mrugacz, M.; Kaczmarski, M.; Bakunowicz-Łazarczyk, A.; Żelazowska, B; Wysocka, J. & Minarowska, A. (2006). IL-8 and IFN-gamma in tear fluid of patients with cystic fibrosis. *J Interferon Cytokine Res,* 26, pp. 71-5, ISSN 1079-9907

Mrugacz, M.; Żelazowska, B.; Bakunowicz-Łazarczyk, A.; Kaczmarski, M. & Wysocka, J. 2007. Elevated tear fluid levels of MIP-1α in patients with cystic fibrosis. J Interferon Cytokine Res 27:491-495

Mrugacz M, Żak J, Bakunowicz-Łazarczyk A, Wysocka J, Kaczmarski M. 2007. ICAM-1 expression on conjunctival epithelial cells in patients with cystic fibrosis. *Cytometry B Clin Cytom,* 72, pp. 204-8, ISSN 1009-3591

O'Sullivan, B.P. & Freedman, S.D. (2009). Cystic fibrosis. *Lancet,* 373, pp. 1891-94, ISSN 0140-6736

Pflugfelder, S.C. (2004). Antiinflammatory therapy for dry eye. *Am J Ophthalmol,* 137, pp. 337-342, ISSN 1549-4713

Pisella, P.J.; Brignole, F.; Debbasch, C.; Pharm, D.; Lozato, P.A. & Creuzot-Garcher C. (2000). Flow cytometric analysis of conjunctival epithelium in ocular rosacea and keratoconjunctivitis sicca. *Ophthalmology,* 107, pp. 1841-1849, ISSN 0301-4738

Quinton, P.M. (2008). Cystic fibrosis: impaired bicarbonate secretion and mucoviscidosis. *Lancet,* 372, pp. 415–17, ISSN 0140-6736

Reisin, I.L.; Prat, A.G. & Abraham, E.H. (1994). The cystic fibrosis transmembrane conductance regulator is a dual ATP and chloride channel. *J Biol Chem,* 269, pp. 20584–91, ISSN 0021-9258

Schwachmann, H. & Kulczycki, L.L. (1958). Long term study of 105 patients with cystic fibrosis. Studies made over a 5 to 14 year period. *Am J Dis Child,* 96, pp. 6-15, ISSN 0096-8994

Schwiebert, E.M.; Egan, M.E. & Hwang, T.H. (1995). CFTR regulates outwardly rectifying chloride channels through an autocrine mechanism involving ATP. *Cell,* 81, pp. 1063–73, ISSN 0092-8674

Solomon, A.; Dursun, D. & Liu. Z. (2001). Pro- and anti-inflammatory forms of interleukin-1 in the tear fluid and conjunctiva of patients with dry-eye disease. *Invest Ophthalmol Vis Sci* , 42, pp. 2283-92, ISSN 1552-5783

Stutts, M.J.; Canessa, C.M. & Olsen, J.C. (1995). CFTR as a cAMP-dependent regulator of sodium channels. *Science,* 269, pp. 847–50, ISSN 0036-8075

Turner, H.C.; Bernstein, A. & Candia, O.A. (2002). Presence of CFTR in the conjunctival epithelium. *Curr Eye Res,* 24, pp. 182-7, ISSN 0271-3683

Vankeerberghen, A.; Cuppens, H. & Cassiman, J.J. (2002). The cystic fibrosis transmembrane conductance regulator: an intriguing protein pleiotropic functions. *J Cyst Fibros,* 1, pp. 13–29, ISSN 8755-6863

Verma, M.J.; Lloyd, A.; Rager, H.; Strieter, R.; Kunkel, S.; Taub, D. & Wakefield, D. (1997). Chemokine in acute anterior uveitis. *Curr Eye Res* 16: pp. 1202-1208, ISSN 0271-3683

Walters, S. & Mehta, A. (2007). Epidemiology of cystic fibrosis. In: Hodson M, Geddes DM, Bush A, eds. *Cystic fibrosis,* 3rd ed. London: Edward Arnold Ltd, pp. 21–45, ISBN 10: 0340742089

Yamagami, S.; Miyazaki, D.; Ono, S.J. & Dana, M.R. (1999). Differential chemokine gene expression in corneal trans plant rejection. *Invest Ophthalmol Vis Sci*, 40, pp.2892-2897, ISSN 1552-5783

8

The Genetic Makeup of Azoreans *Versus* Mainland Portugal Population

Cláudia Castelo Branco and Luisa Mota-Vieira
Molecular Genetics and Pathology Unit,
Hospital of Divino Espirito Santo of Ponta Delgada, EPE, Azores
Portugal

1. Introduction

Since the first draft of the human genome we observed a boost in biomedical research. As consequence, nowadays, it is possible to know a person's predisposition to a genetic disease or even how its organism will metabolize a given drug. Although, there is some delay in translating this knowledge to the development and implementation of personalized medicine, there are currently available some successful pharmacogenetic based treatment decisions. One of such example is abacavir, a nucleoside analog reverse transcriptase inhibitor used in treatment of HIV-1 infection. Abacavir hypersensitivity is strongly associated with HLA-B*57:01 allele. Genetic testing before abacavir's prescription is now recommended in clinical guidelines and is practiced in most western countries (Chaponda & Pirmohamed 2011). In a near future, personalized medicine will, most certainly, bring considerable health gains to society.
The new approaches to analyze the human genome, - genome-wide association studies (GWAS; Orange et al., 2011), deep resequencing (1000 Genomes Project Consortium, 2010) and gene expression variability (Li et al., 2010) –, are producing massive data, which are already historic marks in the understanding of the genetic makeup of traits. A good example is the 9p21 genomic region association with coronary artery disease (McPherson et al., 2007; Helgadottir et al., 2007). However, only a small fraction of the heritable variation of complex diseases has been identified. One possible explanation may be that many rare variants, which are not included in the common genotyping platforms, may contribute substantially to the genetic variation of complex diseases. Therefore, researchers are becoming aware that common disease - common variant and common disease - rare variant models (Gorlov et al., 2011; Carvajal-Carmona, 2010; Zhu et al., 2011) will largely contribute to understand the genetic architecture of the populations with a diverse ancestry, such as the Azoreans. Hence, regional and local studies are good approaches to comprehend the genetic specificities of each population.

1.1 Mainland Portugal and Azores populations: historic and demographic data

Portugal, with a population of 10,637,713 inhabitants, is the most western country of the European continent and is bordered by the Atlantic Ocean to the west and south and by Spain to the north and east. The present Portuguese genetic landscape is the outcome of an old and slow process of gene flow, admixture with many different populations and local differentiation. These include the expansion from isolated population nuclei in refuges following the Last Glacial Maximum, the movement of peoples related to the introduction of agriculture, and subsequent Roman and Germanic invaders, which may have influenced the distribution of genetic diversity in the territory (Amaral & Amaral, 1997). Roman settlers strongly influenced Portuguese culture, particularly the Portuguese language, which is derived from Latin. During the 8th century Muslim Moors occupied most of the Iberian Peninsula, contributing also to admixture events observed by the presence of north African paternal lineages in the Portuguese genetic background (Adams et al., 2008; Pereira et al., 2000a). With the establishment of the country in the year 1139, after several wars, Portugal is the oldest European nation-state. In the 15th and 16th centuries, as the result of maritime expeditions, the country established a global empire that included possessions in Africa, Asia, Oceania and South America, becoming the world's major economic, political and military power. Portugal's empire was the first and most long-lived global empire in the world, spanning almost six centuries (Russel-Wood, 1998; Jenkins & Sofos, 1996). During the Portuguese age of discovery, two archipelagos - Madeira and Azores (Figure 1) -, which are

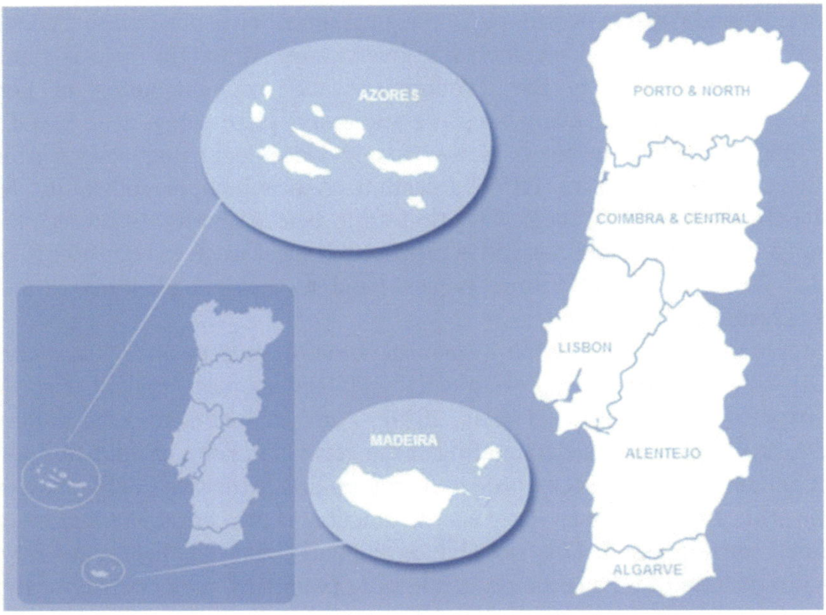

Fig. 1. Portugal's regions map.

currently part of the country's territory, were discovered. The Azores is composed of nine volcanic islands unevenly distributed by three geographic groups: the Eastern group with two islands - São Miguel and Santa Maria -, the Central includes five islands - Terceira, Pico, Faial, São Jorge and Graciosa -, and the Western group with Flores and Corvo. This archipelago has a total area of 2332.74 km^2, unevenly distributed by the nine islands, varying from São Miguel, the largest, with 746.82 km^2 to Corvo, the smallest, with 17.13 km^2. The present-day population is composed of 241,763 inhabitants (National Institute of Statistics - Portugal, 2001 Census), derived from about 27 generations. The majority of the population lives on São Miguel (54.4%). The remainder is unevenly dispersed throughout the other eight islands; for example, Corvo has only 425 individuals. From the total Azorean population, 41.4% are living in the Central group, where Terceira is the most populated of this group (24.9%; 55,833 inhabitants). The first settlers arrived in the mid 15th century and were mainly Portuguese, but the peopling was a slow and difficult process (Mendonça, 1996; Guill, 1993). Someone wrote "...The Azorean settlement was done with people from the interior of mainland Portugal, those who could not swim nor build boats, making impossible the abandonment of the islands...". Historical data report that the Portuguese crown was compelled to give out land and privileges in order to attract people to the islands (Guill, 1993). The first islands to be settled were Santa Maria and São Miguel in 1439 and the last were Flores and Corvo in the beginning of the 16th century. Some early settlers were of foreign origin, including Flemish, Jews, Moorish prisoners and black slaves from Guinea, Cape Verde and São Tomé. In the following centuries, contributions from Spanish, French, Italians, Germans and Scottish also occurred.

2. DNA banking of the healthy Azorean population

Biobanks have become an absolute requirement for biomedical research (Simon et al., 2007; Deplanque et al., 2009) and are defined as collections of samples of human bodily substances that are or can be associated with personal and clinical data. Depending on the purpose of a given biobank, both genetic and health information may be linked with the samples. The location of the Azorean population in the middle of the Atlantic, its geography, socio-cultural characteristics and, finally, the same environmental conditions, make a priori this population a good model to perform population genetic studies. Bering this in mind, the Molecular Genetics and Pathology Unit (UGPM, located at the main Azorean Hospital, Hospital of Divino Espírito Santo of Ponta Delgada, EPE - HDESPD) researchers adopted a strategy that began with the establishment of a DNA bank of the Azorean healthy population. Currently, it comprises a collection of 1558 representative genetic samples obtained from healthy non-family-related adult volunteers. The blood collection counted with the collaboration of the Department of Haematology of HDESPD for São Miguel samples, and municipalities Health Centres (Centro de Saúde de Vila do Porto, Centro de Saúde de Angra do Heroísmo, Centro de Saúde da Praia da Vitória, Centro de Saúde da Calheta, Centro de Saúde de Velas, Centro de Saúde de Santa Cruz da Graciosa, Centro de Saúde da Horta, Centro de Saúde das Lajes, Centro de Saúde da Madalena, Centro de Saúde de São Roque, Centro de Saúde de Santa Cruz das Flores) of volunteers resident in the other eight islands. As part of the research project entitled "Study of the genetic diversity in the Azorean population", the biobank was approved by the local Ethics Committee, and follows the international ethical guidelines, which include informed consent, confidentiality, anonymity of personal data and abandonment option in case of expressed will. To each volunteer was hand-out a leaflet (Figure 2) explaining thoroughly: (1) the purpose of the study; (2) the involvement in the blood donation process and of personal information sharing; (3) the risks and benefits of participation; and (4) the privacy protection measures.

A code number was assigned to each blood sample, identifying it during the whole project's protocol. Only authorized staff at the previously mentioned blood collection facilities had access to the participant's name. After individual's acceptance, written informed consent was signed and, with the help of the team involved, an anonymous blood sample record was filled, providing information regarding the participant's age, sex, birthplace and parental birthplace. As far as São Miguel is concerned, the sample consisted of 7.5mL of blood, while in the other islands only 2.7mL were collected. In order to assure individual ancestral origin, the blood collection was preferably taken from individuals whose parents were born in the same island. A thorough analysis of the parental birthplace revealed a distribution of individuals by four different groups (Table 1).

STUDY OF THE GENETIC DIVERSITY IN THE AZOREAN POPULATION *

This leaflet is intended to inform you about the objectives and goal of the study entitled "**Study of the genetic diversity in the Azorean population**". We aim that after this inf ormation you decide free and clearly whether or not you want to participate. In the affirmative case your participation consists in donating 2.7 mL of blood to the Hospital of Divino Espírito Santo of Ponta Delgada, EPE (HDES) collected in the Health Centre of your residence . Your sample will be used to extract genetic material which will be stored at the Molecular Genetics and Pathology Unit (UGPM) of the HDES.

Why is this study being done?
The purpose of this study is to identify and quantify the genetic variation that is present in the population of the different Azorean islands , analysing t he diversity present in the genetic material (DNA).

Is my participation important?
Yes, your particip ation is very important because this study is only possible if a large number of Azorean blood samples are analyzed. You will contribute to a better understanding of the origin , nature and distribution of genetic disorders in the Azorean.

What should I do to participate?
To participate you have to donate 2,7 ml of blo od for DNA extraction . With the help of a specialized team in the Heath Centre, you will fill an anonymous record of the blood sample , providing information concerning your age, sex, birth place and your parent's birth place.

How will my personal informa tion be kept private?
After your blood sample is collected a code number will be assigned which will identify sample during this project protocol. Only the Heath Centre will have access to your name, thus guaranteeing the anonymous nature of the genetic material and corresponding personal information.

Are there any risks associated with this study?
No, there are no risks associated with this study.

Are there any financial benefits in taking part in this study?
No, there is no financial gratification in taking part in this study.

Do I have to pay to participate in the project?
No, your participation is volunteer and free of any charge.

What will happen to my sample after the study is over?
After this study is over, your sample will be stored at MGPU and used in future studies, following all national and international ethic regulations.

What are my rights as a participant?
You are free to choose if you want to participate or not; no restrictions will be imposed on you.

Who do I call if I have questions or problems?
If you have any concerns or questions relating this project, please contact the MGPU.

Can I leave this project even after I have signed the informed consent?
Yes, you are free to leave the project at any time and we will destroy your sample and personal data. All you need to do is inform your Heath Centre of your intention.

* This study was approved by the Hospital of Divino Espirito Santo of Ponta Delgada, EPE, Ethics Committee.

Fig. 2. Leaflet containing information for participation in the Azores DNA bank.

Parents origin	Samples	
	No.	%
Both parents were born in the same island	1373	88,13
Both parents were born in different Azores islands	70	4,49
Only one parent was born in the Azores islands	59	3,79
No parents born in the Azores islands	56	3,56
Individuals that inhabit the Azores islands	**1558**	**100,00**

Table 1. Parental birthplace analysis of the individuals that compose the Azorean DNA bank.

A total of 1443 individuals (92.6%) presented Azorean parents. Age and sex distribution show an average age of 42 years old, ranging from 18 to 88 years, and the majority of individuals are men (71%, Figure 3). Considering the individuals who both parents were born in the same island (N=1373), the population representativeness varies from 0.2% (Terceira) to 7% (Corvo). The largest sample representation is observed in São Miguel with 64% (Figure 3). The relation between the number of inhabitants and samples in each island

indicates a very high correlation coefficient (r=0.92; $p<0.01$), demonstrating the sample representativeness of the population distribution by all nine Azores islands.
Overall, Azoreans were willing to participate and understood its importance for long-term health gains. Until now, no requests to remove samples have been made. This biobank constitutes a very significant resource for biomedical research in Azoreans, some of them described below.

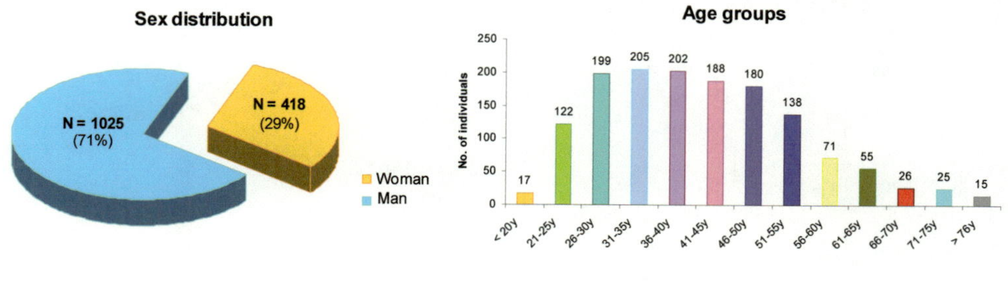

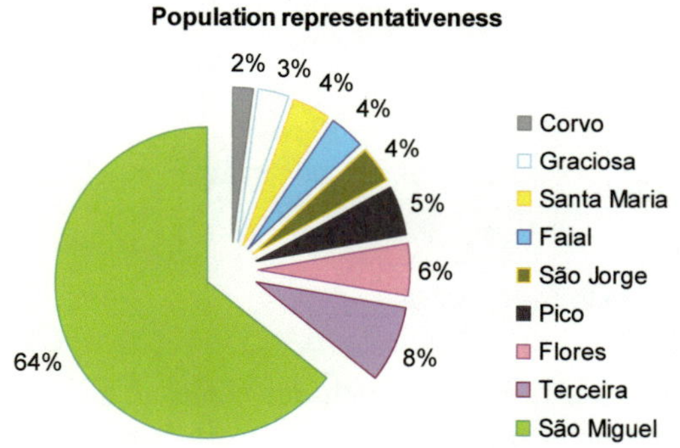

Azores demographic data

Islands	Area (km^2)	Inhabitants
São Miguel	746.82	131,609
Santa Maria	97.10	5578
Terceira	402.20	55,833
Pico	447.00	14,806
Faial	172.43	15,063
São Jorge	237.59	9674
Graciosa	62.00	4780
Flores	142.00	3995
Corvo	17.13	425
Azores	**2332.74**	**241,763**

Fig. 3. DNA bank samples distribution by sex, age and general Azores population representativeness. Calculations were based only in the individuals whose parents were born in the same Azorean island (N=1443).

3. Population studies: knowing the past to predict the future

The plethora of genomic research, produced since the first draft of the human genome (Venter et al., 2001; International Human Genome Sequencing Consortium, 2001), led to the acknowledgment that disease related rare variants with small effects are very difficult to identify (Figure 4) and that common variants implicated in complex diseases are frequently determined by GWAS. Additionally, the Human Genome Project (http://www.genome.gov/ 10001772) also contributed to the understanding of the structure and organization of the genome. Variability is observed through single nucleotide polymorphisms (SNPs), variable number of tandem repeats (VNTRs; e.g. mini and microsatellites), presence or absence of transposable elements (e.g. *Alu* elements) and structural alterations, which include insertions, deletions, duplications, inversions, translocations and copy number variants (CNVs).
The global analysis of population neutral variation is an essential part in the comprehension of the disease related variation, since it has also been subject to evolutionary forces, such as,

genetic drift, mutation, selection and migration. Altogether, the perception of our "roots" and genetic signature has several implications in society's own knowledge, in the design of future genetic studies, as well as, in the healthcare system.

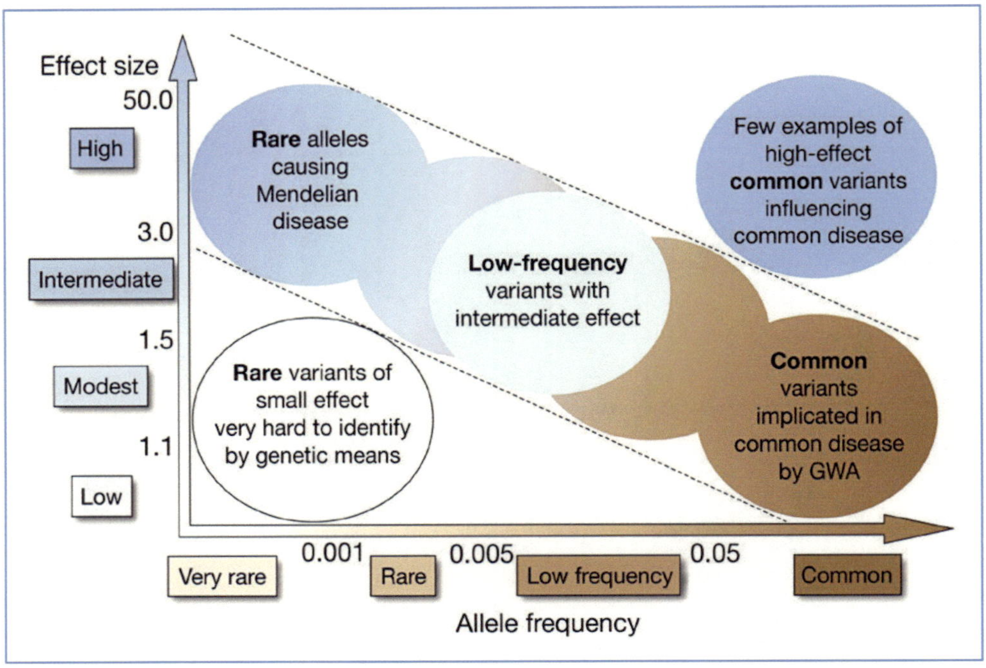

Fig. 4. The frequency spectrum of human disease risk alleles includes alleles at all frequencies from rare to common, with effect sizes from high to low (from Manolio et al., 2009).

3.1 Diversity, ancestry and linkage disequilibrium

The comprehension of how genetic diversity is structured in the human being is not only of anthropological importance, but also of medical relevance with significant implications for human evolution, forensics, genetic diseases and pharmacogenetics (1000 Genomes Project Consortium, 2010; The International HapMap Consortium, 2010; Heard et al., 2010). As more geographic populations are studied with high density genotype arrays it is also becoming apparent that allele frequencies for the relevant disease markers can vary widely. For instance, what is true for Europeans may not be for Africans, such is example the Type 2 Diabetes protective allele with increased frequency in non-Africans compared to Africans (Silander et al., 2009; Kral et al., 2011). These emerging data must be incorporated into a strategy that positions genomic medicine for a clinical role.
To grasp the genetic origins of mainland Portugal and Azorean populations studies on Y-chromosome lineages (Pacheco et al., 2005; Montiel et al., 2005; Beleza et al., 2006; Gonçalves et al., 2005; Fernando et al., 2005), mitochondrial DNA (Pereira et al., 2000b; Santos et al., 2003; Santos et al., 2005; Santos et al., 2008; Santos et al., 2010) and autosomal *Alu* insertion polymorphisms (Branco et al., 2006) were performed. The nonrecombining portion of the Y-chromosome retains a record of the mutational events that occurred along male lineages throughout evolution (Karafet et al., 2008). Presently, new binary polymorphisms reshaped

and increased resolution of the Y-haplogroup tree; however, for comparison purposes old nomenclature was maintained. According to Pacheco et al. (2005), the Azorean population presented nine different haplogroups, most of which are frequent in Europe (Figure 5). Hapogroup J* is the second most frequent in Azores (13.4%), but it is modestly represented in mainland Portugal (6.8%). The other non European haplogroups - N3 and E3a -, which are prevalent in Asia and subSahara, respectively, have been found in Azores (0.6% and 1.2%, respectively) but not in mainland Portugal (Neto et al., 2007). The absence of haplogroup E3a in western Iberia suggests that, despite the massive introductions of African slaves in historical times, there was little admixture between the African males and western Iberian populations (Pereira et al., 2000a). In general, four major haplogroups - P*(xR1b8,R1a,Q3), J*, BR*(xB2b,CE,F1,H,JK) and E*(xE3) - account for the majority of the male lineages in the Azores and mainland Portugal.

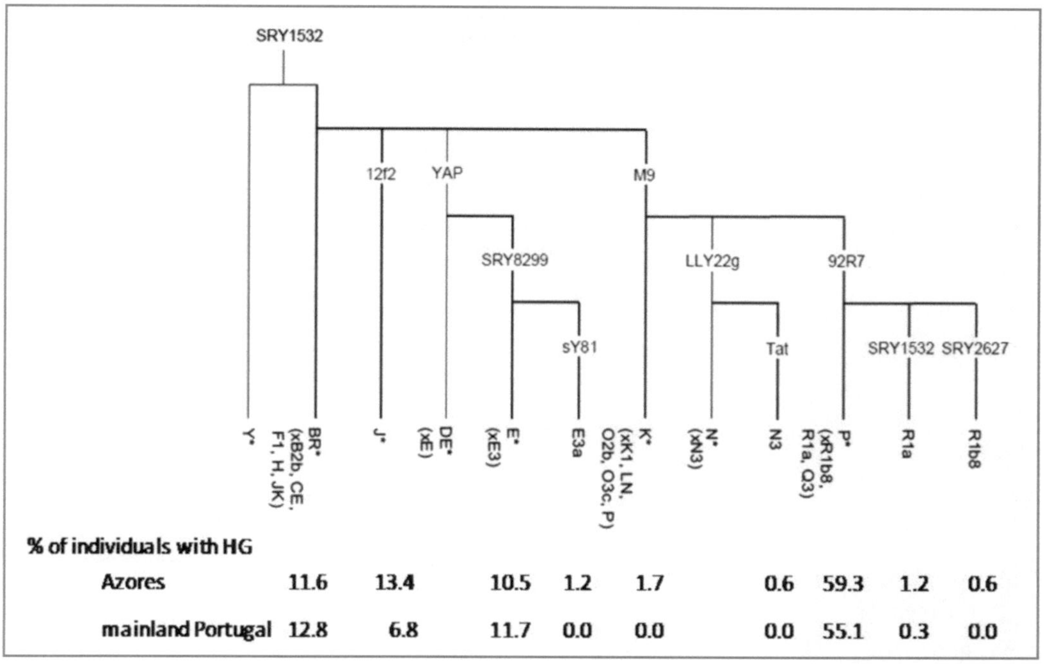

Fig. 5. Phylogenetic tree of the Y-chromosome haplogroups and their percent frequencies in the Azores and mainland Portugal. Numbers of % individuals with HG for mainland Portugal represent average values based on literature reports by Beleza et al. (2006) and Gonçalves et al. (2005).

All studies (Pacheco et al., 2005; Montiel et al., 2005; Beleza et al., 2006; Fernando et al., 2005) report that the main contributors to the genetic origin of the Azores are, as expected, the mainland Portuguese. Moreover, an important contribution of Middle eastern (HG J*) and north African (HG E*(xE3)) populations is observed in both populations. This observation is corroborated by mitochondrial DNA HVRI (hypervariable region I) analysis, where the majority of mtDNA lineages originated from the Iberian peninsula, mainly from mainland Portugal. The presence of Jews in the Azorean Central group is also supported by the mtDNA data (Santos et al., 2003).

Without any doubt, Y-chromosome and mtDNA studies are crucial to address the origin of the population; however, a population loses mtDNA when a woman has only sons and Y-chromosome DNA when a man has only daughters. As a result, these genetic markers may give less correct information on broad ancestry of most genes in a population. A full picture of the histories of populations requires studies of markers in the recombining parts of the nuclear DNA, namely the autosomes. Albeith several types of markers can be used to achieve this purpose, *Alu* insertion polymorphisms present some interesting advantages. These markers arose within the human population as a unique event in evolutionary history, making *Alu* repeats identical by descent from a common ancestor (Batzer & Deininger, 2002). Moreover, the ancestral state, which is absence of the *Alu* insertion, is always known. The allele frequencies for each *Alu* polymorphism in Azoreans and mainland Portugal (Table 2) are very similar to those obtained in other European populations.

		Autosomal *Alu* insertion polymorphisms					
Population	**N**	**TPA-25**	**ACE**	**APO**	**PV92**	**D1**	**B65**
Azores	65						
Frequency		0.592	0.385	0.946	0.208	0.254	0.585
Heterozygosity		0.424	0.485	0.106	0.257	0.348	0.409
HW (*p value*)		0.323	1.000	1.000	0.033	0.524	0.211
Locus diversity		0.493	0.481	0.117	0.343	0.392	0.493
Av. gene diversity		0.383 +/- 0.233					
F_{IS}		0.117					
Portugal	30						
Frequency		0.600	0.367	0.917	0.283	0.233	0.500
Heterozygosity		0.517	0.483	0.034	0.345	0.275	0.483
HW (*p value*)		0.665	1.000	0.073	1.000	0.453	1.000
Locus diversity		0.496	0.480	0.128	0.404	0.370	0.517
Av. gene diversity		0.392 +/- 0.240					
F_{IS}		0.094					

Table 2. *Alu* insertion frequencies, heterozygosity and gene diversity for Azores and mainland Portugal. F_{IS} represents inbreeding coefficient (from Branco et al., 2006).

The evolution of populations is dependent on several mechanisms, such as migration, genetic drift, selection and mutation, all affecting the patterns of diversity of neutral and disease variants. Consequently, the measure of diversity of neutral markers allows the inference of how these processes are shaping the overall signature of a population and has further implications in the general diseases apportionment. Genetic diversity values, based on autosomal STR markers, for Azores (0.788; Branco et al., 2008a; Santos et al., 2009) and mainland Portugal (0.782; Perez-Lezaun et al., 2000) indicate that both populations are very diverse. Studies of HLA markers in mainland (Spinola et al., 2005a; 3 *loci*) and in Azores

(Spinola et al., 2005b; 6 *loci*) demonstrate values of average diversity of 0.92. The results obtained for Azores (Pacheco et al., 2010), based in 7 *loci*, presented a smaller value (0.83). HLA haplotype analysis showed that A*01-B*08-DRB1*03 haplotype, known to be of Indo-European Celtic origin, is present in Centre and North Portugal regions at relatively low frequencies of 3% and 2.2%, respectively. However, this haplotype is the most frequent in São Miguel Island (8%). According to Spínola et al. (2005b), it's presence results from a colonizing event from people originating from the Centre of Portugal.
The patterns of genetic diversity of a population have a direct influence in the linkage disequilibrium (LD) extent, which has been found to improve the knowledge of human evolution and origin, and to identify genes causing disease. Table 3 describes the number of haplotypes, gene diversity and standardized multiallelic disequilibrium coefficient (D'), based on X-linked markers for Azores and mainland Portugal populations (Branco et al., 2008b; Branco et al., 2009).

Populations	HN	GD	D'
Azores			
Western group	93	0.718	0.328
Central group	150	0.690	0.189
Eastern group	207	0.686	0.176
Total	450	0.695	0.142
mainland Portugal	97	0.683	0.226

Table 3. Haplotype number (HN), gene diversity (GD) and standardized multiallelic disequilibrium coefficient (D') for Azorean and mainland Portugal populations (from Branco et al., 2008b).

The Azorean Western group shows a higher genetic diversity (0.718) when compared with the other two groups. Overall, Azoreans and mainland Portuguese do not show extensive LD, as direct consequence of the large genetic diversity of these populations. These data were also corroborated by Silva et al. (2010), based on pairwise linkage of 10 X-chromosome STRs, and Service et al. (2006), who compared levels of LD between several European populations. Finally, both mainland Portuguese and Azoreans constitute admixed and outbred populations.

4. Studies of rare and common genetic diseases

Population genetic architecture can also be revealed by distribution patterns of mutations causing Mendelian disorders. Bering this in mind, the UGPM developed three main research areas, based on the Azorean healthy population. The first encompassed the analysis of mutations causing Gilbert's syndrome (GS) and hereditary haemochromatosis (HH), the second constituted the evaluation of some genetic variants predisposing to complex diseases, namely, congenital heart diseases (CHD) and thrombosis, and, finally, the third included the characterization of variants involved on drug metabolism, particularly, irinotecan and warfarin. The results from these research projects are presented and discussed in this section.

4.1 Gilbert's syndrome

Gilbert syndrome is a mild hereditary unconjugated hyperbilirubinemia without liver dysfunction or hemolytic anemia (Matsui et al., 2010; Zhang et al., 2007). No treatment or long-term medical attention is necessary and it is usually one of the differential diagnoses of liver or hemolytic disease. The primary cause of this syndrome is the accumulation of bilirubin - hyperbilirubinemia -, due to decreased hepatic activity levels of glucoronosyl transferase, an enzyme responsible for glucoronidation reaction (Figure 6; Matsui et al., 2010).

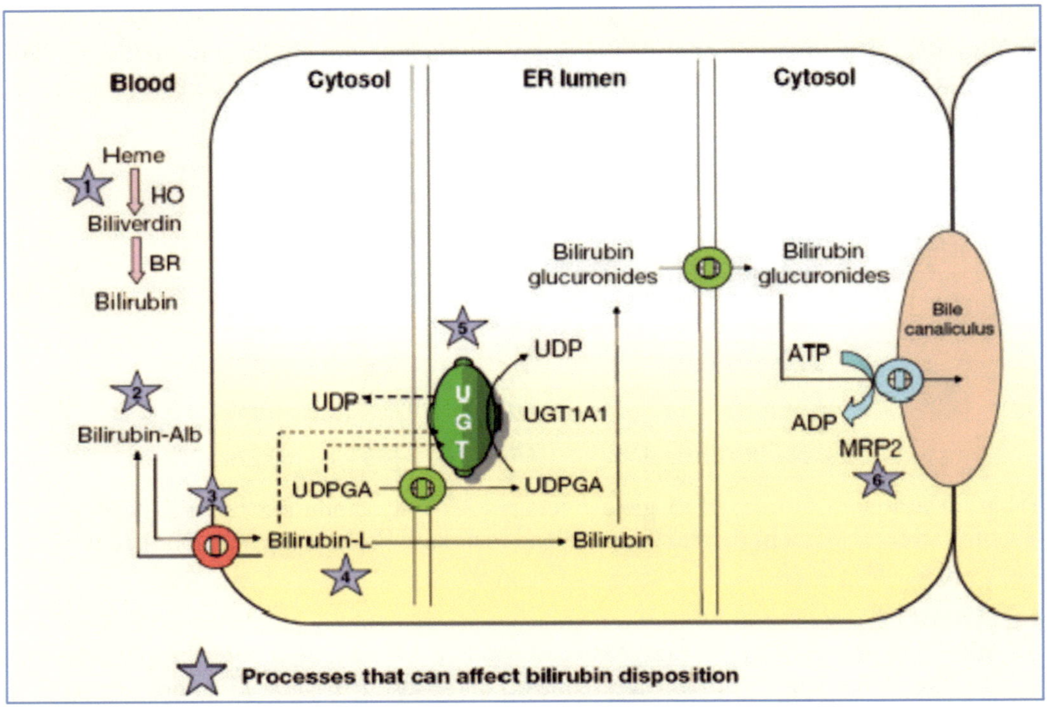

Fig. 6. Bilirubin uptake and processing in the liver cell. The heme initially breaks apart into biliverdin, which is rapidly reduced to bilirubin (1). Bound to albumin, bilirubin is transported from sites of production to hepatic sinusoids (2). At the sinusoidal surface of hepatocytes, bilirubin dissociates from albumin and enters hepatocytes by facilitated diffusion (3). Binding to cytosolic glutathione-*S*-transferases (GSTs) increases net uptake of bilirubin by inhibiting its efflux (4). Bilirubin is converted to mono- and diglucuronide by the action of UGT1A1, which catalyses the transfer of the glucuronic acid moiety from UDP-glucuronic acid (UDPGA) to bilirubin (5). Bilirubin glucuronides are actively transported into bile against a concentration gradient by the ATP-utilizing pump MRP2 (6; Figure from http://www.natap.org/2011/EASL/EASL_83.htm).

Bilirubin has been shown to inhibit DNA synthesis, uncouple oxidative phosphorylation, and inhibit ATPase activity in brain mitochondria (Strassburg, 2010). It also inhibits a variety of different classes of enzymes including dehydrogenases, electron transport proteins, hydrolases, enzymes of RNA synthesis, protein synthesis and carbohydrate metabolism. All toxic effects of bilirubin are reversed by binding to albumin. In fact, albumin plays a vital role in the distribution of bilirubin in the body by keeping the compound in solution and transporting it from sites of production (primarily bone marrow and spleen) to the liver (Strassburg, 2010).

GS is associated with a dinucleotide polymorphism in the TATA box promoter of the UDP glucuronosyltransferase 1 (*UGT1A1*) gene, more precisely the UGT1A1*28 allele (Costa, 2006). In São Miguel Island a group of 67 suspected GS patients and 469 unrelated healthy blood donors were studied (Pacheco et al., 2006; Table 4). The results demonstrated that 65.9% of patients (45 out of 67) and 9.2% controls (43 out of 469) were homozygous for allele *28/*28. The genotype frequency in the control group showed a similar value to the reported to mainland Portugal (9.9%; Gonçalves et al., 2001). Additionally, Oliveira et al. (2007) reported, in a group of healthy individuals, an UGT1A1*28 allele frequency of 28.0%, a value very similar to the obtained in the Azorean control group (29.0%; Pacheco et al., 2009).

UGT1A1			Genotype frequency			
			Suspected GS patients (N=67)		Control group (N=469)	
Alleles		Genotypes	N	%	N	%
*1	A[TA]$_6$TAA	*1*1	4	6.0	237	50.5
*28	A[TA]$_7$TAA	*1*28	18	29.9	186	39.7
*36	A[TA]$_5$TAA	*1*36	-	-	2	0.4
*37	A[TA]$_8$TAA	*1*37	-	-	1	0.2
		*28*28	45	65.9	43	9.2

Table 4. Genotype frequencies of *UGT1A1* variants in suspected GS patients and control group in São Miguel islanders (adapted from Pacheco et al., 2006).

A molecular study based in a cohort of 120 Portuguese patients with the clinical diagnosis of Gilbert syndrome demonstrated that 110 individuals were homozygous for the UGT1A1*28 allele (*28/*28), and one patient was a compound heterozygote for two different insertions *28/*37. The remaining 9 patients were heterozygous, *1/*28 (Costa et al., 2006). The analysis of the control group allowed the identification of alleles characteristic of African populations, *36 (0.2%) and *37 (0.1%), which corroborates previous data on the Azorean and mainland Portuguese genetic background.

4.2 Hereditary hemachromatosis

Hereditary haemochromatosis (HH) is an inherited disorder characterized by accumulation of iron. The phenotypic condition was uncommon and typically diagnosed only when significant complications had ensued. The transmission mode is autosomal recessive and the disease manifests more commonly in males than in females, where natural iron losses are greater (Pietrangelo, 2004; Griffiths, 2007). In HH, gradual deposition of iron occurs in the liver and in a number of other tissues including the pancreas, joints, skin and heart. Disease manifestations include hepatic fibrosis, diabetes mellitus, arthropathy, pigmentation, cardiomyopathy and hypogonadotrophic hypogonadism. Fatigue and arthralgia are common early symptoms and painful arthropathy is a considerable cause of morbidity. However, it is iron toxicity within the liver which increases mortality in patients with HH. Cirrhosis of the liver is associated with significantly reduced survival and there is a 200-fold increased risk of hepatocellular carcinoma (Pietrangelo, 2004; Griffiths, 2007; Swinkels et al., 2006).

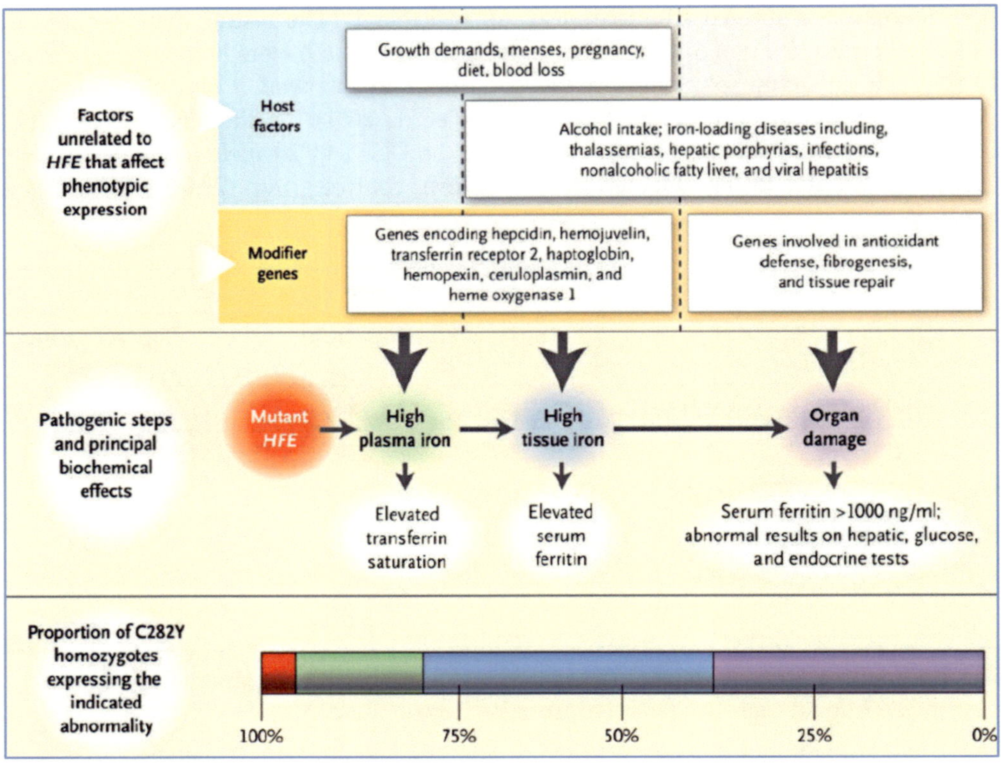

Fig. 8. *HFE* -related Hereditary Hemochromatosis (adapted from Pietrangelo, 2004).

The *HFE* gene encodes an HLA-A class 1-like protein and is located on 6p21.3, 4 megabases (Mb) telomeric to the human leukocyte antigen region (HLA). Two *HFE* mutations - C282Y (845 G>A) and H63D (187 C>G) - are significantly correlated with HH (Feder et al., 1996). The majority (60% to 90%) of clinically diagnosed probands are homozygous for C282Y, and 5% are compound heterozygous for C282Y and H63D.

The C282Y allele frequency in São Miguel population is 5.01%, a similar frequency (5.8%; de Fez et al., 2005; Gomes et al., 2007) to the obtained in the north of mainland Portugal, but statistically different from that observed in the south populations (0.9%; Cardoso et al., 2001). Contrary to this C282Y decreasing gradient, the H63D presents an even country distribution (Figure 10), with values of 17.88% and 20.36% for mainland and São Miguel Island, respectively.

Because C282Y mutation seems to have originated by chance on a HLA-A*03-B*07 haplotype in an individual from northwestern Europe and early spread, by Celts or Vikings (Milman & Pedersen, 2003; Distante et al., 2004), in many countries including Portugal, the background of this mutation was assessed in São Miguel islanders (Gomes et al., 2007). Four non-ancestral HLA haplotypes were associated with C282Y: A*01-B*35, A*02-B*44, A*02-B*55 and A*24-B*15, contrary to mainland, where the C282Y occurred mainly on the ancestral haplotype HLA-A*03-B*07 (Cruz et al., 2006). In addition, the C282Y mutation was also identified in two HLA A*03 bearing: A*03-B*27 and A*03-B*50. These results evidence that C282Y mutation was introduced in the Azorean population by individuals with genetic background other than Celts or Vikings.

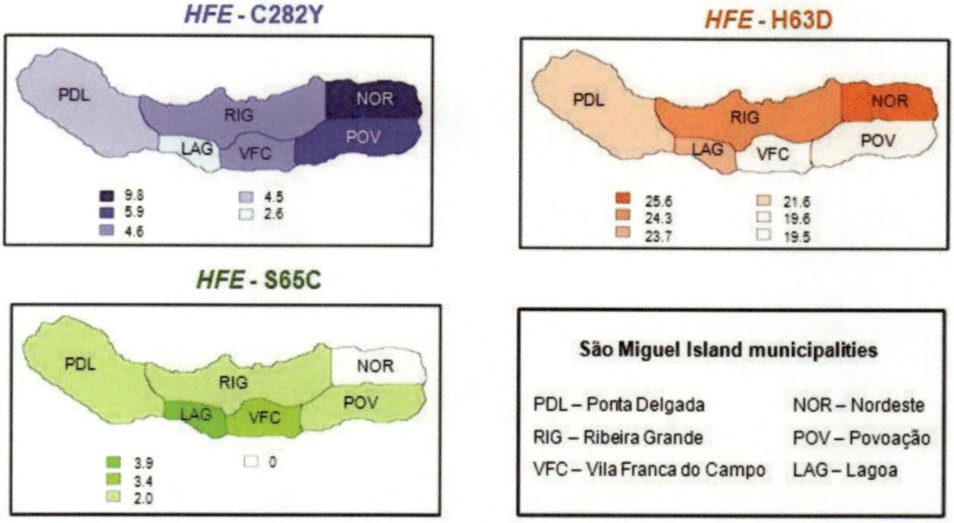

Fig. 9. Geographic distribution of *HFE* mutations in São Miguel Island. Frequency values are expressed in percentage.

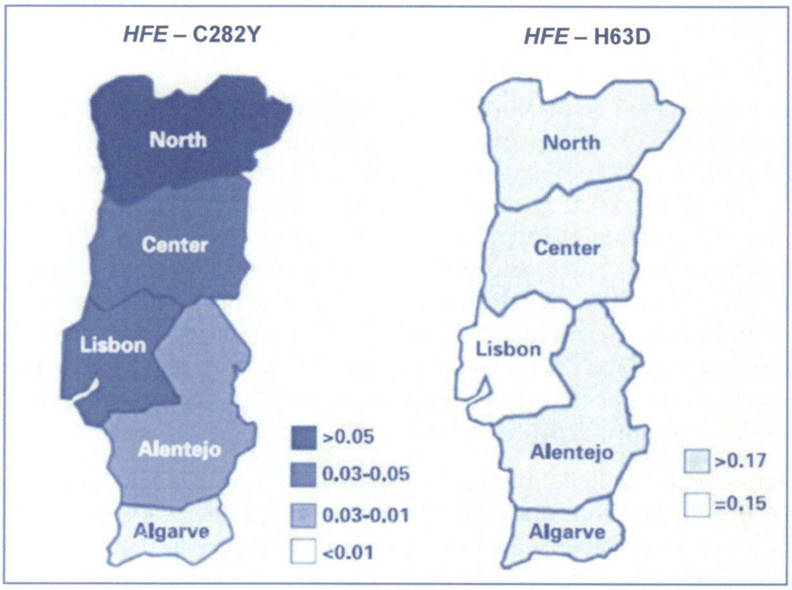

Fig. 10. Geographical distribution of the allelic frequencies of the C282Y and H63D *HFE* mutations in five Portuguese regions. (adapted from Cardoso et al., 2001).

4.3 Congenital heart disease

The evaluation of genetic variants predisposing to complex diseases in Azores began with the characterization congenital heart diseases (CHD). Congenital malformations of the heart and great vessels are among the most frequent of all clinically significant birth defects, with a major contribution to paediatric morbidity, mortality and healthcare costs.

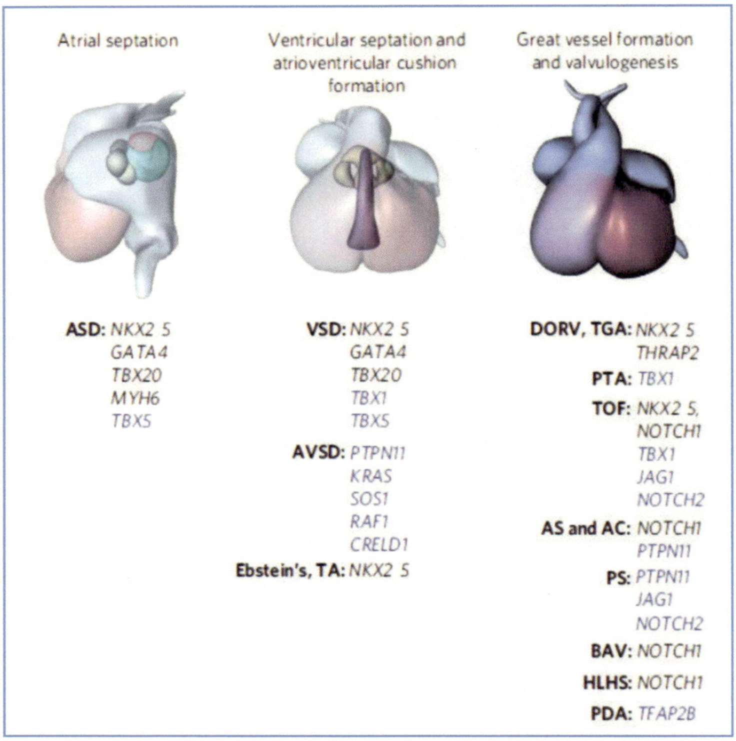

Fig. 11. Three major classes of developmental defects are indicated: defects in atrial septation, in ventricular or atrioventricular septation, and in the great vessels. The types of congenital heart disease that occur within each class are indicated, with the associated mutated genes listed. AC, aortic coarctation; AS, aortic stenosis; ASD, atrial septal defect; AVSD, atrioventricular septal defect; BAV, bicuspid aortic valve; DORV, double outlet right ventricle; Ebstein's, Ebstein's anomaly of the tricuspid valve; HLHS, hypoplastic left heart syndrome; HRHS, hypoplastic right heart; IAA, interrupted aortic arch; MA, mitral atresia; MS, mitral stenosis; PDA, patent ductus arteriosus; PS, pulmonary artery stenosis; PTA, persistent truncus arteriosus; TA, tricuspid atresia; TAPVR, total anomalous pulmonary venous return; TGA, transposition of the great arteries; TOF, tetralogy of Fallot; VSD, ventricular septal defect (From Bruneau, 2008).

Population based epidemiologic studies indicate a prevalence of CHD ranging from 3.23 to 12.23 *per* 1000 live births (Dolk et al., 2011; Bruneau, 2008; Engelfriet et al., 2005). This wide variation in the reported values is mainly due to the difference in the methodologies used, but a number of other factors, such as consanguinity, ethnic background, environmental pollutants and access to healthcare also contribute to this variation (Becker et al., 2001; Nabulsi et al. 2003; Botto et al., 2001). In 2006, the first study on the prevalence of CHD in children born alive in São Miguel Island from January 1992 to December 2001 was carried out by Cymbron et al. (2006). Based on the Azorean Registry of CHD, which includes complete clinical and personal information, 189 patients were diagnosed. During this 10-year period, the average prevalence of CHD is 9.16 *per* 1000 live births placing Azores in the 10 European regions with higher prevalence of CHD (Table 5).

Countries	Total births	N	Prevalence (*per* 1000 births)
Austria	62,667	960	15.32
Malta	23,668	348	14.70
Switzerland	42,874	576	13.43
Germany	124,952	1457	11.66
Poland	206,170	2304	11.18
Norway	346,838	3538	10.20
São Miguel Island	**20,634**	**189**	**9.16**
Denmark	32,003	291	9.09
France	343,715	2853	8.30
Ukraine	25,835	201	7.78
UK	951,001	6497	6.83
Italy	431,727	2944	6.82
Belgium	182,467	1212	6.64
Ireland	215,021	1423	6.62
Netherlands	119,104	732	6.15
Spain	194,234	1080	5.56
Croatia	33,933	182	5.36
Total	3,356,843	26,787	7.97

Table 5. Prevalence of CHG in European countries and São Miguel Island (adapted from Dolk et al., 2011). The period of time analysed was from 2000 to 2005, with the exception of São Miguel Island (1992 to 2001). No data for mainland Portugal is available.

Considering that half of the São Miguel population lives in small rural localities (range from 309 - 7407 inhabitants for Lomba de São Pedro and Rabo de Peixe, respectively) and the internal migration is reduced, aspects that increase endogamy and inbreeding, a structured family questionnaire to the parents with CHD children was performed. The questionnaire included *i*) questions for CHD risk factors - maternal diabetes mellitus, alcohol and drug abuse by the mother during pregnancy, viral infections of the fetus and genetic conditions -, *ii*) queries concerning the number of family members affected with CHD and parental consanguinity, and *iii*) a detailed family history to construct the ascending genealogy until the 3th generation. Results revealed a relatively high number of multiplex families (44;

40.37%, Table 6) and a significantly high value of consanguinity (9.17%). Half of the consanguineous families (5 out of 109 total families) are multiplex. In addition, 36 out of 44 multiplex families are endogamous (81.8%; Table 7).
The data suggest that genetic factors may be responsible for the development of CHD in São Miguel Island. Familial aggregation, which is of great interest for understanding the genes involved in these complex pathologies, is evident.

	Families (N=109)	
Parameters	**No.**	**%**
Type of family:		
Simplex	65	59.63
Multiplex	44	40.37
Parental consanguinity:		
With	10	9.17
Without	99	90.83

Table 6. Parental consanguinity evaluation in CHD families from São Miguel Island.

No. affected individuals *per* multiplex family	No. families	Consanguinity		Distribution of families according to grandparental (GP) endogamy				
				Same locality			Different localities	Do not know
		With	Without	Four GP	Three GF	Two GP	All GP	
2	26	3	23	5	5	10	3	3
3	16	1	15	4	3	7	1	1
4	1	0	1	-	-	1	-	-
5	1	1	0	1	-	-	-	-
Total	**44**	**5**	**39**	**10**	**8**	**18**	**4**	**4**

Table 7. Analysis of consanguinity and grandparental endogamy in multiplex families from São Miguel Island.

Research has implicated both folate deficiency and genetic variation in folate pathway genes with birth defects, including CHD (Lee et al., 2005). Some studies suggest that polymorphisms in the methylenetetrahydrofolate reductase (*MTHFR*) gene may be implicated in cardiac defects development. In mainland Portugal, Marinho et al. (2009) reported a higher prevalence of the 677T allele in tetralogy of Fallot (TF) compared to the control group (OR=1.675; 95% CI [1.022- 2.743]; p=0.05). The 677TT genotype increased by 4.856 the risk for this congenital disease (95% CI [1.308-12.448]; p=0.028), suggesting that *MTHFR* can be considered a susceptibility gene for TF. Cabral et al. (2008) genotyped two polymorphisms, C677T and A1298C, in *MTHFR* in CHD children (N=95) and respective mothers (N=89), as well as in the control group (N=469; Table 8). No significant differences were obtained between all studied groups, indicating that in São Miguel Island *MTHFR* C677T and A1298C polymorphisms are not the main cause of CHD development. Currently, further genetic studies, based on functional candidate genes, in the Azorean population are on-going.

Variants	Allele frequency (%)		Genotype frequency (%)		
MTHFR - C677T	**C**	**T**	**CC**	**CT**	**TT**
Control group (N=469)	58.32	41.68	34.54	47.55	17.91
CHD children (N=95)	57.89	42.11	29.47	56.84	13.68
Mothers of CHD children (N=89)	62.92	37.08	39.33	47.19	13.48
MTHFR - A1298C	**A**	**C**	**AA**	**AC**	**CC**
Control group (N=469)	75.16	24.84	56.29	37.74	5.97
CHD children (N=95)	57.89	42.11	58.95	40.00	1.05
Mothers of CHD children (N=89)	62.92	37.08	49.44	44.94	5.62

Table 8. Allele and genotype frequencies for *MTHFR* C677T and A1298C polymorphisms in the São Miguel CHD study.

4.4 Thrombosis

In February 2007, the National Geographic Portugal magazine published a special issue dedicated to cardiovascular diseases. Based on the Euro Heart Survey 2006, the number of deaths *per* 100,000 inhabitants in 2004, due to CVD, places Portugal with higher values (390) compared with south-western European countries like Spain (290), France (262) and Belgium (364). In a similar analysis, performed within Portugal regions, the Azores archipelago clearly stands out with the highest value (116.9), followed by Lisbon (84.8). Family based investigation tends to have biased relative risk estimation, because oversampling of affected individuals is normally present. Therefore, the genetic characterization of disease variants in the general population is important to correct this potential bias. Since thrombosis is a common cause of CVD, Branco et al. (2009) analysed four polymorphisms in three thrombotic risk genes - *F5* (G1691A), *F2* (G20210A) and *MTHFR* (C677T, A1298C), in 469 healthy blood donors from São Miguel Island. Figure 12 shows allele frequencies in Caucasian populations, including São Miguel, for the above mentioned polymorphisms.

Comparison of allele frequencies for thrombotic risk factors between São Miguel and mainland Portugal (Mansilha et al., 2006) revealed statistically significant differences (χ^2, p<0.001; Table 9) for *F5* - 1691A, justifying the need to perform regional biomedical research to ultimately benefit the patient.

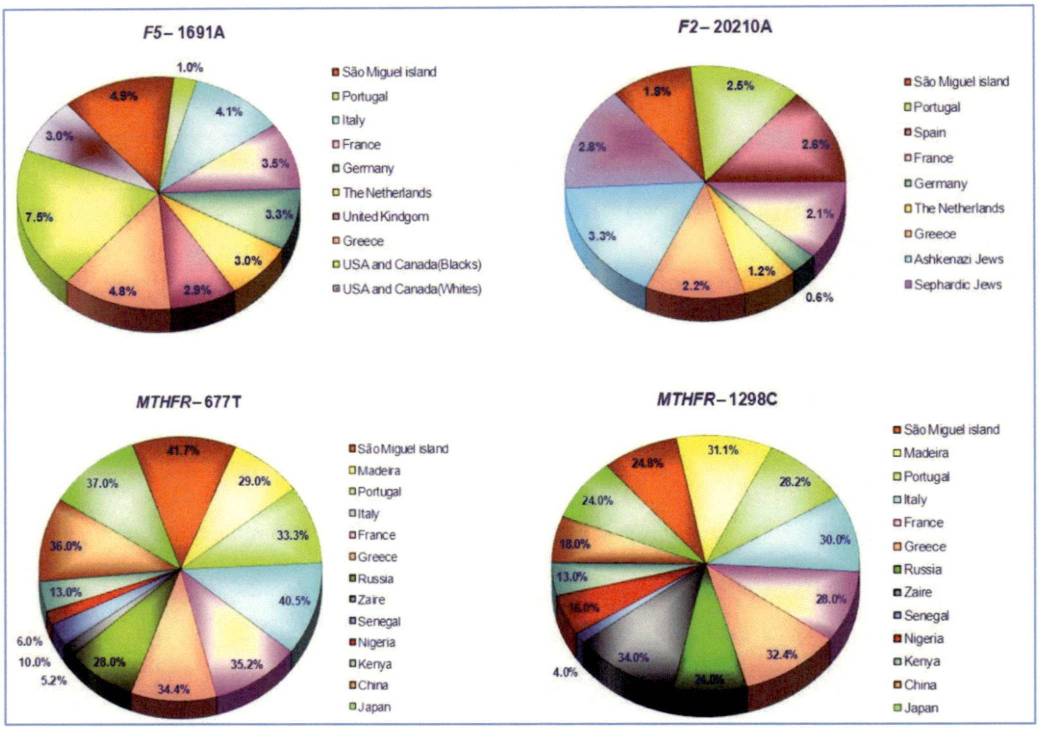

Fig. 12. Allele frequencies of the thrombotic risk factors - *F5* (1691A), *F2* (20210A) and *MTHFR* (677T, 1298C) - in different populations, including São Miguel (adapted from Branco et al., 2009).

	Allele frequency (%)			
Populations	***F5* (1691A)**	***F2* (20210A)**	***MTHFR* (677T)**	***MTHFR* (1298C)**
São Miguel Island	4.9	1.8	41.7	24.8
mainland Portugal	1.0	2.5	33.3	28.2

Table 9. Comparison between thrombotic genetic risk variants frequency between Azoreans and mainland Portugal.

Twenty-two different genetic profiles for *F5*, *F2* and *MTHFR* (order in genotype profile) were observed in São Miguel's population (Figure 13). The frequency of individuals who present a wild-type genotype for all polymorphisms (GG GG CC AA; 11.7%) was almost half of the major profile (GG GG CT AA; 22.4%), differing in heterozygosity for *MTHFR* 677CT. No heterozygous or homozygous profiles for all four variants were observed. Almawi et al. (2004) reported an OR of 10.5 (95% CI [4.3-25.3]) or 6.3 (95% CI [1.5-26.0]) for joint occurrence of the *F5*-G1691A or *F2*-G20210A with *MTHFR*-677TT genotype, respectively, enhancing the risk for deep vein thrombosis (DVT). Based on this criterion, fifteen (3.2%, *F5/MTHFR*) and two individuals (0.4%, *F2/MTHFR*) would have higher risk for DVT development (Figure 13 - asterisk character).

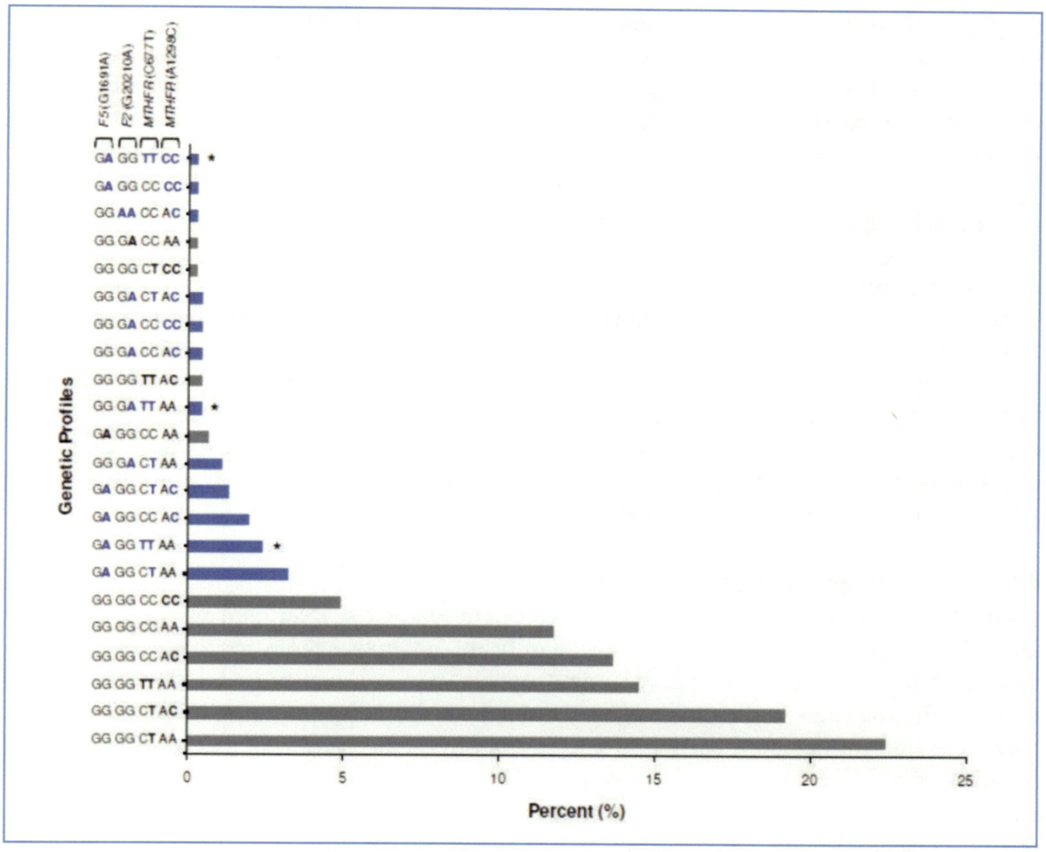

Fig. 13. Combined genotypes for thrombotic risk factors - *F5*, *F2* and *MTHFR* - in São Miguel population. Twenty-two different genetic profiles were obtained. Bold characters (blue and black) indicate nucleotide changes compared to the wild-type allele. Blue bars represent profiles with increase genetic predisposition to thrombosis. The asterisk (*) represents the combination of the *F5*-G1691A or *F2*-G20210A with *MTHFR*-677TT genotype (adapted from Branco et al., 2009).

Taken together, 12.4% (58 out of 469) of São Miguel islanders have increased genetic predisposition to thrombosis. No general population profile analysis for mainland Portugal is reported in the literature, and, consequently, no comparison was performed. These results are corroborated by further CVD studies, where 2 genomic regions associated with CVD risk, *USF1* and 9p21 were evaluated (Correia et al., 2010). Preliminary results, based on haplotype inference, showed that *USF1* "CCGCC" (0.288) and "CTGCT" (0.346) are the two most frequent haplotypes in Azoreans, which, according to Komulainen et al. (2006), correspond to the protective and high risk haplotype in females, respectively. In 9p21 region, the risk haplotype "TGGGCGCGC", associated with CHD in Europeans (Silander et al., 2009), is the most frequent (0.414). Analysis of homozygosity patterns for risk genotypes showed similar frequencies for *USF1* (12.4%) and 9p21 region (14.7%), indicating that, despite recombination, homozygosity must be taken in consideration when performing risk profile studies. Collectively, the data suggest that there is a considerable genetic risk for CVD in Azoreans, evidencing the need to carry out regional genetic studies with the aim to improve and complement health strategies adopted by the decision makers of each country. Further genetic studies on CVD are on-going.

4.5 Pharmacogenetics of irinotecan and warfarin

In the last 50 years, fundamental developments in pharmacology and genetics led to important improvements in personalized medicine based on pharmacogenetics and pharmacogenomics. Pharmacogenomics uses a whole genome approach to investigate or predict drug responses, or to relate the application of these technologies to drug discovery, while pharmacogenetics is the study of the clinically relevant inherited differences in drug response that can be in part explained by genetic variations. Pharmacogenetic analysis contributes to reduce adverse drug reactions (ADRs) or to maximize drug efficiency. Variants involved in drug metabolism of two commonly prescribed drugs, irinotecan and warfarin, were studied in Azoreans and mainland Portugal.

4.5.1 Pharmacogenetics of irinotecan

Irinotecan, an antineoplastic-prodrug, is widely used for the treatment of colorectal, lung and other cancers. The most clinically significant adverse events for patients receiving irinotecan-based therapy are diarrhea, neutropenia, nausea, vomiting and alopecia (Kehrer et al., 2001; Marques & Ikediobi, 2010; Lankisch et al., 2008; Fujiwara & Minami, 2010). Irinotecan can induce both early and late forms of diarrhea and requires dose adjustment based on severity of diarrhea. Also, sepsis related death following severe neutropenia has been reported in irinotecan treated patients. The active metabolite SN-38 is responsible for the pharmacological and toxic effect of irinotecan. SN-38, is a topoisomerase I inhibitor generated by hydrolysis of irinotecan by carboxylesterases (Figure 14). SN-38 is subsequently glucuronidated by uridine diphosphate glucuronosyltransferase 1As (UGT1As) to form an inactive metabolite, SN-38G (Marques & Ikediobi, 2010; Fujiwara & Minami, 2010).

The human UDP-glucuronosyltransferase 1A gene *locus* is organized to generate enzymes, which share a carboxyterminal portion and are unique at their aminoterminal variable region. Expression is tissue-specific and overlapping substrate specificities include a broad spectrum of endogenous and xenobiotic compounds, as well as many therapeutic drugs targeted for detoxification and elimination by glucuronidation. The absence of glucuronidation leads to fatal hyperbilirubinemia (Marsh & Hoskins, 2010; Zhang et al., 2007). Genetic variants and haplotypes have been identified as risk factors for unwanted drug effects of cancer treatment with irinotecan. Since variants in *UGT1A1*, *UGT1A6* and *UGT1A7* are related to irinotecan toxicity, these were studied in 469 individuals from São Miguel Island by Pacheco et al. (2009). Haplotype analysis revealed that H3 (Table 10), which includes all low activity allelic variants of the three UGT isoforms, accounts for 23.5% of the population, suggesting that those individuals have reduced glucuronidation activity due to the combination of UGT1A1*28, UGT1A6*2 and UGT1A7*3 alleles.

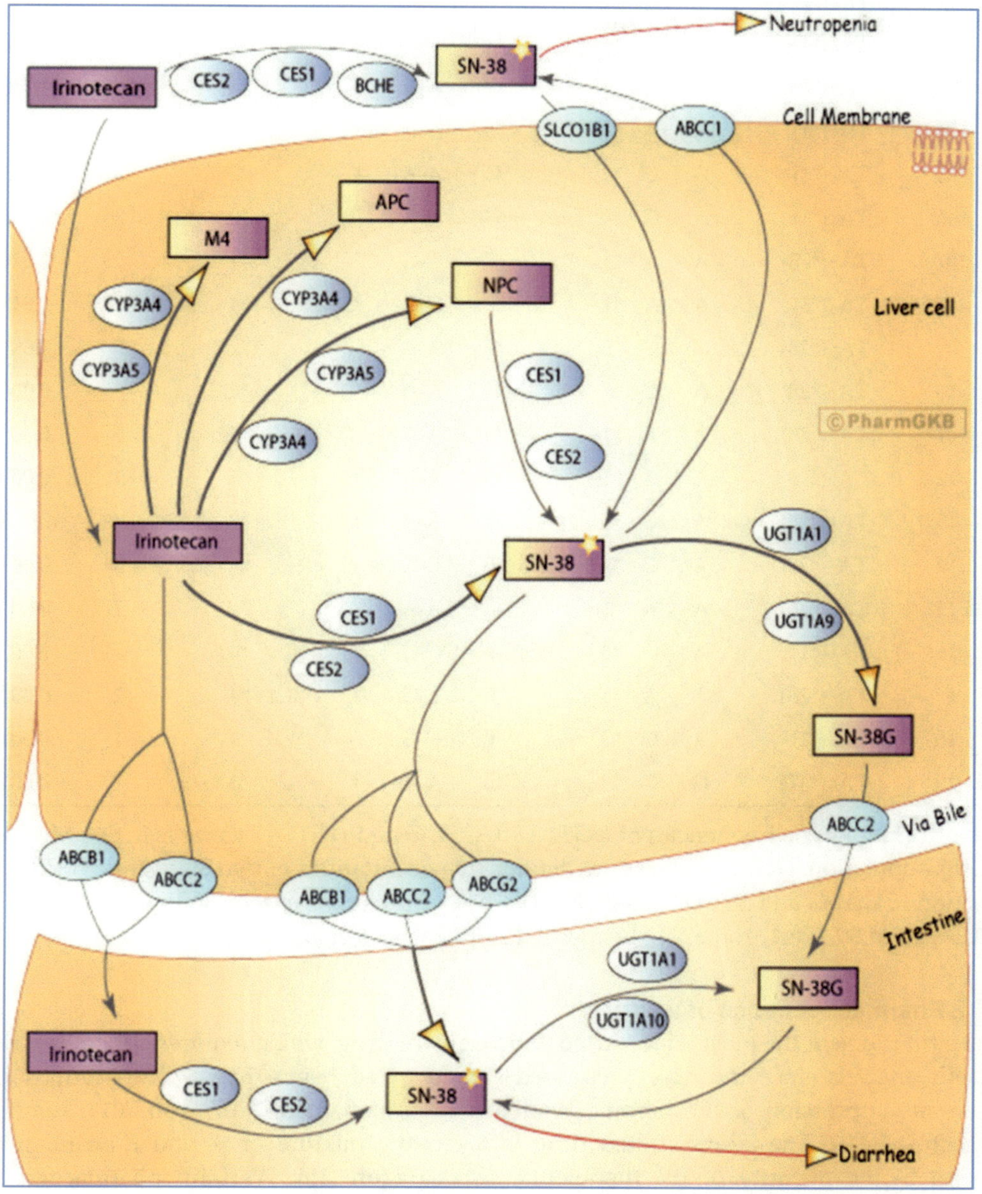

Fig. 14. Irinotecan pathway indicating tissue specific involvement of genes in the irinotecan metabolism. PharmGKB copyright. Available at http://www.pharmgkb.org/search/pathway/irinotecan/liver.jsp.

Haplotype (H)	*UGT1A* genes									Haplotype frequency	
	UGT1A1	*UGT1A6*			*UGT1A7*						
	A[TA]$_n$TAA	541	552	541/552	387	391/392	622	387/391/392/622		N	(2N=938)
01	TA_6 (*1)	A	A	*1	T	C-G	T	*1		296	0.316
02	TA_6 (*1)	A	A	*1	G	A-A	T	*2		225	0.240
03	TA_7 (*28)	G	C	*2	G	A-A	C	*3		220	0.235
04	TA_6 (*1)	A	A	*1	G	A-A	C	*3		65	0.069
05	TA_6 (*1)	G	C	*2	G	A-A	C	*3		31	0.033
06	TA_6 (*1)	A	C	*3	G	A-A	T	*2		26	0.028
07	TA_7 (*28)	A	A	*1	T	C-G	T	*1		23	0.024
08	TA_6 (*1)	A	A	*1	T	C-G	C	*4		17	0.018
09	TA_7 (*28)	G	C	*2	G	A-A	T	*2		7	0.007
10	TA_7 (*28)	A	C	*3	G	A-A	T	*2		6	0.006
11	TA_7 (*28)	A	A	*1	G	A-A	T	*2		5	0.005
12	TA_7 (*28)	A	A	*1	G	A-A	C	*3		5	0.005
13	TA_7 (*28)	A	C	*3	G	A-A	C	*3		3	0.003
14	TA_7 (*28)	A	C	*3	T	C-G	C	*4		3	0.003
15	TA_5 (*36)	A	A	*1	G	A-A	T	*2		2	0.002
16	TA_6 (*1)	A	C	*3	T	C-G	C	*4		2	0.002
17	TA_7 (*28)	A	A	*1	T	C-G	C	*4		2	0.002
18	TA_6 (*1)	A	C	*3	T	C-G	T	*1		1	0.001
19	TA_8 (*37)	G	C	*2	G	A-A	C	*3		1	0.001

Table 10. Haplotype frequencies of *UGT1A1, UGT1A6* and *UGT1A7* variants in São Miguel Island population. *UGT1A6* alleles are defined by permutations of two SNPs (nucleotide positions 541A>G and 552A>C) and *UGT1A7* by permutations of four SNPs (387T>G, 391C>A and 392G>A, and 622T>C; adapted from Pacheco et al., 2009).

4.5.2 Pharmacogenetics of warfarin

Warfarin is one of the most widely used anticoagulant drug, which requires a thorough risk-benefit analysis since the dose prescribed should avoid hemorrhagic complications and achieves suppression of thrombosis (Wadelius & Pirmohamed, 2007; You 2011; Limdi & Veenstra, 2008). The administrated drug is a racemic mixture of S- and R-enantiomers, having S- the majority of the therapeutic effect (Figure 15). Warfarin pharmacogenetic studies demonstrated that variants in the *CYP2C9* (Cytochrome P450 2C9) and *VKORC1* (Vitamin K epoxide reductase complex subunit 1) genes account for approximately 50-60% of drug dosing variability (Finkelman et al., 2011). The remaining variability can be explained by clinical and environmental factors (age, sex, diet, concomitant drugs, body mass index), which in conjunction with genetics are used, in warfarin dosing algorithms, as an advice for the best dose prescription. Cytochrome P450 2C9 is the major enzyme responsible for metabolising the active S-enantiomer. Although there are many polymorphisms in *CYP2C9*, the most clinically relevant variants are: *CYP2C9**1 (Arg144/Ile359, wild-type), *CYP2C9**2 (Arg144Cys) and *CYP2C9**3 (Ile359Leu). These last two are associated with decreased metabolic efficiency of the CYP2C9 enzyme and increased risk of bleeding when administrated initial dosages of warfarin (Yasar et al., 1999). Considering *VKCORC1*, a G>A variation at position 1639 in the gene's promoter region results in decreased mRNA transcription and increased sensitivity to warfarin inhibition of hepatic synthesis of functional vitamin K-dependent coagulation factors. Rieder et al. (2005) studied *VKORC1* polymorphisms and classified individuals according to warfarin dose requirements into distinct groups: high (GG), intermediate (GA) and low (AA). Recently, the U.S. Food and Drug Administration (FDA) added to the warfarin product label dosing recommendations stratified by combined *CYP2C9* and *VKORC1* genotypes (http://www.fda.gov/drugs/scienceresearch/researchareas/pharmacogenetics/ucm083378.htm).

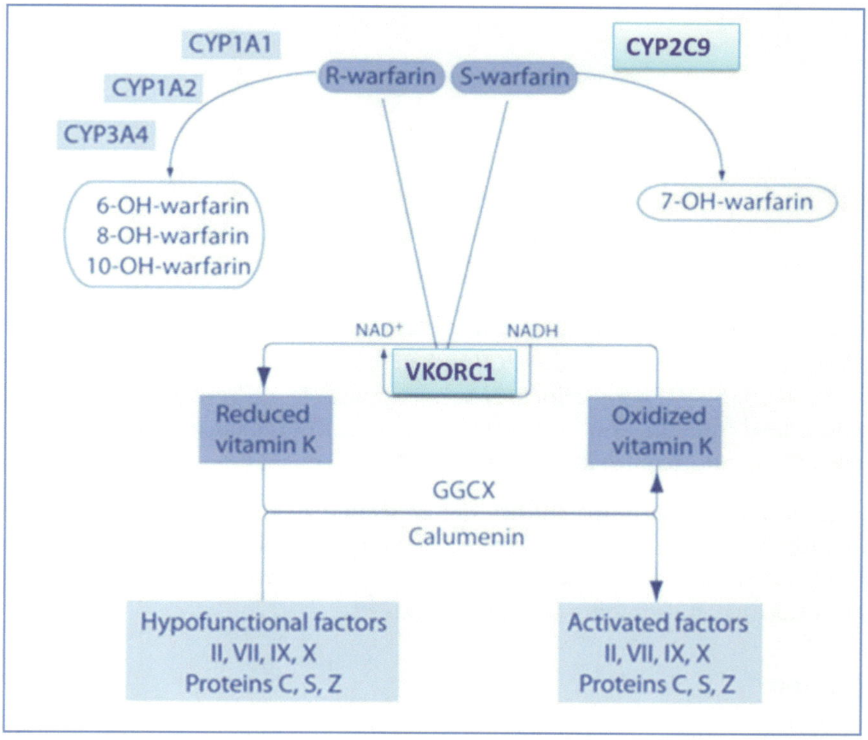

Fig. 15. Warfarin pharmacokinetic and pharmacodynamic pathway. Warfarin is administered as a racemic admixture of R- and S-enantiomers. The more potent S-enantiomer is metabolized principally by CYP2C9. The pharmacological effect of warfarin is mediated by the inhibition of vitamin K epoxide reductase complex 1 (VKORC1). This results in decreased concentrations of activated clotting factors (II, VII, IX and X) producing therapeutic anticoagulation (adapted from Božina 2010).

Comparison of separate genotypes for *CYP2C9* and *VKORC1* between mainland Portugal (Jorge et al., 2010) and the Azores (Pereirinha et al., 2009, personal communication) populations revealed no significant differences (Table 11). In the Azores population no individuals with *CYP2C9*-*3*3 genotype were identified, however a higher frequency of *CYP2C9*-*2*3 was observed when compared to mainland. The joint analysis of *CYP2C9* and *VKORC1*, in Azoreans, showed that around 12% of individuals need low doses of warfarin, if treatment is started (Table 11; blue characters).

CYP2C9			*VKORC1*			*CYP2C9/VKORC1*		
Genotype	Frequency (%)		Genotype	Frequency (%)		Genotype	Frequency (%)	
	Azores	m. Portugal		Azores	m. Portugal		Azores	m. Portugal
*1/*1	57.6	64.0	GG	30.0	33.0	*1*1-GG	17.1	NA
*1/*2	25.3	22.0	GA	56.5	50.5	*1*1-GA	34.1	NA
*1/*3	8.2	9.0	AA	13.5	16.5	*1*2-GG	7.0	NA
*2/*2	5.3	3.3				*1*3-GG	2.4	NA
*2/*3	3.5	1.1				*1*1-AA	6.4	NA
*3/*3	0	1.1				*1*2-GA	13.5	NA
						*1*3-GA	4.1	NA
						*2*2-GG	1.8	NA
						*2*3-GG	1.8	NA
						*1*2-AA	4.7	NA
						*1*3-AA	1.8	NA
						*2*2-AA	0.6	NA
						*2*2-GA	2.9	NA
						*2*3-GA	1.8	NA

Table 11. Genotype frequencies of *CYP2C9* and *VKORC1* variants in Azores (N=170) and mainland Portugal (N=91) populations. **NA**- not applicable; no joint analysis of both genes has been described for mainland Portugal populations. Blue characters represent individuals who would require low doses of warfarin.

Overall, irinotecan and warfarin studies demonstrated that the Azores population shows significant differences on allele frequencies of pharmacogenetic variants, which must be taken in consideration when treating patients. These results have a high impact on the physicians' decisions in managing patient's treatment.

5. Conclusion

Genomic medicine, which uses the individual information to provide better healthcare, has been considerably developed since the Human Genome Project. One of its current challenges is the identification of risk alleles for multifactorial diseases and the study of their frequency in different populations. In summary, both the Azores and mainland Portugal populations are outbred with high genetic diversity, relative gene flow among its individuals, and without extensive LD. Nevertheless, the islanders have a particular genetic makeup evidenced by the African and Asian traits, and by the differences in terms of common diseases apportionment compared to mainland. Biomedical investigation has been the driving force in improving practices in patient care, based on new drugs, diagnostic methods, medical instruments and services. The genetic research performed in the Azorean population allowed the implementation of molecular diagnosis in the main Hospital of the archipelago, as well as a faster and most costly effective response to clinicians, benefiting the patient and, ultimately, the Azorean Health System.

6. Aknowledgments

The authors would like to express their gratitude to UGPM collaborators, previous (Ainhoa Balagué, Ann Lismond, Bernardo Peixoto, Cidália Gomes, Ester Cabrol, Felipe Serrano, Francesc Sigalat, Helena Polena, Laura de Fez, Marta São Bento, Nicholas Bruffaerts, Paula Pacheco, Raquel Palla, Silvia Lino, Teresa Cymbron) and current (Maria José Brilhante, Maria Manuela Correia, Rita Cabral Veloso, Tânia Pereirinha), who contributed to the scientific research presented in this book chapter. Moreover, the work was not possible without the contribution of blood donors and health professionals involved in building the Azorean DNA bank. Thanks to the funding agencies, Fundação para a Ciência e a Tecnologia (FCT, Portuguese Ministry of Science; funded research projects: POCTI/ESP/49236/2002, SFRH/BD/12254/2003, POCI/SALMMO/58413/2004), Direcção Regional da Ciência, Tecnologia e Comunicações (DRCTC, Azorean Government; funded research projects: M1.2.1/I/003/2005, M1.2.1/I/002/2008, M2.1.2/F/003/2007), Fundação Luso-Americana para o Desenvolvimento (FLAD) and Fundação Calouste Gulbenkian (FCG) are also obliged.

7. Databases and Websites of interest

1000 Genomes Project	http://www.1000genomes.org/
ALFRED - Allele Frequency Database	http://alfred.med.yale.edu/alfred/index.asp
Copy Number Variation Project	http://www.sanger.ac.uk/humgen/cnv
Cytochrome P450 database	http://bioinformatics.charite.de/supercyp/
DrugBank database	http://www.drugbank.ca/
European Directory DNA Diagnostic Laboratories	http://www.eddnal.com/
Ensembl Database	http://www.ensembl.org/index.html
Food and Drug Administration - FDA	http://www.fda.gov/default.htm
Human Gene Mutation Database	http://www.hgmd.cf.ac.uk/ac/index.php
Human Genome Project	http://www.genome.gov/10001772
Human Genome Variation Database	http://hgvbase.cgb.ki.se
Human Variome Project	http://www.humanvariomeproject.org/
IMGT/HLA Database	http://www.ebi.ac.uk/imgt/hla
mtDB - Human Mitochondrial Genome Database	http://www.mtdb.igp.uu.se/
National Centre for Biotechnology Information	http://www.ncbi.nlm.nih.gov
National Human Genome Research	http://www.genome.gov/

Institute (NIHGRI)	
Online Mendelian Inheritance in Man	http://www.ncbi.nlm.nih.gov/sites/entrez?db=OMIM
Orphanet	http://www.orphanet.pt/
Pharmacogenetics of Membrane Transporters Database	http://pharmacogenetics.ucsf.edu/
Rare diseases database	http://www.rarediseases.org/
Single Nucleotide Polymorphism Database	http://www.ncbi.nlm.nih.gov/projects/SNP
The International HapMap Project	http://www.hapmap.org
The Pharmacogenomics Knowledge Base	http://www.pharmgkb.org/
Y-Chromosome Consortium	http://ycc.biosci.arizona.edu

8. References

1000 Genomes Project Consortium, Durbin RM, Abecasis GR, Altshuler DL, Auton A, Brooks LD, Durbin RM, Gibbs RA, Hurles ME &McVean GA. (2010). A map of human genome variation from population-scale sequencing. *Nature*, 467: 1061-1073.

Adams SM, Bosch E, Balaresque PL, Ballereau SJ, Lee AC, Arroyo E, López-Parra AM, Aler M, Grifo MS, Brion M, Carracedo A, Lavinha J, Martínez-Jarreta B, Quintana-Murci L, Picornell A, Ramon M, Skorecki K, Behar DM, Calafell F & Jobling MA. (2008). The genetic legacy of religious diversity and intolerance: paternal lineages of Christians, Jews, and Muslims in the Iberian Peninsula. *Am J Hum Genet*, 83: 725-36.

Almawi WY, Ameen G, Tamim H, Finan RR & Irani-Hakime N. (2004). Factor V G1691A, prothrombin G20210A and methylenetetrahydrofolate reductase [MTHFR] C677T gene polymorphisms in angiographically documented coronary artery disease. *J Thromb Thrombolysis*, 17: 199-205.

Amaral JF & Amaral AF. (1997). Povos antigos de Portugal. Quetzal (Ed.), Lisbon.

Batzer MA & Deininger PL. (2002). *Alu* repeats and human genomic diversity. *Nat Rev Genet*, 3: 370-379.

Becker SM, Al Halees Z, Molina C & Paterson RM. (2001). Consanguinity and congenital heart disease in Saudi Arabia. *Am J Med Genet*, 99: 8–13.

Beleza S, Gusmão L, Lopes A, Alves C, Gomes I, Giouzeli M, Calafell F, Carracedo A & Amorim A. (2006). Micro-phylogeographic and demographic history of Portuguese male lineages. *Ann Hum Genet*, 70: 181-194.

Botto LD, Correa A & Erickson JD. (2001). Racial and temporal variations in the prevalence of heart defects. *Pediatrics*, 107: 1–8.

Božina N. (2010). The pharmacogenetics of warfarin in clinical practice. *Biochemia Medica*, 20: 33–44.

Branco CC, Cabrol E, São Bento M, Gomes CT, Cabral R, Vicente AM, Pacheco PR & Mota-Vieira L. (2008b). Evaluation of linkage disequilibrium on the Xq13.3 region: comparison between the Azores Islands and mainland Portugal. *Am J Hum Biol*, 20: 364-366.

Branco CC, Pacheco PR, Cabrol E, Cabral R, Vicente AM & Mota Vieira L. (2009). Linkage disequilibrium and diversity for three genomic regions in Azoreans and mainland Portuguese. *Genet Mol Biol,* 32: 220-226.

Branco CC, Palla R, Lino S, Pacheco PR, Cabral R, de Fez L, Peixoto BR & Mota-Vieira L. (2006). Assessment of the Azorean ancestry by *Alu* insertion polymorphisms. *Am J Hum Biol,* 18: 223-226.

Branco CC, Pereirinha T, Cabral R, Pacheco PR & Mota-Vieira L. (2009). Thrombotic genetic risk factors and warfarin pharmacogenetic variants in São Miguel's healthy population (Azores). *Thromb J,* 7:9.

Branco CC, São Bento M, Gomes CT, Cabral R, Pacheco PR & Mota Vieira L. (2008a). Azores Islands: genetic origin, gene flow and diversity patterns. *Ann Hum Biol,* 35: 65-74.

Bruneau BG. (2008). The developmental genetics of congenital heart disease. *Nature,* 451: 943-948.

Cabral R, Tejero F, de Fez L, Pacheco PR, Branco CC, Duarte CP, Anjos R & Mota-Vieira L. (2008). *MTHFR* gene polymorphisms as a risk factor for congenital heart disease in São Miguel Island, Azores (Portugal). *Eur J Hum Genet,* 16 Suppl.: P06.050.

Cardoso CS, Oliveira P, Porto G, Oberkanins C, Mascarenhas M, Rodrigues P, Kury F & de Sousa M. (2001). Comparative study of the two more frequent *HFE* mutations (C282Y and H63D): significant different allelic frequencies between the North and South of Portugal. *Eur J Hum Genet,* 9: 843-848.

Carvajal-Carmona LG. (2010). Challenges in the identification and use of rare disease-associated predisposition variants. *Curr Opin Genet Dev,* 20: 277-281.

Castro R, Rivera I, Ravasco P, Jakobs C, Blom HJ, Camilo ME & de Almeida IT. (2003). 5,10 - Methylenetetrahydrofolate reductase 677C>T and 1298A>C mutations are genetic determinants of elevated homocysteine. *QJM,* 96: 297-303.

Chaponda M & Pirmohamed M. (2011). Hypersensitivity reactions to HIV therapy. Br *J Clin Pharmacol,* 71: 659-671.

Correia M, Bruffaerts N, Balagué A, Pereirinha T, Branco CC & Mota-Vieira L. (2010). Study of 9p21 genomic region and *USF1* gene associated with predisposition to cardiovascular diseases in Azorean healthy population. 60th Annual Meeting of American Society of Human Genetics, Washington, USA. PN699. (http://www.ashg.org/cgi-bin/2010/showdetail.pl?absno=21437).

Costa E, Vieira E, Martins M, Saraiva J, Cancela E, Costa M, Bauerle R, Freitas T, Carvalho JR, Santos-Silva E, Barbot J & Dos Santos R. (2006). Analysis of the UDP-glucuronosyltransferase gene in Portuguese patients with a clinical diagnosis of Gilbert and Crigler-Najjar syndromes. *Blood Cells Mol Dis,* 36: 91-97.

Costa E. (2006). Hematologically important mutations: bilirubin UDP-glucuronosyltransferase gene mutations in Gilbert and Crigler-Najjar syndromes. *Blood Cells Mol Dis,* 36: 77-80.

Couto AR, Peixoto MJ, Garrett F, Laranjeira F, Cipriano T & Armas JB. (2003). Linkage disequilibrium between S65C *HFE* mutation and HLA-A29-B44 haplotype in Terceira Island, Azores. *Hum Immunol,* 64: 625-628.

Cruz E, Vieira J, Almeida S, Lacerda R, Gartner A, Cardoso CS, Alves H & Porto G. (2006). A study of 82 extended HLA haplotypes in *HFE*-C282Y homozygous hemochromatosis subjects: relationship to the genetic control of CD8+ T-lymphocyte numbers and severity of iron overload. *BMC Med Genet,* 7: 16.

Cymbron T, Anjos R, Cabral R, Macedo C, Pereira Duarte C & Mota-Vieira L. (2006). Epidemiological characterization of congenital heart disease in São Miguel Island, Azores, Portugal. *Community Genet*, 9: 107-112.

de Fez L, Cabral R, Branco CC, Pacheco PR, Peixoto BR & Mota-Vieira L. (2005). *HFE* mutations in the São Miguel's population: genetic frequencies and geographic distribution. *Eur J Hum Genet*, 13 Suppl.: P1220.

Deplanque D, Birraux G, Bertoye PH & Postaire E. (2009).Collections of human biological samples for scientific purposes. Why do current regulation need to be clarified and how? *Therapie*, 64: 259-267.

Distante S, Robson KJ, Graham-Campbell J, Arnaiz-Villena A, Brissot P & Worwood M. (2004). The origin and spread of the HFE-C282Y haemochromatosis mutation. *Hum Genet*, 115: 269-279.

Dolk H, Loane M & Garne E. (2011). European Surveillance of Congenital Anomalies (EUROCAT) Working Group. Congenital heart defects in Europe: prevalence and perinatal mortality, 2000 to 2005. Circulation, 123: 841-849.

Engelfriet P, Boersma E, Oechslin E, Tijssen J, Gatzoulis MA, Thilén U, Kaemmerer H, Moons P, Meijboom F, Popelová J, Laforest V, Hirsch R, Daliento L, Thaulow E & Mulder B. (2005). The spectrum of adult congenital heart disease in Europe: morbidity and mortality in a 5 year follow-up period. The Euro Heart Survey on adult congenital heart disease. *Eur Heart J*, 26: 2325-2333.

Feder JN, Penny DM, Irrinki A, Lee VK, Lebron JA, Watson N, Tsuchihashi Z, Sigal E, Bjorkman PJ & Schatzman RC. (1998). The hemochromatosis gene product complexes with the transferrin receptor and lowers its affinity for ligand binding. *Proc Natl Acad Sci USA*, 95: 1472-1477.

Fernando O, Mota P, Lima M, Silva C, Montiel R, Amorim A & Prata MJ. (2005). Peopling of the Azores Islands (Portugal): Data from the Y-chromosome. *Hum Biol*, 77: 189-199.

Finkelman BS, Gage BF, Johnson JA, Brensinger CM & Kimmel SE. (2011). Genetic warfarin dosing: tables versus algorithms. *J Am Coll Cardiol*, 57: 612-618.

Fujiwara Y & Minami H. (2010). An overview of the recent progress in irinotecan pharmacogenetics. *Pharmacogenomics*, 11: 391-406.

Gomes CT, Pacheco PR, São Bento M, Cabral R, Branco CC & Mota-Vieira L. (2007). A multiple founder effect of HFE C282Y mutation explains the hereditary hemochromatosis in Azorean island of São Miguel (Portugal). *Am J Hum Genet*, 81 Suppl.: P1310.

Gonçalves E, Bento MC, Relvas L, Ribeiro ML & Tamagnini GP. (2001). Síndroma de Gilbert - frequência do genótipo UGT1A1 (TA)7/(TA)7 numa amostra da população portuguesa. *GE- J Port Gastrenterol*, 8: 250-253.

Gonçalves R, Freitas A, Branco M, Rosa A, Fernandes AT, Zhivotovsky LA, Underhill PA, Kivisild T & Brehm A. (2005). Y-chromosome lineages from Portugal, Madeira and Açores record elements of Sephardim and Berber ancestry. *Ann Hum Genet*, 69: 443-454.

Gorlov IP, Gorlova OY, Frazier ML, Spitz MR & Amos CI. (2011). Evolutionary evidence of the effect of rare variants on disease etiology. *Clin Genet*, 79: 199-206.

Griffiths WJ. (2007). Review article: the genetic basis of haemochromatosis. *Aliment Pharmacol Ther*, 26: 331-342.

Guill JH. (1993). A history of the Azores Islands, Vol 5 California: Division of Golden Shield International Publications Cooperation. 662 pp.

Heard E, Tishkoff S, Todd JA, Vidal M, Wagner GP, Wang J, Weigel D & Young R. (2010). Ten years of genetics and genomics: what have we achieved and where are we heading? *Nat Rev Genet*, 11: 723-733.

Helgadottir A, Thorleifsson G, Manolescu A, Gretarsdottir S, Blondal T, Jonasdottir A, Jonasdottir A, Sigurdsson A, Baker A, Palsson A, Masson G, Gudbjartsson DF, Magnusson KP, Andersen K, Levey AI, Backman VM, Matthiasdottir S, Jonsdottir T, Palsson S, Einarsdottir H, Gunnarsdottir S, Gylfason A, Vaccarino V, Hooper WC, Reilly MP, Granger CB, Austin H, Rader DJ, Shah SH, Quyyumi AA, Gulcher JR, Thorgeirsson G, Thorsteinsdottir U, Kong A & Stefansson K. (2007). A common variant on chromosome 9p21 affects the risk of myocardial infarction. *Science*, 316: 1491-1493.

International Human Genome Sequencing Consortium (2001). Initial sequencing and analysis of the human genome. *Nature*, 409: 860–921.

Jenkins B & Sofos SA. (1996). Nation and identity in contemporary Europe. Routledge. p.145.

Jorge E, Pêgo JM, Baptista R, Lourenço M, Marques I, Correia A, Monteiro P, Antunes F & Providência LA. (2010). Genetic characterization of warfarin sensitivity in a population of cardiovascular patients on chronic anticoagulation. *Rev Port Cardiol*, 29: 1831-1838.

Karafet TM, Mendez FL, Meilerman MB, Underhill PA, Zegura SL & Hammer MF. (2008). New binary polymorphisms reshape and increase resolution of the human Y chromosomal haplogroup tree. *Genome Res*, 18:830-838.

Kehrer DF, Sparreboom A, Verweij J, de Bruijn P, Nierop CA, van de Schraaf J, Ruijgrok EJ & de Jonge MJ. (2001). Modulation of irinotecan-induced diarrhea by cotreatment with neomycin in cancer patients. *Clin Cancer Res*, 7: 1136-1141.

Komulainen K, Alanne M, Auro K, Kilpikari R, Pajukanta P, Saarela J, Ellonen P, Salminen K, Kulathinal S, Kuulasmaa K, Silander K, Salomaa V, Perola M & Peltonen L. (2006). Risk alleles of USF1 gene predict cardiovascular disease of women in two prospective studies. *PLoS Genet*, 2: e69.

Kral BG, Mathias RA, Suktitipat B, Ruczinski I, Vaidya D, Yanek LR, Quyyumi AA, Patel RS, Zafari AM, Vaccarino V, Hauser ER, Kraus WE, Becker LC & Becker DM. (2011). A common variant in the CDKN2B gene on chromosome 9p21 protects against coronary artery disease in Americans of African ancestry. *J Hum Genet*, 56: 224-229.

Lankisch TO, Schulz C, Zwingers T, Erichsen TJ, Manns MP, Heinemann V & Strassburg CP. (2008). Gilbert's Syndrome and irinotecan toxicity: combination with UDP-glucuronosyltransferase 1A7 variants increases risk. *Cancer Epidemiol Biomarkers Prev*, 17: 695-701.

Lee CN, Su YN, Cheng WF, Lin MT, Wang JK, Wu MH & Hsieh FJ. (2005). Association of the C677T methylenetetrahydrofolate reductase mutation with congenital heart diseases. *Acta Obstet Gynecol Scand*, 84: 1134-1140.

Li J, Liu Y, Kim T, Min R & Zhang Z. (2010). Gene expression variability within and between human populations and implications toward disease susceptibility. *PLoS Comput Biol*, 6: e1000910.

Limdi NA & Veenstra DL. (2008). Warfarin pharmacogenetics. *Pharmacotherapy*, 28: 1084-1097.

Manolio TA, Collins FS, Cox NJ, Goldstein DB, Hindorff LA, Hunter DJ, McCarthy MI, Ramos EM, Cardon LR, Chakravarti A, Cho JH, Guttmacher AE, Kong A, Kruglyak L, Mardis E, Rotimi CN, Slatkin M, Valle D, Whittemore AS, Boehnke M, Clark AG, Eichler EE, Gibson G, Haines JL, Mackay TF, McCarroll SA &Visscher PM. (2009). Finding the missing heritability of complex diseases. *Nature*, 461: 747-753.

Mansilha A, Araújo F, Severo M, Sampaio SM, Toledo T & Albuquerque R. (2006). Combined factor V Leiden (R506Q) and prothrombin G20210A genotyping in young patients presenting with deep venous thrombosis. *Phlebology*, 21: 24-27.

Marinho C, Alho I, Guerra A, Rego C, Areias J & Bicho M. (2009). The methylenetetrahydrofolate reductase gene variant (C677T) as a susceptibility gene for tetralogy of Fallot. *Rev Port Cardiol*, 28: 809-812.

Marques SC & Ikediobi ON. (2010). The clinical application of *UGT1A1* pharmacogenetic testing: gene-environment interactions. *Hum Genomics*, 4: 238-249.

Marsh S & Hoskins JM. (2010). Irinotecan pharmacogenomics. *Pharmacogenomics*, 11: 1003-1010.

Matsui K, Maruo Y, Sato H & Takeuchi Y. (2010). Combined effect of regulatory polymorphisms on transcription of UGT1A1 as a cause of Gilbert syndrome. *BMC Gastroenterol*, 10: 57.

McPherson R, Pertsemlidis A, Kavaslar N, Stewart A, Roberts R, Cox DR, Hinds DA, Pennacchio LA, Tybjaerg-Hansen A, Folsom AR, Boerwinkle E, Hobbs HH & Cohen JC. (2007). A common allele on chromosome 9 associated with coronary heart disease. *Science*, 316: 1488-1491.

Mendonça L. (1996). História dos Açores - Visão geral (sécs. XV-XIX). Centro de Apoio Tecnológico à Educação, Ponta Delgada, Azores. 196 pp.

Milman N & Pedersen P. (2003). Evidence that the Cys282Tyr mutation of the *HFE* gene originated from a population in Southern Scandinavia and spread with the Vikings. *Clinical Genetics*, 64: 36-47.

Montiel R, Bettencourt C, Silva C, Santos C, Prata MJ & Lima M. (2005). Analysis of Y-chromosome variability and its comparison with mtDNA variability reveals different demographic histories between islands in the Azores Archipelago (Portugal). *Ann Hum Genet*, 69: 135-144.

Nabulsi MM, Tamim H, Sabbagh M, Obeid MY, Yunis KA & Bitar FF. (2003). Parental consanguinity and congenital heart malformation in a developing country. *Am J Med Genet*, 116: 342–347.

Neto D, Montiel R, Bettencourt C, Santos C, Prata MJ & Lima M. (2007). The African contribution to the present-day population of the Azores Islands (Portugal): analysis of the Y-chromosome haplogroup E. *Am J Hum Biol*, 19: 854-860.

Oliveira E, Marsh S, van Booven DJ, Amorim A, Prata MJ & McLeod HL. (2007). Pharmacogenetically relevant polymorphisms in Portugal. *Pharmacogenomics*, 8: 703-712.

Orange JS, Glessner JT, Resnick E, Sullivan KE, Lucas M, Ferry B, Kim CE, Hou C, Wang F, Chiavacci R, Kugathasan S, Sleasman JW, Baldassano R, Perez EE, Chapel H, Cunningham-Rundles C & Hakonarson H. (2011). Genome-wide association identifies diverse causes of common variable immunodeficiency. *J Allergy Clin Immunol*, Apr 15. [Epub ahead of print]

Pacheco PR, Branco CC, Cabral R, Costa S, Araujo AL, Peixoto BR, Mendonca P & Mota-Vieira L. (2005). The Y-chromosomal heritage of the Azores Islands population. *Ann Hum Genet*, 69: 145-156.

Pacheco PR, Branco CC, Gomes CT, Cabral R & Mota-Vieira L. (2010). HLA Class I and II profiles in São Miguel Island (Azores): genetic diversity and linkage disequilibrium. *BMC Res Notes* 3: 134.

Pacheco PR, Brilhante MJ, Ballart C, Sigalat F, Polena H, Cabral R, Branco CC & Mota-Vieira L. (2009). *UGT1A1, UGT1A6* and *UGT1A7* genetic analysis: repercussion for irinotecan pharmacogenetics in the São Miguel Island Population (Azores, Portugal). *Mol Diagn Ther*, 13: 261-268.

Pacheco PR, Gomes C, Cabral R, Branco CC & Mota-Vieira L. (2006). Analysis of the *UGT1A1* promoter polymorphism in São Miguel population (Azores, Portugal). *Eur J Hum Genet* 14 Suppl.: P1159.

Pereira L, Prata MJ & Amorim A. (2000b). Diversity of mtDNA lineages in Portugal: not a genetic edge of European variation. *Ann Hum Genet*, 64: 491-506.

Pereira L, Prata MJ, Jobling MA, Carracedo A & Amorim A. (2000a). Clinal variation of YAP+ Y-chromosome frequencies in western Iberia. *Hum Biol*, 72: 937-944.

Pereirinha T, Branco CC, Pacheco PR, Brilhante MJ, Cabral R & Mota Vieira L. (2009). Warfarin pharmacogenetic profiles in the Azorean population (Portugal). 4th International Congress - Genetics of Complex Diseases and Isolated Populations, Trieste, Italy, oral communication.

Perez-Lezaun A, Calafell F, Clarimon J, Bosch E, Mateu E, Gusmão L, Amorim A, Benchemsi N & Bertranpetit J. (2000). Allele frequencies of 13 short tandem repeats in population samples from the Iberian Peninsula and northern Africa. *Int J Legal Med*, 113: 208-214.

Pietrangelo A. (2004). Hereditary Hemochromatosis — A New Look at an Old Disease. *N Engl J Med*, 350: 2383-2397.

Rieder MJ, Reiner AP, Gage BF, Nickerson DA, Eby CS, McLeod HL, Blough DK, Thummel KE, Veenstra DL & Rettie AE. (2005). Effect of *VKORC1* haplotypes on transcriptional regulation and warfarin dose. *N Engl J Med*, 352: 2285-2293.

Russel-Wood AJR. (1998). The Portuguese Empire, 1415–1808: A World on the Move. Baltimore, The Johns Hopkins University Press.

Santos C, Alvarez L, Aluja MP, Bruges-Armas J, Lima M. (2009). Genetic structure of the Azores Islands: a study using 15 autosomal short tandem repeat loci. *Coll Antropol*, 33:991-999.

Santos C, Fregel R, Cabrera VM, González AM, Larruga JM & Lima M. (2010). Mitochondrial DNA patterns in the Macaronesia islands: Variation within and among archipelagos. *Am J Phys Anthropol*, 141: 610-619.

Santos C, Lima M, Montiel R, Angles N, Pires L, Abade A & Aluja MP. (2003). Genetic structure and origin of peopling in the Azores Islands (Portugal): The view from mtDNA. *Ann Hum Genet*, 67: 433-456.

Santos C, Montiel R, Arruda A, Alvarez L, Aluja MP & Lima M. (2008). Mutation patterns of mtDNA: empirical inferences for the coding region. *BMC Evol Biol*, 8: 167.

Santos C, Montiel R, Sierra B, Bettencourt C, Fernandez E, Alvarez L, Lima M, Abade A & Aluja MP. (2005). Understanding differences between phylogenetic and pedigree-derived mtDNA mutation rate: a model using families from the Azores Islands (Portugal). *Mol Biol Evol*, 22: 1490-1505.

Service S, DeYoung J, Karayiorgou M Roos, JL, Pretorious H, Bedoya G, Ospina J, Ruiz-Linares A, Macedo A, Palha JA, Heutink P, Aulchenko Y, Oostra B, van Duijn C, Jarvelin MR, Varilo T, Peddle L, Rahman P, Piras G, Monne M, Murray S, Galver L, Peltonen L, Sabatti C, Collins A & Freimer N. (2006). Magnitude and distribution of linkage disequilibrium in population isolates and implications for genome-wide association studies. *Nat Genet*, 38: 556-560.

Silander K, Tang H, Myles S, Jakkula E, Timpson NJ, Cavalli-Sforza L & Peltonen L. (2009). Worldwide patterns of haplotype diversity at 9p21.3, a locus associated with type 2 diabetes and coronary heart disease. *Genome Med*, 1: 51.

Silva F, Pereira R, Gusmão L, Santos C, Amorim A, Prata MJ, Bettencourt C, Lourenço P & Lima M. (2010). Genetic profiling of the Azores Islands (Portugal): data from 10 X-chromosome STRs. *Am J Hum Biol*, 22: 221-223.

Simon J, Paslack R, Robienski J, Cooper DN, Goebel JW & Krawczak M. (2007). A legal framework for biobanking: the German experience. *Eur J Hum Genet*, 15: 528-532.

Spínola H, Brehm A, Bettencourt B, Middleton D & Bruges-Armas J. (2005b). HLA class I and II polymorphisms in Azores show different settlements in Oriental and Central islands. *Tissue Antigens*, 66: 217-230.

Spinola H, Middleton D & Brehm A. (2005a). HLA genes in Portugal inferred from sequence based typing. In the crossroad between Europe and Africa. *Tissue Antigens*. 66: 26-36.

Strassburg CP. (2010). Hyperbilirubinemia syndromes (Gilbert-Meulengracht, Crigler-Najjar, Dubin-Johnson, and Rotor syndrome). *Best Pract Res Clin Gastroenterol*, 24: 555-571.

Swinkels DW, Janssen MC, Bergmans J & Marx JJ. (2006). Hereditary hemochromatosis: genetic complexity and new diagnostic approaches. *Clin Chem*, 52: 950-968.

The International HapMap Consortium. (2010). Integrating common and rare genetic variation in diverse human populations. *Nature*, 467: 52-58.

Venter JC, et al. (2001). The sequence of the human genome. *Science*, 291: 1304–1351.

Wadelius M & Pirmohamed M. (2007). Pharmacogenetics of warfarin: current status and future challenges. *Pharmacogenomics J*, 7: 99-111.

Yasar Ü, Eliasson E, Dahl ML, Johansson I, Ingelman-Sundberg M & Sjöqvist F. (1999). Validation of methods for CYP2C9 genotyping: frequencies of mutant alleles in a Swedish population. *Biochem Biophys Res Commun*, 254: 628-631.

You JH. (2010). Pharmacoeconomic evaluation of warfarin pharmacogenomics. *Expert Opin Pharmacother*, 12: 435-441.

Zhang D, Zhang D, Cui D, Gambardella J, Ma L, Barros A, Wang L, Fu Y, Rahematpura S, Nielsen J, Donegan M, Zhang H & Humphreys WG. (2007). Characterization of the UDP glucuronosyltransferase activity of human liver microsomes genotyped for the UGT1A1*28 polymorphism. *Drug Metab Dispos*, 35: 2270-2280.

Zhu Q, Ge D, Maia JM, Zhu M, Petrovski S, Dickson SP, Heinzen EL, Shianna KV & Goldstein DB. (2011) A Genome-wide Comparison of the Functional Properties of Rare and Common Genetic Variants in Humans. *Am J Hum Genet*, 88: 458-468.

9

Double-Factor Preimplantation Genetic Diagnosis: Preliminary Results

Obradors A[1,2,3], Rius M[2], Daina G[2], Cuzzi JF[4], Martínez-Pasarell O[5], Fernández E[6], López O[5], Polo A[5], Séculi JL[7], Gartner S[8], Oliver-Bonet M[2], Benet J[1,2] and Navarro J[1,2]

1. Introduction

Preimplantation Genetic Diagnosis (PGD) was first employed successfully for a monogenic disease detection almost 20 years ago (Handyside *et al.*, 1990). PGD was also applied to screen for chromosomal abnormalities in couples at risk of aneuploidy (i.e., Preimplantation Genetic Screening: PGS) six years later (Munne and Weier, 1996, Verlinsky *et al.*, 1996, Verlinsky *et al.*, 1996). Currently, both approaches have been extensively used worldwide with more than 2,000 scientific publications.

Briefly, PGS aims for the selection of euploid embryos to transfer, aiming to increase their implantation rate. FISH for 9 chromosomes is mostly the technique applied in PGS. It seems, however, that according to recent publications PGS may not be useful (Staessen *et al.*, 2004, Staessen *et al.*, 2008, Hardarson *et al.*, 2008, Mastenbroek *et al.*, 2007). In fact, analyzing the latest data presented by the European Society of Human Reproduction and Embryology (E.S.R.H.E.), on average just 27.4% of the transferred PGS-selected embryos implant (3,926 positive heartbeats / 14,325 transferred embryos)(Harper *et al.*, 2010). On the other hand, after 167,192 ART cycles in Europe using ICSI, the pregnancy rate is 29.8% (Andersen *et al.*, 2008). Obviously, PGS patients differ from ICSI patients since the first ones suffer from repetitive implantation failure (RIF) or have an advanced maternal age (AMA), but the low implantation rate obtained in these patients still remains as a problematic issue.

But, also referring to the E.S.H.R.E. data, the implantation rate in patients undergoing PGD for a monogenic disease, in which the maternal age is not at risk of producing aneuploid

[1]*Càtedra de Recerca Eugin-UAB*
[2]*Unitat de Biologia Cel.lular i Genètica Mèdica, Facultat de Medicina, Universitat Autònoma de Barcelona; 08193; Bellaterra, Spain.*
[3]*Clínica EUGIN. Travessera de les Corts 322, Barcelona, Spain.*
[4]*Departamento de Genetica, Faculdade de Medicina de Ribeirão Preto, CNPq Schorlarship, Universidade de São Paulo, Brazil.*
[5]*Unitat de Reproducció Assistida. Fundació Puigvert. Hospital Sant Pau. Barcelona, Spain.*
[6]*Laboratorio de Reproducción Asistida, Hospital Quirón, Avenida Europa 16; Pozuelo de Alarcón; 28224, Madrid, Spain.*
[7]*Servei de Pneumologia, Hospital Sant Joan de Deu, Barcelona, Spain.*
[8]*Servei de Fibrosi Quística, Hospital Materno Infantil, La Vall d'Hebrón, Barcelona, Spain.*

gametes, is 15.2% (1067 positive heartbeats /7,035 transferred embryos) (Harper *et al.*, 2010). It appears clear, then, that an increase of the implantation rate would not only be advantageous for the PGS patients but also for the PGD ones.

In PGS patients, in order to increase the implantation rate, comprehensive chromosomal analysis techniques have been proposed to completely karyotype the embryo to be transferred. One of these techniques is Comparative Genomic Hybridization (CGH), which has been applied widely in PGS (Keskintepe *et al.*, 2007, Sher *et al.*, 2007, Voullaire *et al.*, 2002, Wells *et al.*, 2002, Wilton, 2005), achieving up to a 74%-80% rate of implantation. Two different cells can be analyzed by CGH-PGS, the first polar body (1PB) and the blastomere (BL). Both options have their advantages and disadvantages; the use of 1PB-CGH permits the diagnosis of the cell within the same IVF cycle, as the CGH procedure requires up to 4 working days, but the result obtained only reflects indirect information about the oocyte, despite it being known that it is during the first meiotic division when most embryonic aneuploidies occur (Hassold and Hunt, 2001, Nicolaidis and Petersen, 1998). On the other hand, BL-CGH gives information about the embryo directly, but it cannot be analyzed during the same IVF cycle and, therefore, involves a cryopreservation step followed by a defrost step of euploid embryos prior to transfer.

Other techniques that allow for a full karyotype analysis and that are potentially useful to increase implantation in PGS patients are array-CGH or SNP-array, which permits a diagnosis within the IVF cycle and investigates the embryo directly, as it is applied to blastomeres. So far, several publications have tested the efficiency of array-CGH on single cells with promising results (Fiegler *et al.*, 2007, Hu *et al.*, 2004, Le Caignec *et al.*, 2006, Wells *et al.*, 2004, Handyside *et al.*, 2009). Recently, it has been applied clinically after blastomere or polar body biopsy, obtaining six pregnancies (Hellani *et al.*, 2008, Fishel *et al.*, 2009). Although array-CGH is a capable technique, more research must be done to validate it and monitor any increase in the implantation rate. Toward this aim, the ESHRE PGS Task Force have proposed a multicenter randomized control trial to assess the possible positive effect on implantation of the PGS on polar body using a 24-chromosome detecting technique as array-CGH (Geraedts *et al.*, 2009).

Now considering the enhancement of the implantation rate on patients undergoing PGD for a monogenic disease (PGD-patients), several approaches have been published with this aim. A methodology called Cell Recycling, i.e., FISH analysis of a blastomere and posterior PCR amplification of the very same cell, was described as a possible option for selected the embryos both genetically and cytogenetically (Thornhill *et al.*, 1994), but it was demonstrated that the protocol increased the allele drop-out (ADO) rate, thus reducing its diagnostic robustness (Rechitsky *et al.*, 1996).

Another approach is the Double-Factor PGD (DF-PGD) where the 1PB is analyzed using CGH and a single blastomere of the produced embryo is biopsied in order to diagnose the monogenic disease. This method permits the double selection of the embryos for being free of the family disease plus having originated from a potentially euploid oocyte. In addition, as 1PB-CGH is used, the diagnosis is performed within the same IVF cycle, avoiding the need of cryopreservation. The DF-PGD has been previously applied on two couples, carriers of cystic fibrosis and von Hippel-Lindau syndrome, respectively, achieving the birth of three healthy children (Obradors *et al.*, 2008, Obradors *et al.*, 2009).

The aims of this work are to assess the feasibility and application of the DF-PGD after two year of experience and ten clinical applications and, moreover, to determine if it is a valuable tool to increase the implantation rate in PGD for monogenic-disease patients.

2. Materials and methods

Patients

Over two years, a total of eight couples affected by a monogenic disease participated in this study after fully understanding the protocol and the signing of an approved-consent form. The results of two of them were previously published (Obradors et al., 2008 and 2009) (Table 1). Two of the couples repeated the DF-PGD clinical protocol after no pregnancy on the first attempt.

The mean age of the patients was 35.1 years old. For comparison proposes, the patients were classified into two groups depending on the maternal age: four patients were classified with advanced maternal age (AMA) (mean age of 39.2 y.o.) and the other 6 patients were ≤ 35 y.o. (mean age of 32.3 y.o.).

Most of the couples (6 out of 8) were unaffected carriers of Cystic Fibrosis (CF, OMIM #219700) with an affected child. Considering the other two couples, one was affected by von Hippel-Lindau syndrome (VHL, OMIM #193300), a dominantly-inherited family cancer syndrome, and the other couple was an unaffected carrier of Angelman Syndrome (AS; OMIM #105830).

A summary of the mutations affecting each couple can be also found in Table 1.

Monogenic disease detection protocol

In order to minimize misdiagnosis and increase protocol robustness, two independent diagnoses were performed. A direct diagnosis of the causative mutation and an indirect diagnosis using informative Small Tandem Repeats (STRs) were optimized for each couple. The causative mutation detection, mostly point-mutations, was achieved after two rounds of nested-PCR amplification of a region surrounding the mutation using specific primers designer using the Primer3 website (http://frodo.wi.mit.edu) (Table 2). After PCR amplification, the mutant site was interrogated using the MiniSequencing Reaction (Snapshot Multiplex Kit, Applied Biosystems; CA, USA). During the reaction, a mutation-specific primer anneals a base before the point-mutation site; then, a polymerase incorporates a single ddNTP fluorescently labeled (Fiorentino *et al.*, 2003). The product of the reaction (1μL) is analyzed in a DNA sequencer in order to detect the presence or absence of the causative mutation.

In order to detect mutations involving short deletions, such as ΔF508 mutation in the CFTR gene which is causative of Cystic Fibrosis (CF), where three nucleotides are deleted in the mutant allele, a pair of fluorescent primers was designed to anneal on both sides of the deletion in order to detect the fragment analysis variation, between the alleles. After PCR amplification of genomic DNA of a CF carrier and analysis on a DNA sequencer, two different peaks appear, a wild-type peak at 94 bp followed by the mutant peak at 91 bp.

As commented upon before, an indirect diagnosis using STRs was also applied. A minimum of four STRs were found surrounding each of the genes causatives of the diseases. The STRs were chosen using the NCBI database (http://www.ncbi.nlm.nih.gov/mapview) according to the following criteria: to contain a tetranucleotide repetition core, to be located as close as possible to the gene (upstream or downstream) and to have the highest heterozygosity value. Once they were chosen, the fluorescent dyes of the forward primers of each STR were selected in order to avoid overlapping of the expected allele size for all STRs of the same disease, so they could be amplified and simultaneously analyzed if required.

Couple	Maternal age	Disease	Gene	Mutation	Direct detection	Indirect detection
Obradors et al. 2009	30	Von Hippel-Lindau, Dominant	VHL	P: R161Q	MiniSequencing	D3S1675 D3S1537
A	32	Cystic Fibrosis, Recessive	CFTR	P: dF508 M: dF508	Fragment analysis	INTRAGENIC D7S1799 D7S1817 D7S3025 D7S2847
A'	32	Cystic Fibrosis, Recessive	CFTR	P: dF508 M: dF508	Fragment analysis	INTRAGENIC D7S1799 D7S1817 D7S3025 D7S2847
B	32	Cystic Fibrosis, Recessive	CFTR	P: dF508 M: dF508	Fragment analysis	INTRAGENIC
C	33	Cystic Fibrosis, Recessive	CFTR	P: 712-1GtoT M: dF508	MiniSequencing and Fragment analysis	D7S1799 D7S3025 D7S2847
Obradors et al. 2008	35	Cystic Fibrosis, Recessive	CFTR	P: 3408C>A M:3849+10Kb (CtoT)	MiniSequencing	INTRAGENIC D7S1799
D	37	Angelman Syndrome, Dominant	UBE3A	M: K109X	MiniSequencing	D15S817 D15S1513
E	38	Cystic Fibrosis, Recessive	CFTR	P:1811+1.6KbAtoG M:2711delT	MiniSequencing	D7S1799 D7S1817
F	41	Cystic Fibrosis, Recessive	CFTR	P: dF508 M:dF508	Fragment analysis	INTRAGENIC D7S1799 D7S2847
F'	41	Cystic Fibrosis, Recessive	CFTR	P: dF508 M:dF508	Fragment analysis	INTRAGENIC D7S1799 D7S2847

Table 1. Diseases and causative mutations of the eight couples included in the present DF-PGP program. The mutation detection methods and the informative STRs to perform direct and indirect analysis, respectively, are also included. The dF508 mutation is detected by the 3-bp difference between the mutant and the wild-type alleles

To assess the diagnostic utility of the STRs, genomic DNA extracted from peripheral blood or from buccal cells was obtained from each member of the couple. The STRs were classified as being 100% informative if the both in the couple were both heterozygote, or to be partially informative if one of the couple was homozygote and the other one heterozygote for the same STR or, finally, not informative if both were homozygote. In order to detect which of the couple's alleles were linked to their mutated copy of the gene, DNA from an affected child or first-degree relatives was also analyzed.

With the aim of avoiding misdiagnosis due to the recombination process between the selected STRs and the gene of interest, a minimum of two 100% or partially informative

Primer	Forward (5′-3′)	Reverse (5′-3′)
K109X-outer	GCCTAGAATGTTTGGCTGTTT	CTCTTCCAATAACACGGATTAAA
K109X-inner	GAACTTTTTGCAACAGAGTAAACA	ATCCTCTCTTTCTCTACATAATTCAAG
K109X-miniseq	AGATGTGACTTACTTAACAGAAGAG	-
dF508	6FAM-TGGAGCCTTCAGAGGGTAAA	TGGGTAGTGTGAAGGGTTCAT
712-1 G to T-outer	TGTTAGTTTCTAGGGGTGGAAGA	AAAGGAGCGATCCACACG
712-1 G to T-inner	GACACCTGTTTTTGCTGTGC	AAATGTGCCAATGCAAGTCC
1811+1.6Kb-outer	AAAGTTTTGCCATTGGTTTTT	AAAGATGAAGACACAGTTCCCATA
1811+1.6Kb-inner	TTGTGTGCTGAATACAATTTTCTTT	AAAGATGAAGACACAGTTCCCATA
1811+1.6Kb-miniseq	AGAGAATCCTATGTACTTGAGAT	-
2711delT-outer	GGAGAGCATACCAGCAGTGA	AAGCACCAAATTAGCACAAAA
2711delT-inner	TTCGATATATTACTGTCCACAAGAGC	AAGCACCAAATTAGCACAAAA
D15S1513	6FAM-GAACTGGGGAAAATCAGGAT	ACACATTTTAAGCCAGCAGC
D15S817	6FAM-GCACCAATAGGCTAGACACG	AGCTTTACATGGCATGTGGT
D7S2847	HEX-TCACCTTCAGAAAGTATTGCC	TGAGGTGTTTCTCCAAGCTC
D7S3052	6FAM-AGTGAGACTAGCAGATGTACTTGG	GCCTCCCCATTTCATCTATT
INTRA	HEX-CAAGTCTTTCACTGATCTTC	TGAGCAGTTCTTAATAGATAA

Table 2. Sequences of the primers used in this study. The underlined primers were also used as MiniSequencing primers, as their 3′ end hybridizes a base before the point-mutation. The other primers' sequences are cited in the previous applications of DF-PGD.

STRs located on each side of the gene (upstream and downstream) were selected for the PGD protocol, or in the case of intragenic STRs, a single STR was considered.

Once both the STRs and the mutation-specific primers were chosen, the PGD protocols were optimized using genomic DNA from one of the patients. Briefly, a multiplex PCR containing the fluorescent primers for the STRs amplification, plus the first-round unlabeled primers for mutation detection was applied in most of the cases. When optimizing the dF508 CF mutation, its primers were fluorescently labeled in order to detect the deletion, as described before. Between 0.5-1 μL of product of this PCR multiplex was used as a template for the second round of amplification of the mutation-specific primers. One microliter of the PCR amplification product was used in a DNA sequencer to assess STRs efficiency on the multiplex, whereas agarose gel analysis was enough to detect to correct amplification of the mutation-specific loci.

When the multiplex was efficient in genomic DNA, it was tested in whole genome-amplified (WGA) single cells, usually cultured fibroblast. The Multiple Displacement Amplification (MDA) (Genomiphi, HE Healthcare; Buckinghamshire, UK) was used following the manufacturer's protocol, but with a previous step of alkaline lysis of the single cell, as described before (Obradors et al., 2008 and 2009, Spits et al., 2006). Finally, and in order to describe the allele drop-out (ADO) rate, 30 patients' lymphocytes were amplified with the optimized protocol.

In order to minimize the presence of contamination due to exogenous DNA, all PCR mixes which included primers, Taq polymerase and buffers were performed on a sterile hood. While the target DNA, i.e., MDA products, PCR amplicons after a first-round amplification and DNA extracted from peripheral blood or from buccal cells were introduced into a separate sterile hood in another room.

A report, the informative study report, including the STRs analyzed, the mutation detection procedure and ADO rate described for each couple, was sent to the IVF centers, which scheduled a date for the PGD case according to the patient's stimulation cycle.

3. First polar body comparative genomic hybrydization

The 1PB-CGH procedure has been extensively described previously by our group (Obradors et al., 2008 and 2009). Briefly, the 1PB was washed four times with sterile PBS/0.1%PVP, in order to avoid potential contamination from cumulus cells, and it was then placed in a 0.2mL PCR tube. Cell lysis (1 µl of sodium dodecyl sulfate (17 µM) and 2 µl of proteinase K (125 µg/ml)) was required to facilitate the cell genomic-DNA liberation. Afterwards, the cellular DNA was amplified by means of DOP-PCR, a WGA technique described to produce a sufficient amount of DNA to perform a CGH (Telenius *et al.*, 1992, Voullaire *et al.*, 1999, Wells *et al.*, 1999). Briefly, the DOP-PCR reaction tubes contained 1X Buffer, 2 µmol/l DOP primer (CCGACTCGAGNNNNNNATGTGG), 0.2 mmol/l dNTP and 2.5U of SuperTaq Plus polymerase (Ambion, USA) in a final volume of 50 µl. The tubes were placed in a thermocycler and underwent the following program: 94°C for 4.5 min; eight cycles of 95°C for 30s, 30°C for 1.5 min and 72°C for 3 min; 40 cycles of 95°C for 30s, 56°C for 1 min and 72°C for 3 min with a final extension step of 72°C for 8 min. After DOP-PCR amplification, fluorescent labeling with Spectrum-Red of the DOP-PCR product was performed by the Nick Translation Kit, following the manufacturer's indications (Vysis; Downers Grove, USA). With the purpose of obtaining reference DNA to compare with the 1PB (test DNA), between twelve to fifteen tubes containing three euploid female fibroblasts each were lysated and amplified like the 1PBs, but labeled with Spectrum-Green instead. The reference DNA produced from these twelve to fifteen cells was mixed in a single tube, kept at -20°C and used as reference DNA when required. The resulting reference-DNA mix avoids intrinsic cell-dependent amplification differences that could bias the CGH results and provides an intense homogeneous fluorescent signal.

Both test and reference DNA co-precipitated with Cot-1-DNA, which blocks repetitive DNA sequences such as telomeres and centromeres. The resulting cytogenetic probe hybridized during 44 hours into a slide of euploid lymphocyte metaphases. After that, the slide was washed to remove unspecific hybridization and analyzed using an epifluorescence microscope. Ten lymphocyte metaphases were captured and karyotyped using the Metasystem's software to obtain a CGH profile. When the fluorescence ratio (test/reference) of a CGH profile for a specific chromosome, reported by the software, was < 0.8, the chromosome was lost in the DNA test, whereas when the ratio is > 1.2, a chromosome gain was present (Wells et al., 1999).

Potentially artifactually gained or lost chromosomes (i.e., Chromosomes 17, 19 and 22) were discarded from analysis when all three chromosomes were simultaneously gained or lost in the same cell; if not, they were considered as being real aneuploidies.

In the present work, no distinction between chromosome or chromatid gain or loss has been considered because, in our experience, after analyzing 1PBs and their corresponding MII using CGH and FISH, respectively, the CGH-loss or CGH-gain profiles on the 1PBs were indistinguishably equivalent to losses or gains of either chromosome or chromatid in the MIIs (Gutiérrez-Mateo, et al., 2004).

4. Double-factor pgd clinical schedule

Exhaustive information about the methodology and schedule, based on the following timetable (Figure 1), of the Double-Factor PGD (DF-PGD) clinical application performed in the families included in this work has been previously published (Obradors et al., 2008 and 2009). On Day 0, retrieved oocytes were cleaned of cumulus cells to avoid cellular contamination during the PGD case. Following the IVF center's protocol, ICSI was performed on all MII oocytes, and immediately afterwards, the 1PB was biopsied using the partial zone dissection (PZD) procedure and washed four times with sterile PBS/0.1PVS as described above. In the cases, when the IVF center was located close to the lab (i.e., Barcelona), the cell lysis and DOP-PCR were done on Day 0; on the other hand, for cases located far from our lab (i.e., Madrid), the 1PB arrived in our lab in Bellaterra on Day +1, when the CGH protocol started. On the afternoon of Day +1, the CGH was placed to hybridize for 44 hours, thus, until the morning of Day +3. On Day +3, the CGH started to be analyzed; in general, a skilled technician took 1 hour to obtain a result for each CGH, so depending on the number of 1PBs it may last until Day +4. Also on Day +3, developing embryos reached the 6-8-cell stage and a single blastomere is biopsied using the same hole produced during the 1PB biopsy, but in order to increase the size of the hole, PZD or acid Tyrodes was used. Again, if the IVF center was located close to the lab (i.e., Barcelona), the PCR protocol started on Day +3, thus achieving the monogenic diagnosis results on Day +4. For IVF centers located in Madrid, the blastomere arrived on Day +4.

Late on Day +4, after the results from the DF-PGD were obtained, a written report was sent to the IVF center indicating not only the embryos free of each particular monogenic family disease, but also the results obtained after the complete cytogenetic analyses of the whole female chromosome complement. At that point, embryos free from the monogenic family pathology that were derived from oocytes that were predicted to be euploid and with a good morphological appearance can be selected and transferred. As is habitual in PGD, the family has been informed that performing a prenatal diagnosis in case of pregnancy would be recommended.

5. Results

First polar body and blastomere obtainment

After ovary stimulation and follicular puncture, 146 oocytes were obtained from the 10 DF-PGD clinical cases presented (mean of 14.6 per couple). One-hundred-thirty-two of them (90.4%) were at the MII stage, thus containing the 1PB, and were inseminated using the couple's spermatozoids by ICSI. Immediately there after, the 1PBs were biopsied, obtaining 112 1PBs; therefore, the 1PBs biopsy efficiency was 84.8% (112/132). The oocytes were incubated at 37°C and checked for fecundation on Day +1. A total of 92 showed morphological signs of fecundation, obtaining a fecundation rate prior to the 1PB biopsy of 69.7%. As established in the IVF centers, embryos were checked for satisfactory division and quality on Day +2. On Day +3, 81 of the 92 (88%) fertilized oocytes did develop to 6-8-cell-stage embryos (mean of 8.1 embryos per cycle) and a single blastomere was biopsied.

Blastomere biopsy was achieved in all embryos (100%), hence 81 blastomeres were acquired. A summary of the cells obtained can be found in Tables 3 and 5.

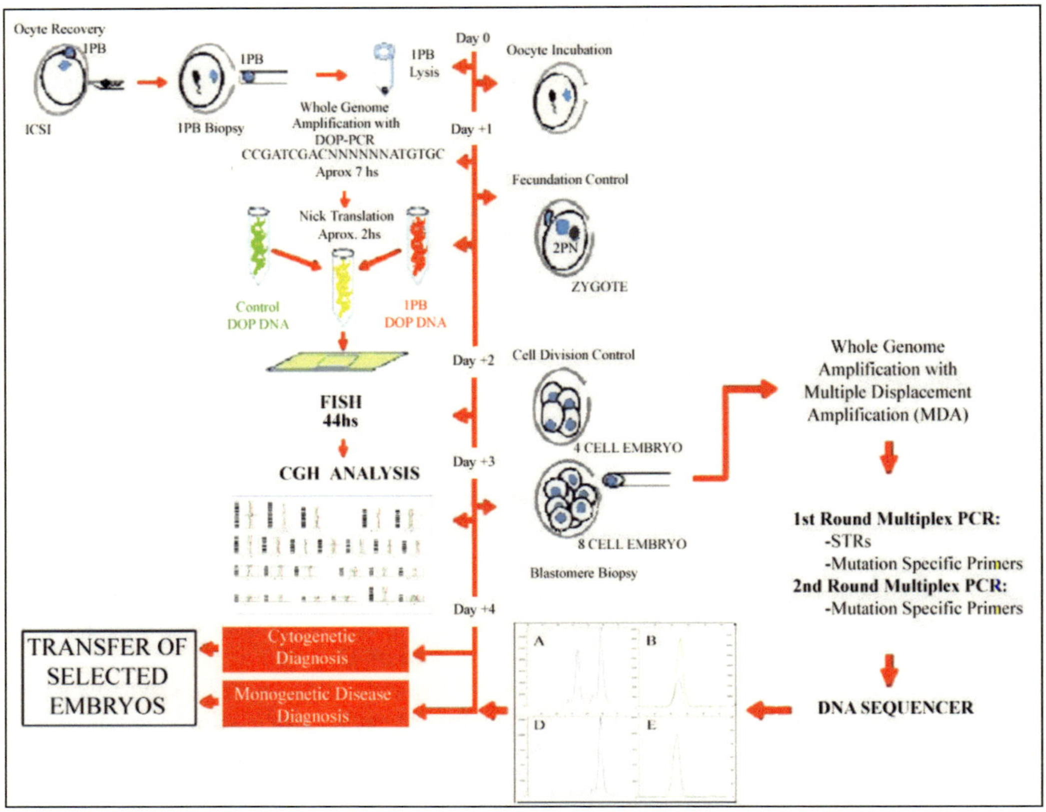

Fig. 1. Illustration showing the DF-PGD timing combined with the IVF procedure.

First polar body cgh results

Analyzable CGH profiles were obtained in 83 of the 112 1PB-CGHs performed, resulting in a CGH success of 74.1%. The remaining 29 1PB-CGHs, in which poor WGA amplification field were observed on the agarose gel, were not analyzable due to a faint hybridization was obtained. Probably it was due to the corresponding 1PB was fragmented or with bad morphology.

Thirty-five of the 1PBs were diagnosed as euploid, whereas the remaining 54.2% (45 out of 83) were aneuploid (Tables 3 and 4). No differences in the incidence of aneuploidy were observed between the two maternal age groups (56% in ≤ 35 years vs. 51.5% in > 35 years).

Aneuploidies involving from one to nine chromosomes were observed. All the 23 chromosomes were involved in aneuploidy. The chromosomes that most frequently were found to be aneuploid were Chromosomes 19 (eleven times), 18 and 16 (nine times), 1 (eight times) (Figure 2). No differences were observed concerning chromosome size, as from the 109 chromosomes involved in aneuploidy, 57 (52.3%) and 52 (47.7%) were classified into the A-C groups or into the D-G groups, respectively.

Only eight out the 45 aneuploid (17.8%) 1PBs would have been fully diagnosed using a FISH analysis for 9 chromosomes (13, 15, 16, 17, 18, 21, 22, X and Y), and a total of 20 (44.4%) of the aneuploid 1PBs would have been diagnosed incorrectly as being euploid (Figure 3). The remaining 17 1PBs (37.8%) would have been diagnosed as being aneuploid, but not all the chromosomal aneuploidies present would have been detected.

Couple	Maternal age	Oocytes retrieved	MII oocytes	1PB	Successful 1PB biopsy %	Analyzable 1PB-CGH	CGH Success %	EUPLOID 1PBs	ANEUPLOIDS 1PBs	ANEUPLOIDY RATE %
Obradors et al. 2009	30	12	12	10	100	12	100	8	1	11.1
A	32	16	16	13	81.25	13	92.3	3	9	75
A'	32	23	17	15	88.2	8	53.3	3	5	62.5
B	32	13	11	9	81.8	5	55.6	1	8	88.8
C	33	11	11	9	81.8	7	77.8	4	3	42.8
Obradors et al. 2008	35	6	5	5	100	5	100	3	2	60
D	37	7	5	5	100	3	100	1	2	66.7
E	38	33	32	23	71.9	13	56.5	4	9	69.2
F	41	11	11	11	100	11	100	7	4	80
F'	41	14	12	12	100	6	50	4	2	33.3
TOTAL	34.75	146	132	112	86.4	83	72.8%	38	45	54.2

Table 3. Summary of the oocytes retrieved from the eight couples included in the present DF-PGP program and cytogenetic results obtained after the 1PB-CGH analysis.

Monogenic disease detection results

All 81 blastomeres (a mean of 8.1 blastomeres per cycle) were amplified using MDA followed by a patient-specific mutation and STR detection multiplex-PCR as described. Six out of the 81 blastomeres (7.4%) did not provide a diagnostic result and thus were classified as non-diagnosed. Hence, as informative diagnostic result was notified in 92.6% of the blastomeres. Allele drop-out (ADO) affected 15.4% of the analyzed loci, and the PCR amplification efficiency was 93.3%.

Globally, of the 75 diagnosed blastomeres, 20 (26.1%) were homozygote wild-type, 21 (28%) homozygote mutant and the remanding 34 (45.3%) were diagnosed as heterozygote (Table 5). These ratios were not statistically different from the expected Mendelian inheritance rates.

Considering the studied monogenic diseases, 45 out of the 75 embryos were diagnosed as being non-affected (i.e., wild-type homozygotes in VHL and AS diseases, and both wild-type homozygotes and heterozygotes in CF).

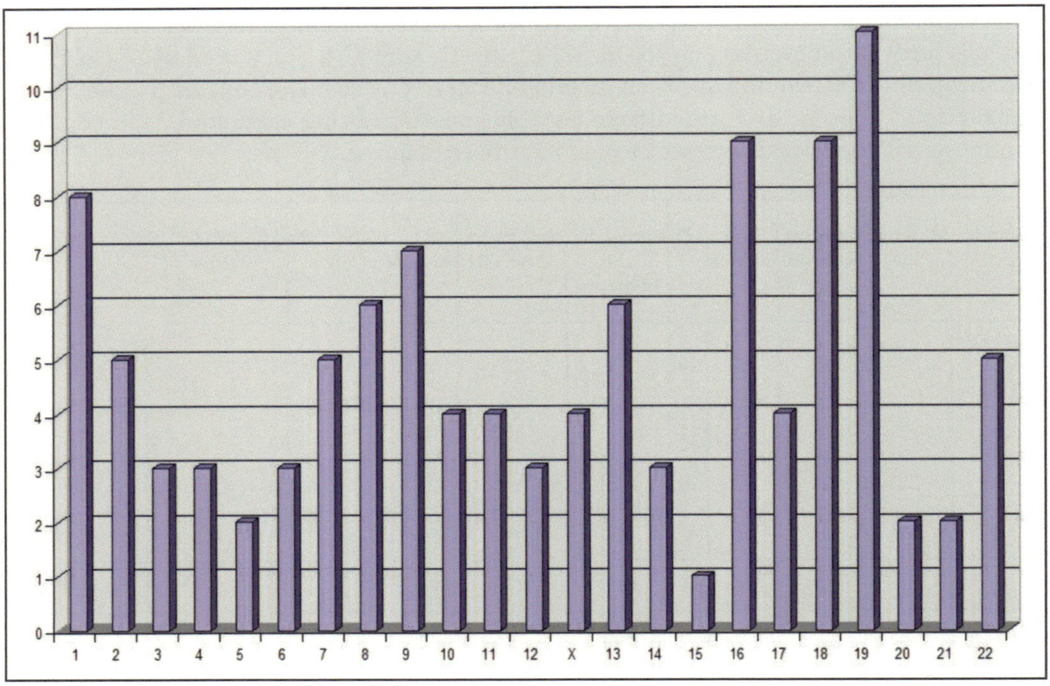

Fig. 2. Incidence of aneuploid chromosomes found in the 1PB-CGH results of the couples included in the present DF-PGP program.

Double-factor dgp outcome and implantation rate versus pgd

Of the 45 embryos free of the disease, in 35 the 1PB-CGH result was available, with the result that 20 of them (57.1%) originated from an aneuploid oocyte and the rest, 15 (42.9%), were potentially euploid. These 15 embryos, free of the monogenic disease and potentially euploid, were tagged as DF-PGD-transferable embryos. No informative 1PB-CGH profiles were obtained from the remaining 10 embryos free of the disease, so only the monogenic-disease diagnosis was performed; they were classified as conventional PGD-transferable embryos.

Consequently, 56 embryos were DF-PGD non-transferable, due to being undiagnosed or affected by the corresponding monogenic disease (6 embryos and 30 embryos, respectively), or due to having originated from aneuploid 1PBs (20 embryos) (Table 6).

On Day +5, according to embryo-quality criteria, nine out of the 15 and eight out of the nine DF-PGD-transferable and conventional PGD-transferable embryos were transferred to nine patients, respectively. Four of them received only DF-PGD-transferable embryos, two received only conventional PGD-transferable embryos and the remaining three patients received both types (Table 6).

Four pregnancies were confirmed with both the hCG test and positive fetal heartbeat. None of the pregnancies involved patients receiving simultaneously both types of embryos (DF-PGD-transferable embryos and conventional PGD-transferable embryos). A pregnancy which turned into the birth of a healthy girl was achieved in one of the patients with just PGD-transferable embryos transferred, and two pregnancies were achieved from the patients receiving only DF-PGD-transferable embryos, which resulted in the birth of three healthy children (one singleton and twins).

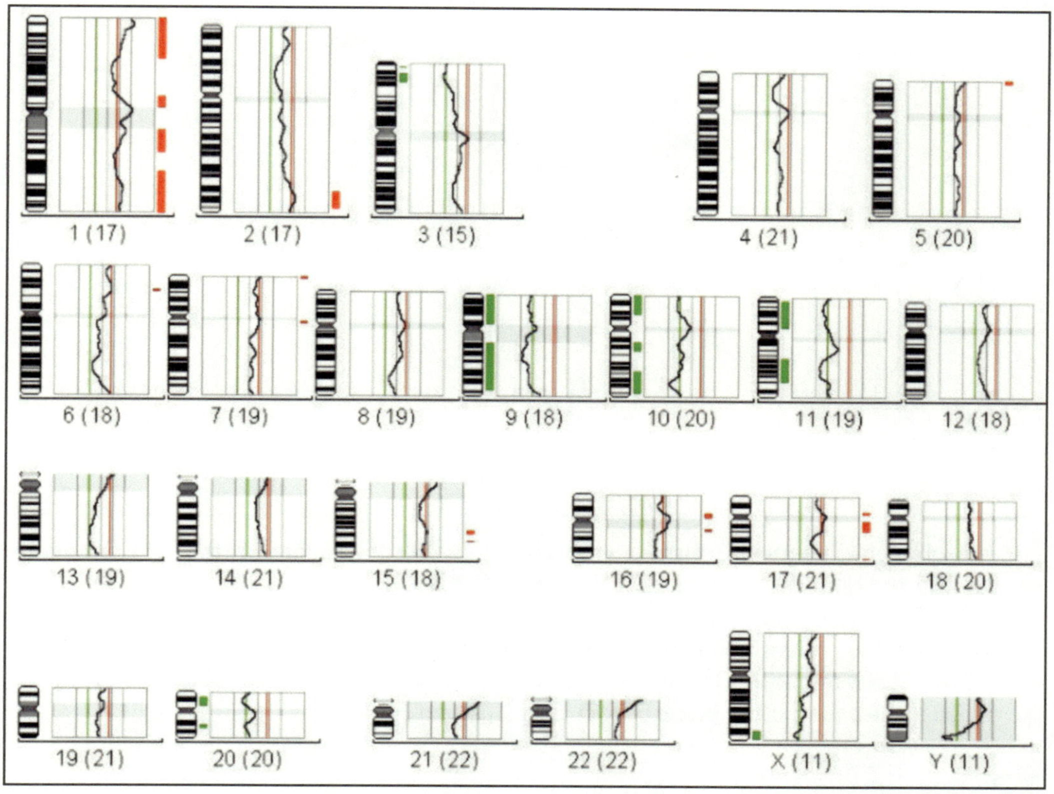

Fig. 3. Comparative Genomic Hybridization profile of 1PB#1 from Patient D, indicating a gain of Chromosome 1 and a loss of Chromosomes 9, 10 and 11. The 1PB would have been misdiagnoses as euploid if instead of CGH; a nine-chromosome FISH would have been used.

Due to most of the embryos were either at the morula stage or degenerated on Day +6, it was totally impossible to isolate blastomeres from the rejected embryos in order to perform a confirmation of both diagnoses.

Prenatal diagnosis has been performed on two out of three pregnancies, according to the parents' decision. In Couple C, an embryo diagnosed as a healthy homozygote turned out to be carrier of one of the copies of the mutation due to ADO of the mutant allele; consequently, the girl delivered was a healthy heterozygote, but a carrier of CF (Figure 4).

Taking into consideration the implantation rate for the two types of embryos, one out of eight embryos healthy for the monogenic disease but undiagnosed for aneuploidies (i.e., PGD-transferable embryos) did implant, achieving an implantation rate of 12.5%, whereas three out of nine healthy embryos diagnosed as potentially euploid (DF-PGD transferable embryos) did implant, meaning an implantation rate of 33.3%. The differences between the groups are not significant for Fisher's test (p= 0.576).

Considering maternal age, none of the six embryos transferred into patients with AMA (mean age of 39.2 y.o.) did implant, whereas four out of the eleven embryos transferred into the patient without AMA (mean age of 32.3 y.o.) implanted. These differences are found to be significantly different (p= 0.03).

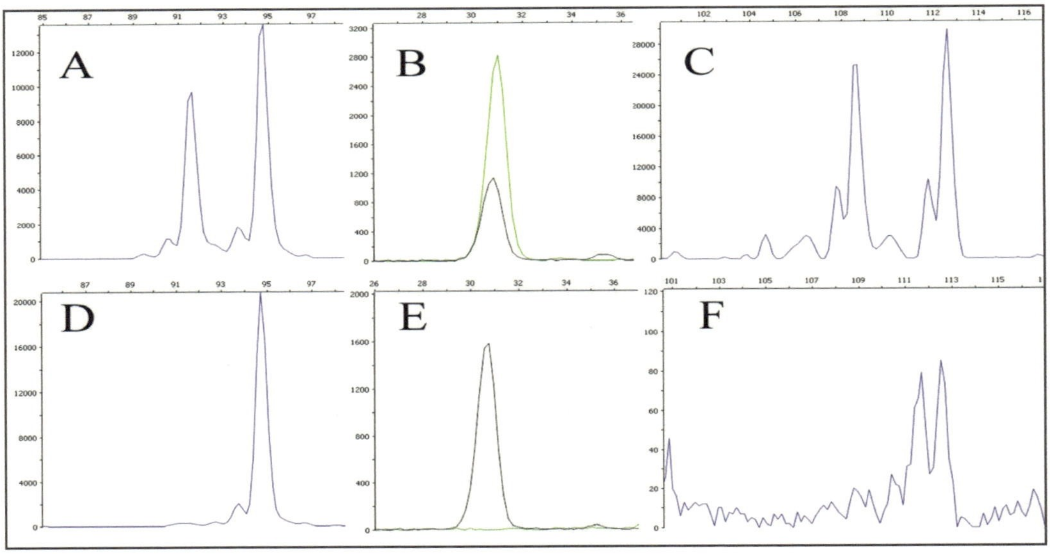

Fig. 4. Monogenic diagnosis results of embryos #4 and #5 of Patient C, carrier of CF. Embryo #4 was affected of both mutation, dF508 (A) and 712GtoC (B), and confirmed with the STR D7S3025 (C), whereas Embryo #5 (D, E, F) was free of both mutations. Embryo #5 was transferred to the patient, achieving a pregnancy. Prenatal diagnosis showed that the foetus carried the dF508 mutation. Therefore, two ADO events occurred in that blastomere, one in the dF508 locus and another in the STR D7S3025 (D and F).

6. Discussion

The embryo implantation rate is one of the most important values in IVF as long as the take-home-baby rate as the major aim of the clinicians is to achieve pregnancy in their IVF patients. Preimplantation Genetic Screening (PGS) appeared to satisfy this demand. It is well documented that aneuploidy affects between 50%-65% of first-trimester abortions (Hassold and Jacobs, 1984, Menasha *et al.*, 2005). Therefore, a positive selection of euploid embryos to transfer should be a useful tool towards an increase of their implantation rate. However, it has been proved that, apart of embryonic mosaicism, the screening of embryos for a limited number of chromosomes is insufficient Steassen et al., 2004 and 2008; Hardarson et al., 2008; Mastenbroek et al., 2007) and that a complete karyotype analysis may be needed to obtain satisfactory results (Sher et al., 2007).

Comparative Genomic Hybridization (CGH) and array-CGH are the main techniques used for comprehensive aneuploidy screening of embryos. The array-CGH has been tested lately for single cells and even applied clinically on blastomeres and on polar bodies, obtaining six pregnancies in nine couples with a clinical history of up to thirteen previous IVF failures (Hellani et al., 2009). One of the main advantages of array-CGH versus conventional CGH is that it is less labour-intensive, more informative and plus it allows embryo diagnosis on Day 4. On the other hand, its main drawback is the cost of the array-CGHs and the consequent processing and analysis equipment required. Thus, in anticipation of more studies of both economic and technical viability of the array-CGH, conventional CGH has been continuously applied with the objective of enhancing the implantation rate with implantation rate up to 68.9% Keskintepe, et al., 2002).

Aiming to contribute on the increase of the implantation rate, even in patients without a previous clinical history of IVF failure or AMA, our group introduced the Double-Factor PGD (DF-PGD), which allows for the selection of potentially euploid embryos with 1PB-CGH and moreover free of the corresponding family monogenic Obradors et al., 2008 and 2009). In the present manuscript we are including results obtained after two years of the application of DF-PGD.

Considering the DF-PGD protocol referred to here, one single blastomere was biopsied from all 81 6-8-cell embryos on Day 3, as recommended by the ESHRE PGD consortium in order not to compromise embryo viability (Thornhill *et al.*, 2005). All 81 blastomeres (a mean of 8.1 blastomeres per cycle) were amplified using MDA prior to PCR amplification with an efficiency rate of 92.59%, similar to the large series of MDA applications previously published, which analyzed 88 and 49 single cells, respectively (Burlet *et al.*, 2006, Renwick *et al.*, 2006). One of the main concerns about MDA is its high ADO rate, which, according to the same cited studies, affects between 25%-27% of the heterozygote cells. In this work, and also analyzing a comparable number of cells, the ADO rate obtained was appreciably low (15.4%). Despite that, on one of the patients (Couple E), the ADO rate found after analyzing their embryos was considerably higher (50%), most probably due to intrinsical problems with this case in particular, as blastomeres quality or transportation issues. If the data from this couple is not included for the ADO rate calculation, its value becomes 11.5%, similar to the obtained from unamplified single cells, and also close to the recommended for the ESHRE PGD consortium Thornhill et al., 2005). The differences in the ADO rates showed in this results compared with the previously published using MDA could be explained by the differences in the size of the PCR amplicons and the type or quality of the amplified cells (Wells, 2004). Unfortunately, and despite the low ADO rate, a misdiagnosis occurred affecting a healthy cystic fibrosis (CF) carrier who was wrongly diagnosed as being a wild-type homozygote.

In that particular case, the family carried two different CF mutations (ΔF508 and 712-1G to T); moreover, they were fully informative for one STR and semi-informative for two more STRs (only informative for one of the progenitors). After MDA and PCR amplification, the analysis showed wild-type alleles for both mutations, failure of amplification on the full informative STR and consistent results on the other two STRs, thus the embryo was diagnosed as being free of both CF mutations. Pregnancy was achieved in this couple, and following the group's recommendation, prenatal diagnosis was performed showing a foetus carrier of the ΔF508 mutation. Hence, two ADO events did occur in that cell, one affecting the ΔF508 mutation site and the other on the semi-informative STR linked to the ΔF508 mutation. This result may indicate that the blastomere analyzed probably was insufficiently lysed. Nevertheless, prenatal diagnosis is mandatory in all PGD cases in order to avoid improbable, but possible misdiagnosis.

In a recent publication, the ESHRE PGS Task Force has aimed for a proof of principle study by a multicentre RCT of the positive effect of implantation of the 1PB and 2PB analysis in the same IVF cycle using a whole chromosome analysis technique as CGH-array (Geraedts et al., 2009) in order to overpass the mosaicism issue and detected all the possible aneuploidies without the requirement of embryo cryopreservation.

In the present study, we have applied a similar approach to the PGS Task Force, also using polar body analysis with a fully comprehensive technique (1PB-CGH). In this case we have decided not the analyze the 2PB in order to avoid an additional second manipulation of the oocytes, after the 1PB biopsy has been performed and due to the first polar body's chromosomal material losing its quality progressively through time (Durban *et al.*, 1998). We also considered inappropriate to wait, at least two hours, for the 2PB extrusion and to perform the biopsy of both polar bodies at the same time. It is obvious that exclusively analyzing the 1PB, meiotic errors produced during second meiotic division remain undetected (Kuliev *et al.*, 2005). Considering that the incidence of the female origin of aneuploidies has been widely described mainly due to errors in the first meiotic division (Hassold and Hunt, 2001, Nicolaidis and Petersen, 1998), we decided that our DF-PGD approach was more than appropriate neither the oocyte nor the embryo was compromised.

A total of 115 1PBs were biopsied from their corresponding oocytes on Day 0, but only 77 of them were analyzed by CGH since the producing embryo was diagnosed as being affected by the monogenic disease. Surprisingly, 54.2% of the 1PBs were aneuploid. This high rate is similar to that previously described in CGH studies of 1PBs-oocytes doublets of IVF patients Gutiérrez-Mateo et al., 2004 a and b). It is noteworthy that the patients that underwent this study were selected for monogenic disease detection, not for sterility problems, so the fact that their aneuploidy rate is similar to that of IVF patients emphasizes the importance of aneuploidy screening even in patients without fertility problems. Moreover, after dividing the patients into two age groups, ≤35 or >35 years old, a similar rate of aneuploidy was found between them (56% vs. 51.5%, respectively). These results, although higher, are comparable to the ones obtained on a previous study of our group after analysis, with CGH, 1PB-MII doublets from 53 IVF donors with a mean age of 26.1 years old (Obradors *et al.*, 2010). The study shows that, despite being produced by young women, 32.1% of the analyzed oocytes were aneuploid. Moreover, it demonstrates that almost 40% of the donors had at least one aneuploid oocyte.

This high aneuploidy rate found in young fertile women, concordant with that described in this manuscript, may be explained due to the ovarian stimulation process (Weghofer *et al.*, 2008, Weghofer *et al.*, 2008). This suggests that not only aged patients may benefit from aneuploidy screening with CGH, but also younger women without sterility problems.

Almost half of the detected aneuploid 1PBs (44.4%), some of them containing up to 4 chromosome abnormalities (such as 1PB#1 from Patient D), would have been diagnosed as being completely euploid if a nine-chromosome (13, 15, 16, 17, 18, 21, 22, X and Y) FISH had been used instead of CGH. This means that even performing an exhaustive FISH aneuploidy screening, almost half of the aneuploid embryos could still have been transferred into the patient's uterus, despite their intrinsic impossibilities to develop a pregnancy.

Consequently, in order to increase the implantation rate, not only a partial chromosome screening must be performed but also it must be done using a full-chromosome analysis technique such as CGH.

Referring to the data presented here, from the 45 developing embryos healthy for their specific monogenic disease, 20 of them originated from a potentially aneuploid oocyte diagnosed with 1PB-CGH, whereas 15 of them were diagnosed as being potentially euploid (tagged as DF-PGD transferable embryos). In the remaining ten embryos, no CGH results had been obtained, and they were classified as PGD transferable embryos.

Nine out of fifteen and eight out of ten embryos were transferred to the patients from the DF-PGD-transferable and PGD-transferable groups, respectively. Three patients (A', B, and E) received both types of embryos. Three from the nine and one out of the eight transferred embryos from each group implanted and developed into the birth of four healthy children. In none of the patients receiving both types of embryos did implantation occur. Also, none of the patients with AMA (mean age of 39.2 y.o.) became pregnant although six embryos were transferred; on the other hand, the four pregnancies achieved did occur in younger patients after transferring 11 embryos. These differences are found to be significantly different (p= 0.03), and may be explained by other factors, rather than aneuploidy, that might affect the implantation rate in aged women like gynecological or immunological aspects, although more studies are required to reach clear conclusions.

Therefore, the implantation rate was 33.3% in the embryos doubly selected (DF-PGD transferable embryos) and 12.5% in the embryos selected as being of the monogenic disease but not screened for aneuploidy, a value that is very similar to the average value (15.2%) obtained in the last ESHRE Consortium Steering Committee recompilation (Harper et al., 2010). Despite the differences between the implantation rates of the DF-DGP transferred embryos being two times higher that the DGP transferred embryos are promising, these differences were not significant. Most probably, the reduced number of clinical applications presented in this work is not enough to have major differences.

In conclusion, although the DF-PGD-selected embryos did not obtain a significant increase of implantation compared with embryos undiagnosed for aneuploidy, it seems clear that comprehensive aneuploidy screening of oocytes using a PGD protocol might benefit the clinical outcome of their corresponding embryo. Therefore, in order to increase the implantation of embryos selected that are free of a monogenic disease, and until the routine assessment of CGH-array methodology, 1PB-CGH is the preferred technique to positively doubly select potentially euploid embryos.

7. Acknowledgements

This work was supported by the Ministerio de Sanidad y Consumo Fondo de Investigaciόn Sanitaria Instituto de Salud Carlos III (FIS-ISCIII; PI 080012), the Grup de Suport a la Recerca de la Generalitat de Catalunya 2009SGR1107 and by the Càtedra de Recerca EUGIN. The manuscript was read and corrected by Mr. Chuck Simmons, a native English-speaking Instructor of English at the authors' university.

8. References

Handyside AH, Kontogianni EH, Hardy K and Winston RM (1990) Pregnancies from biopsied human preimplantation embryos sexed by Y-specific DNA amplification. Nature 344, 768-770.

Munne S and Weier HU (1996) Simultaneous enumeration of chromosomes 13, 18, 21, X, and Y in interphase cells for preimplantation genetic diagnosis of aneuploidy. Cytogenet Cell Genet 75, 263-270.

Verlinsky Y, Cieslak J, Freidine M, Ivakhnenko V, Wolf G, Kovalinskaya L, White M, Lifchez A, Kaplan B, Moise J *et al.* (1996) Polar body diagnosis of common aneuploidies by FISH. J Assist Reprod Genet 13, 157-162.

Verlinsky Y, Cieslak J, Ivakhnenko V, Lifchez A, Strom C and Kuliev A (1996) Birth of healthy children after preimplantation diagnosis of common aneuploidies by polar body fluorescent in situ hybridization analysis. Preimplantation Genetics Group. Fertil Steril 66, 126-129.

Staessen C, Platteau P, Van Assche E, Michiels A, Tournaye H, Camus M, Devroey P, Liebaers I and Van Steirteghem A (2004) Comparison of blastocyst transfer with or without preimplantation genetic diagnosis for aneuploidy screening in couples with advanced maternal age: a prospective randomized controlled trial. Hum Reprod 19, 2849-2858.

Staessen C, Verpoest W, Donoso P, Haentjens P, Van der Elst J, Liebaers I and Devroey P (2008) Preimplantation genetic screening does not improve delivery rate in women under the age of 36 following single-embryo transfer. Hum Reprod 23, 2818-2825.

Hardarson T, Hanson C, Lundin K, Hillensjo T, Nilsson L, Stevic J, Reismer E, Borg K, Wikland M and Bergh C (2008) Preimplantation genetic screening in women of advanced maternal age caused a decrease in clinical pregnancy rate: a randomized controlled trial. Hum Reprod 23, 2806-2812.

Mastenbroek S, Twisk M, van Echten-Arends J, Sikkema-Raddatz B, Korevaar JC, Verhoeve HR, Vogel NE, Arts EG, de Vries JW, Bossuyt PM *et al.* (2007) In vitro fertilization with preimplantation genetic screening. N Engl J Med 357, 9-17.

Harper JC, Coonen E,De Rycke M, Harton G, Moutou C, Pehlivan T, Traeger-Synodinos J, Van Rij MC and Goossens V (2010) ESHRE PGD Consortium data collection X: cycles from January to December 2007 with pregnancy follow-up to October 2008 Hum Reprod 25 (11), 2685-2707. (instead of Goossens V, Harton G, Moutou C, Scriven PN, Traeger-Synodinos J, Sermon K and Harper JC (2008) ESHRE PGD Consortium data collection VIII: cycles from January to December 2005 with pregnancy follow-up to October 2006. Hum Reprod 23, 2629-2645.)

Andersen AN, Goossens V, Ferraretti AP, Bhattacharya S, Felberbaum R, de Mouzon J and Nygren KG (2008) Assisted reproductive technology in Europe, 2004: results generated from European registers by ESHRE. Hum Reprod 23, 756-771.

Keskintepe L, Sher G and Keskintepe M (2007) Reproductive oocyte/embryo genetic analysis: comparison between fluorescence in-situ hybridization and comparative genomic hybridization. Reprod Biomed Online 15, 303-309.

Sher G, Keskintepe L, Keskintepe M, Ginsburg M, Maassarani G, Yakut T, Baltaci V, Kotze D and Unsal E (2007) Oocyte karyotyping by comparative genomic hybridization [correction of hybrydization] provides a highly reliable method for selecting "competent" embryos, markedly improving in vitro fertilization outcome: a multiphase study. Fertil Steril 87, 1033-1040.

Voullaire L, Wilton L, McBain J, Callaghan T and Williamson R (2002) Chromosome abnormalities identified by comparative genomic hybridization in embryos from women with repeated implantation failure. Mol Hum Reprod 8, 1035-1041.

Wells D, Escudero T, Levy B, Hirschhorn K, Delhanty JD and Munne S (2002) First clinical application of comparative genomic hybridization and polar body testing for preimplantation genetic diagnosis of aneuploidy. Fertil Steril 78, 543-549.

Wilton L (2005) Preimplantation genetic diagnosis and chromosome analysis of blastomeres using comparative genomic hybridization. Hum Reprod Update 11, 33-41.

Hassold T and Hunt P (2001) To err (meiotically) is human: the genesis of human aneuploidy. Nat Rev Genet 2, 280-291.

Nicolaidis P and Petersen MB (1998) Origin and mechanisms of non-disjunction in human autosomal trisomies. Hum Reprod 13, 313-319.

Fiegler H, Geigl JB, Langer S, Rigler D, Porter K, Unger K, Carter NP and Speicher MR (2007) High resolution array-CGH analysis of single cells. Nucleic Acids Res 35, e15.

Hu DG, Webb G and Hussey N (2004) Aneuploidy detection in single cells using DNA array-based comparative genomic hybridization. Mol Hum Reprod 10, 283-289.

Le Caignec C, Spits C, Sermon K, De Rycke M, Thienpont B, Debrock S, Staessen C, Moreau Y, Fryns JP, Van Steirteghem A *et al.* (2006) Single-cell chromosomal imbalances detection by array CGH. Nucleic Acids Res 34, e68.

Wells D, Bermudez M, Steuerwald N, Chu L, Weier U, Cohen J and Munne S (2004) Microarrays for analysis and diagnosis of human embryos. In Papp Z and Rodeck

C (eds) Recent Advances in Prenatal Genetic Diagnosis. Medimond, Bologna, Italy, pp. 9-17.

Handyside AH, Harton GL, Mariani B, Thornhill AR, Affara NA, Shaw MA and Griffin DK (2009) Karyomapping: a Universal Method for Genome Wide Analysis of Genetic Disease based on Mapping Crossovers between Parental Haplotypes. J Med Genet.

Hellani A, Abu-Amero K, Azouri J and El-Akoum S (2008) Successful pregnancies after application of array-comparative genomic hybridization in PGS-aneuploidy screening. Reprod Biomed Online 17, 841-847.

Fishel S, Gordon A, Lynch C, Dowell K, Ndukwe G, Kelada E, Thornton S, Jenner L, Cater E, Brown A *et al.* (2009) Live birth after polar body array comparative genomic hybridization prediction of embryo ploidy-the future of IVF? Fertil Steril.

Geraedts J, Collins J, Gianaroli L, Goossens V, Handyside A, Harper J, Montag M, Repping S and Schmutzler A (2009) What next for preimplantation genetic screening? A polar body approach! Hum Reprod.

Thornhill A, Holding C and Monk M (1994) Recycling the single cell to detect specific chromosomes and to investigate specific gene sequences. Hum Reprod 9, 2150-2155.

Rechitsky S, Freidine M, Verlinsky Y and Strom CM (1996) Allele dropout in sequential PCR and FISH analysis of single cells (cell recycling). J Assist Reprod Genet 13, 115-124.

Obradors A, Fernandez E, Oliver-Bonet M, Rius M, de la Fuente A, Wells D, Benet J and Navarro J (2008) Birth of a healthy boy after a double factor PGD in a couple carrying a genetic disease and at risk for aneuploidy: case report. Hum Reprod 23, 1949-1956.

Obradors A, Fernandez E, Rius M, Oliver-Bonet M, Martinez-Fresno M, Benet J and Navarro J (2009) Outcome of twin babies free of Von Hippel-Lindau disease after a double-factor preimplantation genetic diagnosis: monogenetic mutation analysis and comprehensive aneuploidy screening. Fertil Steril 91, 933 e931-937.

Fiorentino F, Magli MC, Podini D, Ferraretti AP, Nuccitelli A, Vitale N, Baldi M and Gianaroli L (2003) The minisequencing method: an alternative strategy for preimplantation genetic diagnosis of single gene disorders. Mol Hum Reprod 9, 399-410.

Spits C, Le Caignec C, De Rycke M, Van Haute L, Van Steirteghem A, Liebaers I and Sermon K (2006) Optimization and evaluation of single-cell whole-genome multiple displacement amplification. Hum Mutat 27, 496-503.

Gutierrez-Mateo C, Benet J, Wells D, Colls P, Bermudez MG, Sanchez-Garcia JF, Egozcue J, Navarro J and Munne S (2004a) Aneuploidy study of human oocytes first polar body comparative genomic hybridization and metaphase II fluorescence in situ hybridization analysis. Hum Reprod 19, 2859-2868.

Gutierrez-Mateo C, Wells D, Benet J, Sanchez-Garcia JF, Bermudez MG, Belil I, Egozcue J, Munne S and Navarro J (2004b) Reliability of comparative genomic hybridization to detect chromosome abnormalities in first polar bodies and metaphase II oocytes. Hum Reprod 19, 2118-2125.

Telenius H, Carter NP, Bebb CE, Nordenskjold M, Ponder BA and Tunnacliffe A (1992) Degenerate oligonucleotide-primed PCR: general amplification of target DNA by a single degenerate primer. Genomics 13, 718-725.

Voullaire L, Wilton L, Slater H and Williamson R (1999) Detection of aneuploidy in single cells using comparative genomic hybridization. Prenat Diagn 19, 846-851.

Wells D, Sherlock JK, Handyside AH and Delhanty JD (1999) Detailed chromosomal and molecular genetic analysis of single cells by whole genome amplification and comparative genomic hybridisation. Nucleic Acids Res 27, 1214-1218.

Hassold TJ and Jacobs PA (1984) Trisomy in man. Annu Rev Genet 18, 69-97.

Menasha J, Levy B, Hirschhorn K and Kardon NB (2005) Incidence and spectrum of chromosome abnormalities in spontaneous abortions: new insights from a 12-year study. Genet Med 7, 251-263.

Wells D, Alfarawati S and Fragouli E (2008) Use of comprehensive chromosomal screening for embryo assessment: microarrays and CGH. Mol Hum Reprod.

Schoolcraft WB, Fragouli E, Stevens J, Munne S, Katz-Jaffe MG and Wells D (2009) Clinical application of comprehensive chromosomal screening at the blastocyst stage. Fertil Steril.

Fragouli E, Katz-Jaffe M, Alfarawati S, Stevens J, Colls P, Goodall NN, Tormasi S, Gutierrez-Mateo C, Prates R, Schoolcraft WB *et al.* (2009) Comprehensive chromosome screening of polar bodies and blastocysts from couples experiencing repeated implantation failure. Fertil Steril.

Thornhill AR, deDie-Smulders CE, Geraedts JP, Harper JC, Harton GL, Lavery SA, Moutou C, Robinson MD, Schmutzler AG, Scriven PN *et al.* (2005) ESHRE PGD Consortium 'Best practice guidelines for clinical preimplantation genetic diagnosis (PGD) and preimplantation genetic screening (PGS)'. Hum Reprod 20, 35-48.

Burlet P, Frydman N, Gigarel N, Kerbrat V, Tachdjian G, Feyereisen E, Bonnefont JP, Frydman R, Munnich A and Steffann J (2006) Multiple displacement amplification improves PGD for fragile X syndrome. Mol Hum Reprod 12, 647-652.

Renwick PJ, Trussler J, Ostad-Saffari E, Fassihi H, Black C, Braude P, Ogilvie CM and Abbs S (2006) Proof of principle and first cases using preimplantation genetic haplotyping--a paradigm shift for embryo diagnosis. Reprod Biomed Online 13, 110-119.

Wells D (2004) Advances in preimplantation genetic diagnosis. Eur J Obstet Gynecol Reprod Biol 115 Suppl 1, S97-101.

Durban M, Benet J, Sarquella J, Egozcue J and Navarro J (1998) Chromosome studies in first polar bodies from hamster and human oocytes. Hum Reprod 13, 583-587.

Kuliev A, Cieslak J and Verlinsky Y (2005) Frequency and distribution of chromosome abnormalities in human oocytes. Cytogenet Genome Res 111, 193-198.

Fragouli E, Wells D, Doshi A, Gotts S, Harper JC and Delhanty JD (2006) Complete cytogenetic investigation of oocytes from a young cancer patient with the use of comparative genomic hybridisation reveals meiotic errors. Prenat Diagn 26, 71-76.

Fragouli E, Wells D, Thornhill A, Serhal P, Faed MJ, Harper JC and Delhanty JD (2006) Comparative genomic hybridization analysis of human oocytes and polar bodies. Hum Reprod 21, 2319-2328.

Obradors A, Rius M, Cuzzi J, Daina G, Gutierrez-Mateo C, Pujol A, Marina F, Marquez C, Benet J and Navarro J (2010) Errors at mitotic segregation early in oogenesis and at first meiotic division in oocytes from donor females: Comparative genomic hybridization analyses in metaphase II oocytes and their first polar body. Fertil Steril. 93(2), 675-9.

Weghofer A, Munne S, Brannath W, Chen S, Barad D, Cohen J and Gleicher N (2008) The impact of LH-containing gonadotropin stimulation on euploidy rates in preimplantation embryos: antagonist cycles. Fertil Steril.

Weghofer A, Munne S, Brannath W, Chen S, Tomkin G, Cekleniak N, Garrisi M, Barad D, Cohen J and Gleicher N (2008) The impact of LH-containing gonadotropins on diploidy rates in preimplantation embryos: long protocol stimulation. Hum Reprod 23, 499-503.

10

Preimplantation HLA Typing

Semra Kahraman and Cagri Beyazyurek
IVF and Reproductive Genetics Center, İstanbul Memorial Hospital
Turkey

1. Introduction

It has been more than ten years since the first Human Leukocyte Antigen (HLA) matching for Fanconi anemia was reported, allowing successful haemopoietic reconstitution in affected sibling by transplantation of stem cells obtained from HLA-matched offspring (Verlinsky et al., 2000; Verlinsky et al., 2001). Preimplantation Genetic Diagnosis (PGD) in combination with HLA matching is being used to detect a particular gene mutation in an unaffected child who can be an HLA donor for its' sibling. HLA typing without mutation analysis has also been used for acquired diseases (Verlinsky et al., 2004), such as acute myeloid leukemia (AML) and acute lymphoid leukemia (ALL), which require allogenic haemopoietic stem cell transplantation (HSCT) from an HLA identical donor for the cure of the disease. Stem cells in the cord blood from an HLA identical sibling can be used with a much higher success rate than a transplant from alternative donors (Gaziev et al., 2000; Orofino et al., 2003) and are therefore of great therapeutic value for hematopoietic and other life-threatening diseases (Fiorentino et al., 2006; Kahraman et al., 2004, 2007; Verlinsky et al., 2001, 2004; Van de Velde et al., 2004, 2009).

In particular for blood-borne disorders, hematopoietic stem cells (HSC) from HLA-identical siblings provide the highest success rate and current results indicate that about 90% of the cases can be cured successfully after HSC transplantation (Gaziev et al., 2005). Use of cord blood as a stem cell source also results in reduced incidence of graft rejection and other serious complications associated with bone marrow transplantation. However, in most cases a suitable donor cannot be found in the family, and due to a small number of children per family, only one third of patients are able to find an HLA-identical sibling (Costeas, 2004). The probability of having an unaffected child who may also be an HLA match for an affected sibling is only one in five; these families often went through multiple cycles of pregnancy before conceiving an unaffected HLA match. In the remaining patients the only resort is the identification of a matched unrelated donor. However, the probability of finding an HLA matched unrelated donor cord blood from the cord blood units is extremely low. Therefore PGD is a much more attractive option, with this technique, sufficient number of embryos may be tested at one time, increasing the chances of identifying an appropriate match.

More than 2000 healthy children have already been born after PGD and the expanding indications include chromosomal abnormalities, single gene disorders, HLA tissue typing of the embryos, predisposition of adult onset disorders, translocations and cancer predispositions (Simpson 2001; Kuliev et al., 2004; Fiorentino et al., 2004; 2006; Kahraman et al., 2005; 2007; Van de Velde et al., 2004; Kokkali et al., 2007). In fact PGD can be carried out for any disorder in which molecular testing can be performed. A partial list of disorders in which Preimplantation Genetic Diagnosis/HLA typing can be applied is shown in Table 1. Although the majority of these disorders are due to rare genetic defects, the incidence of some, such as β thalassemia, sickle cell anemia and cystic fibrosis are very common in certain parts of the world, such as Mediterranean region which include Turkey, Italy, Greece and Cyprus. Turkey is one of the Mediterranean countries in which thalassemia mutations are commonly seen, with a carrier rate of 2.1% in the population (Aksoy, et al., 1985).

Achondroplasia (FGFR3)	Hyper IgM
Acute Lymphocytic Leukemia (ALL)	Krabbe (GALC)
Acute Myelogenous Leukemia (AML)	Li-Fraumeni Syndrome (TP53)
Alpha-Thalassemia (HBA)	Marfan Syndrome (MFN1)
Alzheimer Early Onset (PSEN1)	Metachromatic Leukodystrophy (ARSA)
Beta-Thalassemia (HBB)	Mucolipidosis 2 (I-Cell)
Charcot-Marie-Tooth	Myotonic Dystrophy
Chronic Granulamatous Disease (CYBB)	Neurofibromatosis (NF1 &NF2)
Chronic Myelogenous Leukemia (CML)	Neiman Pick Type C
Crigler Najjar (UGTIA1)	Phenylketanuria (PKU)
Cystic Fibrosis (CFTR)	Polycystic Kidney Disease (AR-PKD1)
Diamond Blackfan Anemia(DBA-RSP19)	Retinoblastoma
Duchenne Muscular Distrophy (DMD)	Sanflippo A (MPSIIIA)
Fanconi Anemia A,C,F,G	Severe combined immunodeficiency (SCID-XI)
Fragile X (FMR1)	Sickle Cell (HBB)
Gaucher Disease (GBA)	Spinal Muscular Atrophy (SMN1)
Glycogen Storage Disease,type IA	Spinocerebellar Ataxia (SCA-2,SCA-3)
Hemophilia A,B	Tay Sacs (HEXA)
Huntington Disease (HD)	Tuberosclerosis (TSC1)
Hurler Syndrome (MPSI-IDUA)	Wiscott-Aldrich Syndome

Table 1. Some of the current indications of PGD/HLA Typing

According to data collected by the Turkish Association of Thalassemia, the heterozygosity rate may be higher than 10%, particularly in the southern regions of Turkey (Basak et al., 2007). A higher rate of consanguineous marriages in those regions is a factor which further increases the incidence of thalassemia. In addition, thalassemia has a great heterogeneity in Turkey, the total frequency of the 6 most commonly seen mutations is only 69% of the whole mutations. The selection of embryos for HLA typing necessitates the application of ART even though the vast majority of the couples are fertile. The successful outcome of ART cycles is highly dependent on female age and ovarian reserve. This technique is made crucially important by the fact that, the theoretical probability of finding an HLA identical embryo in cases of acquired diseases is 25% (1/4) and the probability of finding both HLA identical and mutation free embryo in cases of single gene disorders no more than 18% (3/16). Using a standard IVF procedure, oocytes or embryos are tested for causative gene mutations simultaneously with HLA alleles, selecting and transferring only those unaffected embryos, which are HLA matched to the affected sibling.

The HLA Complex (Human Leukocyte Antigen) is located on chromosome 6 and represents one of the most polymorphic regions of human genome. Comparative DNA sequence analysis of HLA complex has shown the presence of a high number of alleles in this region. Linked short tandem repeat (STR) markers scattered through the HLA complex were studied to increase the accuracy of the analysis and to detect potential contaminations and crossing over occurrence between HLA genes.

Single cell PCR technique has several pitfalls, such as contamination by extraneous DNA, amplification failure, preferential amplification, and allele drop out (ADO) which is the failure of PCR to amplify one of the two alleles. If ADO occurs, only a single allele is amplified and detected after PCR, giving a heterozygous cell the appearance of homozygosity. This may lead to harmful consequences such as in the case for a dominant disease; failure to amplify the mutant allele may lead to the transfer of affected embryos. The ADO rate and the efficiency of amplification of targeted regions depend on efficient lysis methods (Shirazi et al., 2009) and also the type of cell analyzed. With simultaneous usage of linked STR markers the accuracy of single cell PCR is approximately 98% (Rechitsky et al., 2001). ADO rates in single cells can be decreased by analyzing more than one cell which is possible with blastocyst-stage biopsy. Trophectoderm biopsy is a good alternative to cleavage stage biopsy as it enables the evaluation of approximately 2-5 cells, thus decreasing both the rate of amplification failures and ADO associated with single cell PCR (McArthur et al., 2008; Pangalos et al., 2008). There are many advantages of blastocyst stage biopsy such that; since trophectoderm cells are extra-embryonic tissue, the removal of these cells avoids the risk of affecting the development of the fetus. Also the proportion of the cells that are removed is much lower compared to cleavage stage biopsy. Furthermore, blastocyst stage embryos have a higher implantation potential compared to day-3 or day-4 embryos, so a higher rate of implantation could be achieved by trophectoderm analysis (Kokkali et al., 2007; McArthur et al., 2008).

2. Materials and methods

2.1 Study group

The study group consisted of a total of 188 couples with a total of 362 cycles. Between 2003 and the mid of 2011 at Istanbul Memorial Hospital, ART and Reproductive Genetics Center, 149 couples were referred for both mutation analysis for a specific genetic disorder and HLA typing, while 39 couples were referred for the sole purpose of HLA typing for acquired disorders. The detailed list of diseases can be found in Table 2.

2.2 Pre-clinical work up

First, a haplotype analysis of mother, father and child, and when available of other family members, was performed for each family prior to preimplantation HLA typing. For this, genomic DNA is isolated from peripheral blood samples of father, mother and the affected child. To rule out a possible recombination in the affected child, other family members such as unaffected child, or grandparents' DNA have been added to set up procedure. Figure 1 shows the polymorphic STR markers scattered through HLA region which were used to detect any possible ADO in relation to HLA typing.

	TOTAL	**188 couples**	**362 cycles**
HLA + Mutation testing	β-thalassemia	131	258
	Wiscott Aldrich	3	4
	X-Adrenoleukodystrophy	3	3
	Fanconi Anemia	3	4
	Alpha-Mannosidosis	1	4
	Gaucher Syndrome	1	4
	Hurler Syndrome	2	3
	Hyper IgD	1	1
	Glanzmann Trombasthenia	1	2
	Sickle Cell Anemia	1	1
	Diamond Blackfan Anemia	1	1
	Cd3 Deficiency	1	1
HLA only	Acute Lymphoblastic Leukemia	17	30
	Acute Myeloid Leukemia	11	20
	Diamond Blackfan Anemia	3	11
	Histiocytosis	1	3
	Chronic Myeloid Leukemia	1	2
	Burkitt's Lymfoma	1	2
	Aplastic Anemia	2	2
	Anaplastic Anemia	1	3
	Myelodysplastic Syndrome	1	2
	Non-hodgin Lymfoma	1	1

Table 2. Cycle participations of patients and indications for HLA Typing.

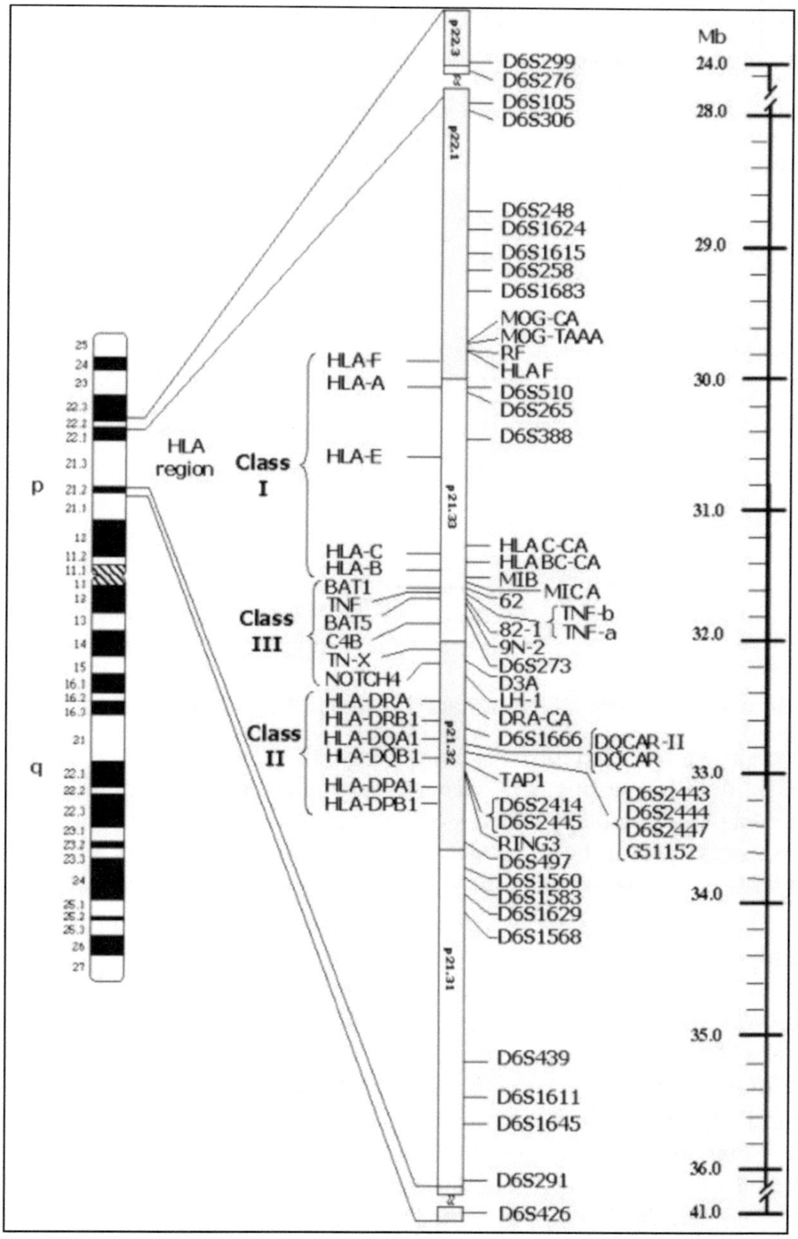

Fig. 1. Polymorphic STR markers used in HLA typing of the embryos.

A panel of 50 different short tandem repeat (STR) markers (figure 1) were tested on genomic DNAs to ensure the presence of enough informative markers (figure 2) to aid the identification of monosomy, trisomy, recombination, allele-drop out (ADO) and uniparental disomy (UPD) of the analyzed chromosomes and regions. For each family at least 12 heterozygous markers spanning the HLA-A, HLA-B, HLA-C, HLA-DR,HLA-DQ regions (HLA Classes I, II, and III) were selected for PGD Study.

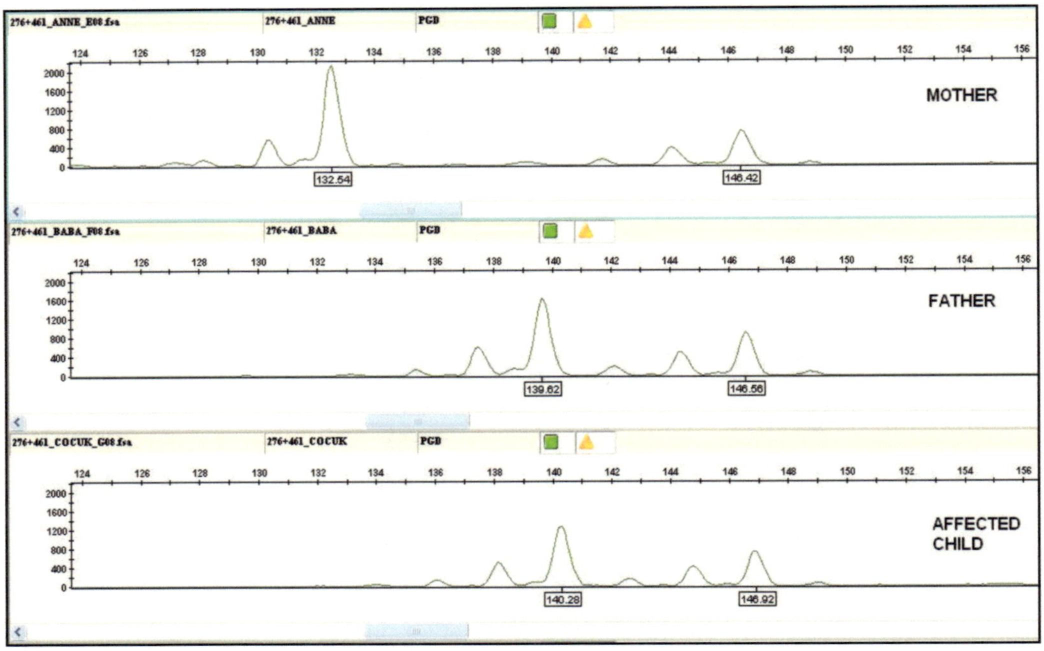

Fig. 2. Identification of informative markers during HLA set up study

The study period was divided into two according to the methods used which included lysis of single cells, mutation testing, polymerase chain reaction (PCR) conditions and primers used in the PGD study. Oocyte collections, inseminations, culture, biopsy and transfer of embryos were performed in Istanbul Memorial Hospital ART unit and all PGD studies and evaluations were performed in Istanbul Memorial Hospital Reproductive Genetics Unit.

2.3 PGD study

The methods can be found elsewhere (Kahraman et al., 2011). In the first period, the alkaline lysis method was used as described previously (Fiorentino et al., 2005). Cells were lysed by incubation at 65C° for 10 minutes in a sterile PCR tube containing 5 µl of lysis buffer (200nmol/1 KOH, 50nmol/1 DDT). The lysis buffer was then neutralized prior to adding the first-round PCR mix which contained all external primers for co-amplification of all selected HLA markers and mutation linked markers. Second-round PCR reaction for each locus was then performed using 2 µl of the first round product.

In the second period, the Proteinase K method was used for lysis of the cells as described previously (Verlinsky et al., 2001). The biopsied single cells were placed into a lysis solution containing 0,5 µl of 10xPCR buffer, 0,5 µl of 1% tween-20, 0,5 µl of 1% triton X-100, 3,5 µl of water, and 0,05 µl of proteinase K. The lysis reaction was as follows: 45 C° for 15 minutes for the lysis of the cells and 96 C° for 20 minutes for inactivation of proteinase K. Although the reaction conditions were different in the two periods, both can be briefly summarized as follows; DNA testing was performed by two rounds of PCR reactions: in the first round, using multiplex PCR which allows simultaneous amplification of HLA regions and mutation-linked markers and in the second round, using singleplex PCR which is a fluorescent PCR with semi or heminested primers. Primer sequences and polymerase chain

reaction conditions used in this study have been reported previously (Verlinsky et al., 2001; Fiorentino et al., 2004; 2005; Rechitsky et al., 2004; Verlinsky et al., 2004).
Between 2003 and 2008, mutation analysis was performed using the minisequencing technique, as described elsewhere (Fiorentino et al., 2003). After middle of 2008 restriction enzyme digestion reactions and subsequently polyacrylamide gel electrophoresis analysis were used (Rechitsky et al., 2004). Since the middle of 2009s, both methods are being used according to preference.

2.4 IVF and embryo biopsy procedure

The stimulation protocols were as outlined previously (Kahraman et al., 2004). Oocyte retrievals were performed 36 h after the injection of rhCG (ovitrel) by transvaginal-ultrasound-guidance. Approximately 2-3 h after oocyte retrieval, cumulus cells were enzymatically removed. Intracytoplasmic sperm injection (ICSI) was applied to metaphase II oocytes. One blastomere was removed from cleavage stage embryos (figure 3a) from an opening made using laser (IodoLaser, Research Instruments). Subsequently, embryo transfer

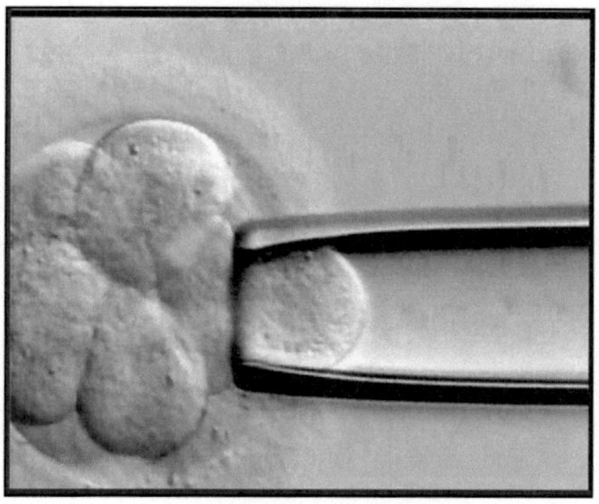

a) Clevage Stage Biopsy

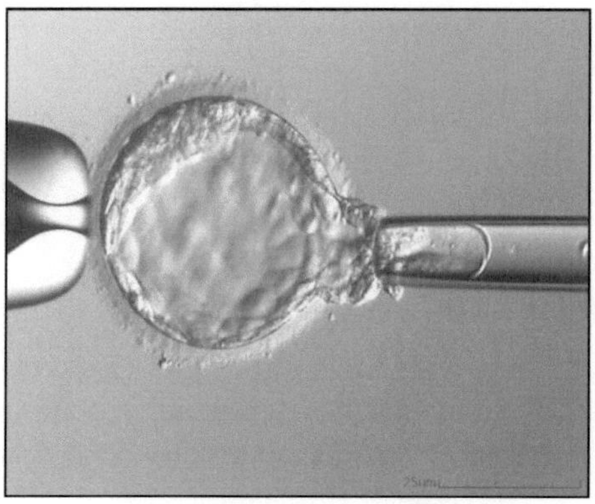

b) Blastocyst Stage Biopsy

Fig. 3. Biopsy Techniques

was performed usually on day-4 but rarely on day-5. Recently, since 2009, trophectoderm tissue biopsies have also been performed. Blastocyst-stage biopsy was performed by making a hole in the zona pellucida on day-3 of embryonic development which allowed the developing trophectoderm cells to protrude after blastulation, facilitating the biopsy. On day-5 post-fertilization, approximately 4-5 cells were excised using laser energy, without loss of inner cell mass (figure 3b). After diagnosis, the embryos was replaced during the same cycle, on day-5 or 6. Pregnancy was first evaluated by serum hCG concentrations assay, 12 days after embryo transfer and clinical pregnancy was diagnosed by ultrasonographic visualization of one or more gestational sacs.

3. Results

In HLA+mutation testing group (Group I), and HLA-only group (Group II), 62.2% and 72.4% of the initiated cycles reached the stage of embryo transfer, respectively. The detailed distribution of indications and overall results for each group was shown in Table 2 and 3.
A full diagnosis was achieved in 91.0% of the biopsied samples. In Group I, 17.8 % of the analyzed embryos were found to be HLA compatible. HLA compatible and disease free embryos were 12.9 % of all diagnosed embryos. In group II, 17.2% of embryos were found to be HLA matched and 71.4% HLA non-matched.

	HLA+mutation testing (Group I)	HLA Only (Group II)	TOTAL
No of patients/cycles	149/286	39/76	188/362
Maternal age, mean	32.0±4.83	33.9±5.65	
Cycles with transfer, %	62.2	72.4	
No of embryos transfered, mean	1.55±0.71	1.56±0.72	
Clinical pregnancy rate per transfer, %	37.6	32.7	
Implantation rate,%	28.9	24.4	
Clinical miscarriages, n	14	3	
No of babies born, n	57	13	
No of succsessful transplantations, n	23	2	25*

*21 children are awaiting an appropriate time for HSC transplantation.

Table 3. Overall clinical results of HLA typing.

The majority of our HLA typing combined with PGD cases were β-Thalassemia carriers (87.9%). The mutations analyzed have high heterogeneity, the most frequent mutation was IVS-I-110 G-A and comprised 46.2% of all mutations. The total frequency of the most frequent 6 mutations were 74.0% (Table 4).
A total of 85 clinical pregnancies (36.5%) were achieved from 233 ET cycles. 5 pregnancies are ongoing. To date, 70 healthy and HLA compatible children have been born. 25 sick children have already been cured with cord blood cell and/or bone marrow transplantation.

21 children are waiting for their newborn siblings to gain sufficient weight and maturity for the donation of stem cells (Table 3). The successful transplantations have been performed for the following indications: β-Thalassemia (n=19), Wiskott Aldrich syndrome (n=2), Glanzmann Disease (n=1), X-Adrenoleukodystrophy (n=1) and acute myeloid leukemia (n=1) and Diamond Blackfan anemia (n=1) (Table 5).

Mutation	Frequency , %
IVS-I-110 G-A	46.2
Cod8 delAA	7.3
Cod39 C-T	6.5
IVS-II-745	5.7
IVS-II-1	4.6
IVS-I-1 G-A	3.8
TOTAL	**74.0**

Table 4. The most frequent Beta-Thalassemia mutations in our sample population

4. Conclusion

This data presents one of the world's largest experiences on preimplantation HLA typing, and the outcome of stem cell transplantation is the largest number available from one center. To date 25 children have been cured with this approach and 21 children are awaiting appropriate time for transplantation. Our results indicate HLA typing with or without mutation analysis is a promising and effective therapeutic tool for curation of an affected sibling.

Indication	Patients, n
Beta-Thalassemia	19
Wiscott-Aldrich	2
Glanzmann disease	1
X-Adrenoleukodystrophy	1
Acute Myeloid Leukemia	1
Diamond Blackfan Anemia	1
TOTAL	**25**

Table 5. The list of diseases and the number of patients who have complete cure after HSCT.

5. Acknowledgements

The authors gratefully acknowledge the contributions of Oleg Verlinsky, Lana Rechitsky and Francesco Fiorentino in design of PGD studies. We gratefully thank the clinical, scientific and laboratory staff of the Memorial Hospital IVF and Genetics Center, in particular, Cumhur Gökhan Ekmekçi, Hüseyin Avni Taç, Neşe Ajredin for their extensive work.

6. References

Aksoy., M., Kutlar, A., Kutlar, F., Dincol, G., Erdem, S., Bastesbihci, S., 1985. Survey on haemoglobin variants, beta thalassaemia, glucose-6-phosphate dehydrogenase deficiency, and haptoglobin types in Turks from western Thrace. J. Med. Genet. 22, 288-290.

Basak, A.N., 2007. The molecular pathology of beta-thalassemia in Turkey: the Boğaziçi university experience. Hemoglobin. 31(2), 233-41.

Costeas PA. 2004 Bone marrow donor registry and availability of HLA matched donors. Abstracts of International Seminar on Preimplantation HLA Typing and Stem Cell Transplantation, 27–28 March, 2004, Limassol, Cyprus, p.9 (http//:www.pgdis.org).

Fiorentino, F., Magli, M.C., Podini, D., Ferraretti, A.P., Nuccitelli, A., Vitale, N., et al., 2003. The minisequencing method: an alternative strategy for preimplantation genetic diagnosis of single gene disorders. Mol. Hum. Reprod. 7, 399-410.

Fiorentino F, Biricik A, Karadayi H, Berkil H, Karlikaya G, Sertyel S, Podini D, Baldi M, Magli MC, Gianaroli L, Kahraman S. 2004 Development and clinical application of a strategy for preimplantation genetic diagnosis of single gene disorders combined with HLA matching. Mol Hum Reprod 10; 445-460.

Fiorentino F, Kahraman S, Karadayi H, Biricik A, Sertyel S, Karlikaya G, et al. 2005 Short tandem repeats haplotyping of the HLA region in preimplantation HLA matching. Eur. J. Hum. Genet. 8, 953-8.

Fiorentino F, Biricik A, Nuccitelli A, De Palma R, Kahraman S, Iacobelli M, Trengia V, Caserta D, Bonu MA, Borini A, Baldi M. 2006 Strategies and clinical outcome of 250 cycles of Preimplantation Genetic Diagnosis for single gene disorders. Hum Reprod. Mar;21(3):670-684.

Gaziev D., Galimberti M., Lucarelli G., Polchi P., Giardini C., Angelucci E., Baronciani D., et al., 2000. Bone marrow transplantation from alternative donors for thalassemia: HLA-phenotypically identical relative and HLA-nonidentical sibling or parent transplants. Bone Marrow Transplant. 25; 815-21.

Gaziev J, Lucarelli G. 2005 Stem cell transplantation for thalassemia. Reproductive BioMedicine Online 10, 111–115.

Kahraman, S., Karlikaya, G., Sertyel, S., Karadayi, H., Findikli, N., 2004. Clinical aspects of preimplantation genetic diagnosis for single gene disorders combined with HLA typing. Reprod. Biomed. Online. 5, 529-32.

Kahraman S, Findikli N. 2005 Effect of Italian referendum on global IVF: a comment from Turkey. Reproductive Biomedicine Online 11; 662-663.

Kahraman S, Findikli N, Karlikaya G, Sertyel S, Karadayi H, Saglam Y, Fiorentino F. 2007 Medical and social perspectives of preimplantation genetic diagnosis for single gene disorders and/or HLA typing. 14, supplement 1, 104-108.

Kahraman S, Beyazyurek C, Ekmekci GC. Seven years of experience on preimplantation HLA typing: a clinical overview of 327 cycles. 2011 Reprod Biomed Online, Accepted in January 2011.

Kokkali G, Traeger-Synodinos J, Vrettou C, Stavrou D, Jones GM, Cram DS, Makrakis E, Trounson AO, Kanavakis E, Pantos K. Blastocyst biopsy versus cleavage stage biopsy and blastocyst transfer for preimplantation genetic diagnosis of beta-thalassaemia: a pilot study. Hum Reprod. 2007 May;22(5):1443-9.

Kuliev A., Verlinsky Y. 2004 Preimplantation HLA typing and stem cell transplantation: report of International meeting, Cyprus, 27-28 March, 2004.

McArthur SJ, Leigh D, Marshall JT, Gee AJ, De Boer KA, Jansen RP. 2008 Blastocyst trophectoderm biopsy and preimplantation genetic diagnosis for familial monogenic disorders and chromosomal translocations. Prenat. Diagn. 5, 434-42.

Orofino, M.G., Argiolu, F., Sanna, M.A., Rosatelli, M.C., Tuveri, T, Scalas M.T, et al., 2003. Fetal HLA typing in β thalassemia implication for hematopoitic stem cell transplantation. Lancet. 362; 41-42.

Pangalos CG, Hagnefelt B, Kokkali G, Pantos K, Konialis CP. 2008 Birth of a healthy histocompatible sibling following preimplantation genetic diagnosis for chronic granulomatous disease at the blastocyst stage coupled to HLA typing. Fetal. Diagn. Ther. 24(4), 334-9.

Rechitsky S, Verlinsky O, Amet T, Rechitsky M, Kouliev T, Strom C, Verlinsky Y, 2001. Reliability of preimplantation diagnosis for single gene disorders. Mol. Cell. Endocrinol 183 (1), 65-68.

Rechitsky, S., Kuliev, A., Tur-Kaspa, I., Morris, R., Verlinsky, Y., 2004. Preimplantation genetic diagnosis with HLA matching. Reprod. Biomed. Online. 2, 210-21.

Simpson JL. 2001 Changing indications for preimplantation genetic diagnosis (PGD) Molecular and Cellular Endocrinology 183 (suppl.1); S69-S75.

Shirazi A, Ahadi AM, Farzaneh D.F. and Sadeghizade, M. 2009 Effect of lysis strategy in accuracy and repeatability of sex determination by single cell polymerase chain reaction method. Journal of Biological Sciences 9, 78-82.

Van de Velde H, Georgiou I, De Rycke M Schots R, Sermon K, Lissens W, Devroey P, Van Steirteghem A, Liebaers I. 2004 Novel universal approach for preimplantation genetic diagnosis of b-thalassemia in combination with HLA matching of embryos. Human Reproduction 19, 700–708.

Van de Velde, H., De Rycke, M., De Man, C., De Hauwere, K., Fiorentino, F., Kahraman, S., et al., 2009. The experience of two European preimplantation genetic diagnosis centres on human leukocyte antigen typing. Hum. Reprod. 3, 732-40.

Verlinsky Y, Rechitsky S, Schoolcraft W, Strom C, Kuliev A. 2000 Designer babies – are they a reality yet? Case report: Simultaneous preimplantation genetic diagnosis for Fanconi anaemia and HLA typing for cord blood transplantation. Reproductive BioMedicine Online 1, 31.

Verlinsky Y, Rechitsky S, Schoolcraft W, Strom C, Kuliev A. 2001 Preimplantation diagnosis for Fanconi anemia combined with HLA matching. Journal of the American Medical Association 285, 3130–3133.

Verlinsky, Y., Rechitsky, S., Sharapova, T., Morris, R., Taranissi, M., Kuliev, A., 2004. Preimplantation HLA testing. JAMA. 291(17), 2079-85.

11

The Contribution of Molecular Techniques in Prenatal Diagnosis and *Post mortem* Fetus with Multiple Malformation

Rejane Gus Kessler[1], Sandra Leistner-Segal[1], Maria Teresa Sanseverino[1], Jose Antonio de Azevedo Magalhaes[2], Mariluce Riegel[1] and Roberto Giugliani[1]

[1]*Medical Genetic Service, Hospital de Clinicas de Porto Alegre*
[2]*Obstetric and Gynecology Service, Hospital de Clinicas de Porto Alegre*
Brazil

1. Introduction

The development of conventional cytogenetic techniques in the 50's leaded to a rapid increase of the knowledge on the etiology of malformation syndromes, being chromosomal anomalies reported as the most common genetic condition in humans (Pena, 1998). Around 2-3% of newborns may have congenital malformations, and from those, just 20% have an established etiology (genetic or environmental), being 80% of these multifactorial or unknown (Stevenson & Hall, 2006). But this is only the tip of the iceberg, as probably half of the human concepts may have some kind of chromosomal defect (A. Boué & J. Boué, 1973), indicating that cytogenetic analysis is fundamental for the investigation of these cases. Since the 70's, prenatal diagnosis for detecting cytogenetic abnormalities has become a routine procedure in many countries, and an important tool for the prevention of birth of handicapped children (A. Milunsky & J. Milunsky, 1998).

Cytogenetic analysis is an important component of invasive prenatal diagnosis as chromosomal abnormalities are detected in about 1 in 200 newborns and constitute a major cause of mental retardation and congenital malformations (Shaffer & Lupski, 2000). Microscopic chromosome analysis of cultured cells has been regarded as the gold standard method for prenatal diagnosis, since its first application to prenatal testing in 1966 by Steele and Breg (Steele & Breg, 1966) and the routine use of chromosome banding analysis in 1970s. Karyotyping has proved to be highly reliable for diagnosis of numerical chromosome abnormalities and structural rearrangements in fetal cells obtained invasively by either amniocentesis in the second trimester of pregnancy, or chorionic villus sampling (CVS) in the first trimester, since the early 1980s. The diagnostic accuracy of karyotyping fetal cells from cultured amniotic fluid (AF) has been found to be 99.4%-99.8%, and that of CVS 97.5-99.6%. However, the main limitation of karyotyping is the requirement of a cell culture, resulting in a period of 10-14 days for obtaining the final results (Bui, 2007). Furthermore, the success of cell culture depends on many factors: very good laboratory conditions for tissue culture, technician's experience, and satisfactory cell growth with good quality of metaphases. Unfortunately, due to failure in one of these steps the whole process becomes jeopardized.

In the early 1980s, as better ultrasonographic imaging became available, the access to fetal blood was improved, and it could be obtained at about 18-20 weeks' gestation from umbilical cord (cordocentesis) (Daffos,et al., 1983). Although blood sample allows rapid karyotyping within 72 hours, the gestational age at collection is already advanced, and in positive cases it would be too late for interruption. Besides, this procedure is associated with higher risk of complications than other prenatal diagnostic and, hence, has been performed only in selected cases (Daffos & Hobbins, 2002).
When a fetus with multiple malformations is detected by ultrasound, the list of possible etiologies is very broad, and the possibility of a chromosomal anomaly is high. However, the result of a karyotype, so important for the clinical evaluation, is not always achieved. In some cases this is caused by the factors explained above, in others, due to death of the fetus before the initiation of any diagnostic investigation. In any case, it is very difficult to provide an appropriate genetic counseling without a karyotype result, and the family remains without information on the fetus condition and the risk for future pregnancies. This is a very unpleasant situation, and trying to find an alternative to decrease the anxiety of those families is the main goal of the strategy described below which involves the application of molecular techniques in different fetal materials to overcome this situation.

2. Methodology

We obtained different tissues from 50 multiple malformation fetuses distributed as: umbilical cord (15), lung (7), amniocytes (14) and paraffin embedded tissues (14). For traditional karyotypes, we used AF, UC and alternative materials from 115 fetuses, also with multiple malformations. The criteria for including the fetus as multiple malformations with indication for chromosomal aberrations were based on the "Catalogue of Unbalanced Chromosome Aberration in Man" (Schinzel, 2001). They are summarized in Table 1.

Cleft palate, cleft lip, or both
Esophageal atresia, TE fistula; anal atresia with fistula
Malrotation of the gut, common mesentery; omphalocele
Malformation of the heart and the great vessels
Malformation of the kidney and urinary tract
Certain brain malformation, particularly holoprosencephaly and agenesis of corpus callosum
Absence or hypoplasia of radius and thumb
Postaxial hexadactyly
Microphtalmia, ocular coloboma
Spina bifida (occipital or lumbar)

Table 1. Common malformations in autosomal chromosomal aberrations

2.1 DNA extraction

The DNA from fresh tissues was extracted as described by Miller (Miller et al., 1988) with slight modifications. Tissue specimens were grinded before addition of the nuclei lysis buffer and 1/10 of the reagent's volume used for blood extraction was used. In a few cases (n=8) a commercial kit was used for DNA extraction. (NucleoSpin®Tissue from Macherey-Nagel).

2.2 DNA extraction from paraffin embedded tissue

This technique was adapted from Andreassen (Andreassen et al., 2004) and Coura (Coura et al., 2005) as follows: Paraffin block was sliced in small pieces between 5-10µ and 5 slices were placed into an ependorff. Xylol (1,5ml) was added and incubated for 30 minutes at 37°C. Tubes were centrifuged at 14.000 rpm for 3 minutes. The supernatant was removed and all steps were repeated once. After the supernatant removal, samples were washed with 70% Ethanol and centrifuged for 3 minutes at 7.200 rpm. This step was repeated twice and samples were left at room temperature for at least 30 minutes. After completely removal of the paraffin, 300 µl of Nuclei Lysis buffer, 20µl of SDS and 20µl of proteinase K were added. Samples were incubated for 3 days at 60°C and on the third day an extra volume of 5µl of proteinase K was added. The remaining steps for DNA precipitation were the same ones as described above for tissue DNA extraction.

2.3 Multiplex ligation-dependent probe amplification (MLPA)

Multiplex ligation-dependent probe amplification (MLPA) is a semiquantitatitive analysis based on polymerase chain reaction (PCR). It possesses many advantages such as high efficiency, simple operation, low cost and has been wildly applied in researches of diseases associated with copy number variation, point mutation and methylation (Zhou & Ren, 2009).

This new multiplex method is able to detect abnormal copy numbers of genomic DNA sequences requiring a minimum of 20ng of human DNA (Schouten et al., 2002). In this technique, it is not the nucleic acid, but the probes added to the samples that are amplified. MLPA allows discrimination of sequences that differ only in a single nucleotide, therefore MLPA can be used for detection of known mutation. It is basically a method to make a nuclei acid sample suitable for multiplex polymerase chain reaction (PCR) with the use of only one pair of primers. In the currently available kits, the products generated by PCR are separated by sequence-type electrophoresis. The thermocycler and sequencing-type electrophoresis equipment that are required, are present in most DNA diagnostic laboratories. Up to 96 samples can be handled simultaneously, 45 DNA sequences, and results can be obtained within 24 hours. One of the currently MLPA kits (P095, MRC-Holland, Amsterdam) is commercially available and contains eight independent probes for each of the chromosomes involved in almost frequent aneupolidies: 13, 18, 21, and X, and four Y-specific probes; and it is used as a rapid prenatal test by several medical centers on a large scale (Schouten et el., 2002). MLPA profiles must be compared with a similar profile obtained from a control DNA sample. Compared with a control reaction, the relative peak area of each amplification product reflects the relative copy number of the target sequence of that probe in the analyzed sample. An aberrant copy number of one or more of the sequences detected by MLPA probes can therefore be detected by a decrease or increase in relative peak area of the amplification products of the probes detecting those sequences.

The length of the amplification product of each probe is different, and ranges in size between 130 and 480 nucleotides. This provides an optimal separation and low background on sequencing type electrophoresis gels. Although performing an MLPA reaction is easy,

the development of new MLPA assays is complex and time-consuming, and the success of the results depends basically on the quality of the DNA extraction.
Briefly the protocol consists of: denaturing 20-500 ng of DNA by heating to 98°C in a thermocycler; adding the MLPA probes and leaving overnight at 60°C for hybridization. For the next step add the ligase and ligase buffer at 54°C for 15 min.(ligation of the two probe parts); inactivate the ligase by heating to 98°C; add PCR primers, dNTPs, and polymerase and start the PCR (amplification of probes). The amplification products are separated by capillary electrophoresis.

2.4 Quantitative Fluorescent-Polymerase Chain Reaction (QF-PCR)

This method uses PCR amplification and fluorescent dye labeled primers targeting highly polymorphic regions of DNA sequence called short tandem repeats (STRs) that are located on the chromosomes of interest (Mansfield, 1993). Each target marker is specific to the chromosome on which it is located, thus the copy number of the STR marker reflects the copy number of the chromosome. Informative STR markers which exhibit a high heterogeneity have been selected so that copy number can be easily determined. A normal diploid sample has the normal complement of two of each of the somatic chromosomes, thus two alleles of a chromosome specific STR are determine by the QF-PCR technique as two peaks in a 1:1 ratio. The observation of an extra STR allele as either a three peak pattern in a 1:1:1 ratio or two peak pattern in a 2:1 ratio is diagnostic of a presence of an additional sequence which in turn may represent an additional chromosome, as in the case of a trisomy.
Amplified products of the QF-PCR technique are analyzed quantitatively on a capillary Genetic Analyzer (ABI 3100) to determine the copy number of the analyzed STRs markers.
The kit used in the study was from ELUCIGENE. The ELUCIGENE QST*R™ range of products are DNA based multiplexed assays for the rapid prenatal determination of aneuploidy status for the three most common autosomal trisomies and the sex chromosomes X and Y. PCR products are observed as a 5 dye labelled system using filter set G5. Filter set G5 detects the 6-FAM (blue), VIC (green), NED (yellow) and PET (red) labelled fragments plus the Size Standard marker labelled with LIZ (orange) on an electrophoretogram in the Genotyper program.
The markers used are described in Tables 2 and 3.

Marker	Location	Observed Heterozygosity	Allele Size Range (bp)	Marker Dye Colour
DXS981	Xq13.1	0.86	225-260	blue
DXS1187	Xq26.2	0.72	122-170	green
HPRT	Xq26.2	0.78	265-300	green
DXS7423	Xq28	0.74	372-388	green
DXYS267	Xq21.3/Yp11.2	0.87	240-280	red
AMEL	Xp22.22/Yp11.2	-	104-110	yellow
DXS6807	Xp22.32	0.70	331-351	blue
DXS1283E	Xp22.31	0.89	292-340	yellow
SRY	Yp11.31	-	244-251	yellow
DYS448	Yq11.223	-	323-381	red

Table 2. X and Y markers in ELUCIGENE QSTRs

Marker	Location	Observed Heterozygosity	Allele Size Range (bp)	Marker Dye Colour
D13S252	13q12.2	0.85	260-330	red
D13S305	13q13.3	0.75	418-470	green
D13S628	13q31.1	0.69	425-472	yellow
D13S634	13q21.33	0.81	355-440	blue
D13S325	13q14.11	0.86	235-320	green
D18S386	18q22.1	0.88	320-407	green
D18S390	18q22.3	0.75	345-400	yellow
D18S391	18q11.31	0.75	196-230	green
D18S535	18q12.3	0.92	450-500	blue
D18S819	18q11.2	0.70	370-450	red
D18S978	18q12.3	0.67	180-230	yellow
D21S11	21q21.1	0.90	220-283	blue
D21S1437	21q21.1	0.84	283-350	blue
D21S1409	21q21.2	0.81	160-220	red
D21S1411	21q22.3	0.93	256-345	yellow
D21S1435	21q21.3	0.75	152-210	blue

Table 3. 13, 18 and 21 markers in ELUCIGENE QSTRs

2.5 PCR Set Up

PCR was performed according to the manufacturer's instruction as described briefly: the thermal cycler is programmed for a single step cycle to activate the DNA polymerase at 95°C, for 15 minutes, linked to an amplification cycling program of 30 seconds at 95°C (denaturation), 1 minute and 30 seconds at 59°C (annealing) and 1 minute and 30 seconds at 72°C (extension) for 26 cycles. This should be linked to a 30 minutes time-delay at 72°C (extension) on the final cycle; sufficient vials should be separated to pre-aliquoted QSTR reaction mix for a number of samples and controls to be run. The vials are centrifuged at 12,000g for 10 seconds; 2.5μl of test DNA is added to a sample vial containing QSTR reaction mix; the 95°C activation program is initiated (step 1). On completion of the amplification program the samples may be stored at room temperature overnight or at 2-8°C up to 7 days before analysis by capillary electrophoresis.

Optimal results can be obtained using an ABI 3100 Genetic Analyzer

We also obtained 115 samples from pregnant women with multiple malformations fetus, for traditional karyotype analysis. The biological samples obtained were: AF, UC and alternative materials, such as urine, cystic hygroma fluid, intraperitoneal or cerebrospinal fluids. AF and alternative materials were cultivated as long term culture, with Amniomax medium, at 37°C, in CO_2 incubator. The blood culture (UC) was processed as short term culture (72hs) following standard cytogenetic procedures.

3. Results

We obtained 50 samples from different fetal materials for molecular techniques analysis, and 115 for traditional karyotyping (AF, UC, or alternative materials). All samples were from multiple malformations fetus without diagnosis.

For the molecular techniques, we first tested all the samples with the MLPA kit P095 and we observed that obtaining genetic profiles from samples containing minimal amounts of DNA can be difficult. Unfortunately, the quantity and quality of DNA was not adequate for this analysis and it was quite difficult to interpret the data obtained (the peak areas tend to be too variable when the DNA quality is not good enough). We then ran all samples again using QF-PCR. The XY test is very sensitive so that even when the quality of DNA was poor we could still determine the presence or absence of a Y chromosome. Thus, for some probands (09 cases), we could only give results for XY and not for autosomes. At times it was not possible to say whether the proband was 45,X or 46,XX since insufficient probes amplified, and the peaks were very weak (Table 4).

Case number	**Chr. 21**	**Chr. 18**	**Chr. 13**	**X/Y**	**Interpretation/comments**	**Traditional Karyotype**
01	2	2	2	XX	No T13, 18, 21 detected	
02	**2**	**2**	**3**	**XY**	**Trisomy 13, meiotic error**	-
03	2	2	2	XY	No T13, 18, 21 detected	
04	2	2	2	XY	No T13, 18, 21 detected	
05	-	-	-	-	Not enough DNA	
06	-	-	-	XY	Very weak peaks	
07	-	-	-	XX	No DNA left	
08	2	2	2	XX	No T13, 18, 21 detected	
09	2	2	2	XY	No T13, 18, 21 detected	
10	2	2	2	XX	No T13, 18, 21 detected	
11	2	2	2	XY	No T13, 18, 21 detected	
12	2	2	2	XY	No T13, 18, 21 detected	
13	-	-	-	XY	Very weak peaks	
14	2	2	2	XX	No T13, 18, 21 detected	
15	2	2	2	XY	No T13, 18, 21 detected	
16	-	-	-	XX	Very weak peaks	
17	-	-	-	XX	Very weak peaks	46,XX
18	2	2	2	XY	No T13, 18, 21 detected	
19	2	2	2	XX	No T13, 18, 21 detected	
20	-	-	-	X/XX?	Very weak peaks	
21	-	-	-	XX	Very weak peaks	
22	-	-	-	XX	Very weak peaks	
23	-	-	-	-	No peaks	
24	-	-	-	XY?	Very weak peaks	
25	-	-	-	X/XX?	Very weak peaks	
26	-	-	-	-	No peaks	
28	-	-	-	-	No peaks	
29	-	-	-	-	No peaks	46,XX
30	-	-	-	-	No peaks	46,XY
31	-	-	-	-	No peaks	**47,XX+21**
32	-	-	-	-	No peaks	
33	-	-	-	-	No peaks	

Case number	Chr. 21	Chr. 18	Chr. 13	X/Y	Interpretation/comments	Traditional Karyotype
37	-	-	-	-	No peaks	
38	-	-	-	-	No peaks	46,XX
39	-	-	-	-	No peaks	**45,X**
40	-	-	-	-	No peaks	46,XY
41	-	-	-	-	No peaks	
42	-	-	-	-	No peaks	
43	-	-	-	-	No peaks	
44	-	-	-	-	No peaks	
45	-	-	-	-	No peaks	
46	-	-	-	-	No peaks	
47	2	3	2	XY	**Trisomy 18, meiotic error**	**47,XY,+18**
48	2	2	2	XX	No T13, 18, 21 detected	46,XX
49	-	-	-	-	No peaks	46,XX
50	-	-	-	XY	Very weak peaks	**47,XY+21**
51	-	-	-	XY	Very weak peaks	**47,XY,+18**
52	2	3	2	XY	**Trisomy 18, meiotic error**	**47,XY,+18**
53	2	2	2	XX	No T13, 18, 21 detected	**47,XX,+mar**
54	2	2	2	XX	No T13, 18, 21 detected	47,XX

Table 4. Results of 50 samples from different tissues analyzes by Q-F PCR

From the 50 cases, we could get partial results in 30. Although we had a very good technique for extracting DNA from paraffin (we've got enough DNA concentrations and relative good quality of DNA), this material showed to be inappropriate for molecular techniques, probably due to the formalin buffer used to embed the tissue at the time of collection. In all those cases we got no detectable peaks.

In one case, the physician was quite sure about the clinical diagnosis of trisomy 13, and when the fetus died, his lung was collected for culture and karyotyping, and also umbilical cord for posterior DNA analysis. The lung culture failed, but we were able to apply QF-PCR in DNA extracted from UC and confirmed the clinical indication. In this case, three peaks were detected with markers D13S252, D13S305, D13S634 and D13S325. For marker D13S628 we observed two peaks being one higher than the other indicating an extra allele.

In two cases, trisomy 18 was detected, confirming the previous karyotyping. In one of the cases, three peaks were detected with marker D18S386 and D18S390, and two peaks, one being higher than the other, with markers D18S535 and D18S391. In the other case, three peaks were detected with marker D18S386, and two peaks detected, again one being higher than the other, with markers D18S391 and D18S978.

From the floating amniocytes that did not adhere to the flask, and were collected at the first medium change (14 cases), we succeeded in extracting DNA and performed QF-PCR. This material would be normally discarded. From those, we were able to obtain eight molecular results from which two did not have a previous successful karyotype.

The best results obtained for molecular analysis were from DNA extracted using a commercial kit as described before (Material and Methods).

From 6 cases of aneuploidies that had previous karyotype, we were able to obtain two confirmations (cases number 47 and 52). On the other hand, for one case (case number 2)

which remained without karyotype, we obtained a positive result through QF-PCR. Case number 53 (table 4) could not be confirmed by molecular analysis because the origin of the extra chromosome marker was unknown and could not hybridize with the probes used. We had no discordant results between the molecular and traditional techniques for those cases were both analyses were performed.

In Table 5, we describe the results from different sources of fetal material for karyotyping in 115 multiple malformation fetuses. When, for some anatomical reason, AF CVS or UC could not be collected, the obstetrician strategy, sometimes for therapeutic reasons, was the collection of alternative fetal material such as bladder drainage. Those biological materials could be also used for karyotying, and although there were few cases available, we had 100% of culture success and karyotyping.

Fetus sample	Number of cases (n)	Culture success (n)	Success rate (%)
AF	87	83	95.5
UC	15	14	93.3
Alternative fluids[a]	13	13	100
TOTAL	115	110	95.6

[a]Bladder (6), cystic hygroma (2), intraperitoneal (2), displastic kidney (1), cystic lung (1), cerebrospinal (1) fluids.

Table 5. Different materials from multiple malformations fetus and success rate of cell cultures

4. Discussion

Cytogenetic analysis is an important tool for detecting chromosome abnormalities, once this is the cause of most common genetic disease in man (Pena, 1998). It has been very useful for prenatal diagnosis, and also in clinical genetics. However the traditional technique has some limitations, and in order to overcome these problems some new molecular and rapid techniques have been developed, such as QF-PCR and MLPA. In our study, we tried to use all possible biological sources obtained form the fetuses to be able to reach a diagnosis for a multiple malformation that could evolve to death, or had already died without any laboratory findings. The main limitation we wanted to overcome was to avoid the situation of leaving a multiple malformation fetus without a final diagnosis or karyotype which is a vital information for genetic counseling and for the family. Thus we tried to apply molecular techniques in postmortem or paraffin-embedded fetal tissues, or even non adhered amniocytes that would be normally discarded after culture.

Karyotyping unconventional fetal samples, when obtaining traditional biological material is difficult, is not a very common approach in most laboratories (Donnenfeld et al., 2001; Gole et al., 1997). Nevertheless, we used this alternative whenever necessary, and achieved 100% success rate on a limited sample of 13 cases (Kessler et al., 2008), being this rate much higher when compared to other studies (Teoh et al., 1996; Donnenfeld, 2001).

There is an ongoing debate whether Rapid Aneuploidy Diagnosis (RAD) should be employed as an adjunct to karyotyping or whether it could be used as a stand-alone test in selected groups of women (Leung et al., 2003; Cirigliano et al., 2006). The controversy is due to residual probability of a chromosome abnormality (both balanced and unbalanced) when RAD demonstrates a normal result. Few studies have estimated the residual risk of a clinically significant chromosome aberration for different indications when RAD results are normal. In a meta-analysis of 12 studies involving invasive tests, the risk of having a chromosome aberration that was not expected to be detected by RAD methods, was estimated to be 0.9% (Leung & Lao, 2005). In our results, from 6 aneuploidies already diagnosed by karyotyping, only two cases (33.3%) were detected by QF-PCR, probably because of poor quality of DNA (mainly in paraffin). On the other hand, a third case detected by QF-PCR, had failed for tissue culture at the time of karyotyping analysis, the result was obtained only using molecular approaches. Little is known about the patients' preference regarding the type of analysis to be performed. However in Sweden a research was made including 6000 women and 70% chose QF-PCR analysis alone (Bui, 2007). In our opinion, the combination of both techniques is safer, in order to overcome the particular limitations of each one. .

MLPA has the same inherent limitations as those of QF-PCR in that it will not detect most structural chromosome aberrations, or balanced rearrangements such as translocations and inversions. Moreover, maternal cell contamination and 69,XXX triploidy will not be diagnosed by MLPA (Bui, 2007). In our study, for example, when a marker chromosome was detected by the traditional karyotype, the molecular techniques were not able to detect it, because the origin of the marker was unknown, so no specific probe could be applied.

Although we developed a good protocol for extracting DNA from paraffin block wax, this material showed to be inappropriate for the molecular techniques used, as demonstrated in other studies which also needed smaller fragments of DNA (Halvarsson et al. 2004). Another study in postmortem tissues embedded in paraffin succeeded to obtain longer amplification fragments of around 300 bp using a specific treatment called pre-PCR restoration (Bonin et al., 2003), thus achieving better results.

Whenever AF was set up for culture, not all amniocytes adhered to the bottom of the flask. After few days, by the first medium change, we observed that there were still a considerable number of floating cells, which could be used to obtain a considerable amount of DNA. We proposed and developed a protocol to extract DNA from those cells in order to guarantee a result independently of the cell culture success, and also to abbreviate the result with molecular techniques. Although we did not succeed as expected, we could obtain results from two cases when cell culture had failed. We could probably improve the success rate of these analyses by extracting DNA with commercial kits rather than in-house techniques in order to obtain better quality DNA, which is essential for the molecular analysis used here.

The need of faster testing methods which do not require cell culture has been recognized by the scientific community to improve pregnancy management and alleviate parental anxiety (Nicolini et al., 2004).

The best results obtained were from the last 8 cases, in which the DNA was extracted using a commercial kit. This is very important information and corroborates the fact that high quality DNA is necessary, from which we can obtain results even with degraded DNA (Roeder et al., 2009).

5. Conclusion

In conclusion, for follow up diagnostic testing, karyotyping has proved to be the gold standard method. This technology has remained essentially unchanged over 30 years, as no new technology has proven to be superior in terms of being able to detect such a wide range of abnormalities with the necessary precision (Slater et al., 2009). Nevertheless, molecular

testing, such as QF-PCR or MLPA, are becoming important alternatives in order to give a rapid result with low cost. Although these molecular techniques have some limitations, we did not find any discordant result, in comparison to traditional karyotype. Nevertheless, the appropriate approach is always performing simultaneously both techniques.
The importance of this study remains in the alternatives we proposed to give a final diagnosis to a multiple malformation fetus. We suggested some approaches to achieve a final laboratory result and deliver to the family the information they need to rebuild their lives, and make plans for their future, with the help of more rapid and efficient technology (RAD) and appropriate genetic counseling.

6. Acknowledgements

This study was supported by institutional (FIPE-HCPA) funds.

7. References

Andreassen C.N., Sorensen F.B., Overgaard J. and Alsner J. (2004). Optimisation and validation of methods to access single nucleotide polymorphisms (SNPs) in Archival histological material. *Radiotherapy and Oncology*, vol. 72, pp.351-356.

Bonin S., Petrera F., Niccolini B. and Stanta G. (2003). PCR analysis in archival postmortem tissues. *Journal of Clinical Patholology: Molecular Pathology*, vol. 56, pp.184-186.

Boué A. and Boué J. (1973). Evaluation des erreurs chromosomiques au moment de la conception, *Biomedicine*, vol. 18, pp.372-377.

Bui T.H. (2007). Prenatal cytogenetic diagnosis: gone FISHing, BAC soon. *Ultrasound in Obstetrics and Gynecology*, vol. 30, pp.247-251,.

Cirigliano V., Voglino G., Marongiu A.,. Canadas M.P, Ordonez E., Lioveras E., Plaja A., Fuster C. and Adinolfi M. (2006).Rapid prenatal diagnosis by QF-PCR:evaluation of 30,000 consecutive clinical samples and future applications. *Annual NY Academy of Sience*, vol. 1075, pp. 288-298.

Coura R., Prolla J.C., Meurer L. and Ashton-Prolla P. (2005). An alternative protocol for DNA extraction from formalin fixed and paraffin wax embedded tissue. *Journal of Clinical Pathology*, vol. 58, pp.894-895.

Daffos F., Capella-Pavlovsky M. and Forestier F.(1983). A new procedure for fetal blood sampling in utero: preliminary results in fifty-three cases.. *American Journal of Obstetrics and Gynecology*, vol. 146, pp. 985-987.

Donnenfeld A.E. Lockwood D. and Lamb A.N. (2001). Prenatal diagnosis from cystic hygroma fluid : The value of fluorescence *in situ* hybridization. *American Journal of Obstetrics and Gynecology* , vol.185 , pp.1004-1008.

Dugoff L. and Hobbins J.C. (2002). Invasive procedures to evaluate the fetus. *Clin Obstet Gynecol*, vol. 45, pp.1039-1053.

Gole L.A., Anandakumar C., Bongso A., Chua T.M., Wong Y.C. and Ratnam S.S.(1997). Analysis of cystic hygroma, ascitic and pleural fluids by conventional lymphocyte culture and fluorescent *in situ* hybridization. *Prenatal Diagnosis*, vol. 17, pp.1151-1157.

Halvarsson B., Lindblom A., Rambech E., Lagerstedt K. and Nilbert M. (2004). Microsatellite instability and/or immunostaining for diagnosis of hereditary nonpolyposis colorectal cancer? *Virchows Archiv* , vol. 444, pp. 134-141.

Kessler R.G., Sanseverino M.T.V., Leistner-Segal S., Magalhães J.A.A. and Giugliani, R. (2008). Prenatal diagnosis of fetal chromosomal abnormalities: Report of an 18-year experience in a Brazilian public hospital. *Genetics and Molecular Biology*, vol.31, no.4, pp.829-833.

Leung W.C. and Lao T.T. (2005). Rapid aneuploidy testing, traditional karyotyping, or both? *Lancet*, vol. 366, pp. 97-98.

Leung W.C., Lau E.T., Lao T.T. and Tang M.H. (2003). Can amnio-polymerase chain reaction alone replace conventional cytogenetic study for women with positive biochemical screening for fetal Down syndrome ? *Obstetric and Gynecology*, vol. 101, pp. 865-861.

Mansfield E.S. (1993). Diagnosis of Down Syndrome and other aneuploidies using quantitative polymerase chain reaction and small tandem repeat polymorphisms. *Human Molecular Genetics*, vol. 2, no.1, pp.43-50.

Miller A.S., Dykes D.D. and Polesky H.F. (1988). A simple salting out procedure for extracting DNA from human nucleated cells. *Nucleic Acids Research*, vol.16, no.3, pp.1215.

Milunsky A. and Milunsky J. (1998).Genetic Counseling: Preconception, Prenatal and Perinatal, In*: Genetic Disorders and the Fetus. Diagnosis, Prevention and Treatment*, Milunsky, A. (Ed.) pp.1-52, The Jonh Hopkins University Press,Boston..

Nicolini U., Lalatta F., Nattacci F., Curcio C. and Bui T.H. (2004). The introduction of Q-F PCR in prenatal diagnosis of fetal aneuploidies: time of reconsideration. *Human Reproduction Update*, vol.10, pp. 541-548.

Pena S.D.J. (1998). Molecular Cytogenetics II: PCR-based diagnosis of chromosomal deletions and microdeletion syndromes. *Genetics and Molecular Biology*, vol.21, no. 4, pp. 453-460.

Roeder A.D., Elsmore P., Greenhalgh M. and McDonald A. (2009). Maximization DNA profiling success from sub-optimal quantities of DNA: a staged approach. *Forensic Science International Genetics*, vol. 3, no.2, pp.128-137.

Schinzel A. (2001) Notes on Clinical Findings in Autosomal Chromosome Aberrations, In: *Catalogue of Unbalanced Chromosome Aberrations in Man,* Schinzel, A. (Ed.), pp.28-34, Walter de Gruyter Press, Berlin, New York.

Schouten J.P., McElgunn C.J., Waaijer R., Zwijnenburg D., Diepvens F. and G. Pals (2002). Relative quantification of 40 nuclei acid sequences by multiplex ligation-dependent probe amplification. *Nucleic Acids Research*, vol. 30, pp. 57.

Shaffer L.G. and Lupski J.R. (2000). Molecular mechanisms for constitutional chromosomal rearrangements in human *Annual Review of Genetics*, vol. 34, pp.297-329,.

Slater H.R., Bruno D.L., Ren H., Pertile M., Schouten J.P. and Choo K.H.A. (2009). Rapid, high throughput prenatal detection of aneuploidy using a novel quantity method (MLPA). *Journal of Medical Genetics* , vol. 40, pp.907-912.

Steele M.W. and Breg W.R.J (1966)..Chromosome analysis of human amniotic-fluid cells, *Lancet*, vol. 19, no.1, pp.383-385.

Stevenson R, and. Hall J.G. (2006). Human Malformation and related Anomalies, Oxford University Press, New York.

Teoh T.G., Ryan G., Johnson J. and E.J. Winsor (1996). The role of fetal karyotyping from unconventional sources. *American Journal of Obstetrics and Gynecology* , vol.175, pp. 873-877.

Zhou D. and Z. Ren (2009). Multiplex ligation-dependent probe amplification and its application. *Zhonghua Yi Xue Yi Chuan Xue Za Zhi*, vol. 26, no. 1, pp. 45-49.

12

Detection of the Most Common Genetic Causes of Male Infertility by Quantitative Fluorescent (QF)-PCR Analysis

Dijana Plaseska-Karanfilska[1], Predrag Noveski[1] and Toso Plaseski[2]
[1]*Macedonian Academy of Sciences and Arts, Research Center for Genetic Engineering and Biotechnology "Georgi D. Efremov", Skopje*
[2]*Clinic of Endocrinology and Metabolic Disorders, Faculty of Medicine, Skopje*
Republic of Macedonia

1. Introduction

Infertility is a major health problem today, affecting about 15% of couples trying to have a child. Impaired fertility of the male factor is causative in 20% of infertile couples and contributory in up to another 30-40%. Infertility already affects about 5-7% of the general male population and may further increase in the future, considering the apparent trend of declining sperm count in industrialized countries. Despite enormous progress in the understanding of human reproductive physiology, the underlying cause of male infertility remains undefined in about 50% of cases, which are referred to as idiopathic infertility (*Ferlin et al., 2006*). Most of the idiopathic cases are likely to be of genetic origin because the number of genes involved in human spermatogenesis is probably over thousands. At present, only few of the genes implicated in the processes of testis determination, testis descent and spermatogenesis have routine clinical importance. These include the cystic fibrosis transmembrane conductance regulator (CFTR) gene, whose mutations cause cystic fibrosis and absence of vas deferens and the androgen receptor (AR) gene, whose mutations cause the androgen insensitivity syndrome and spermatogenic damage.

1.1 Common genetic causes of male infertility

Chromosomal anomalies and microdeletions of the azoospermia factor (AZF) regions of the Y chromosome are the only common known genetic causes of spermatogenic failure. The frequency of these two genetic anomalies increases with the severity of the spermatogenic defect, reaching to an overall 30% (15% karyotype abnormalities and 15% of AZF microdeletions) in azoospermic men.

1.1.1 Sex chromosome aneuploidies

Sex chromosome aneuploidies, such as 47,XXY (Klinefelter's syndrome), 47,XYY and 46,XX males are the most common chromosome anomalies occurring at birth and in the population of infertile males (*Hetch & Hetch, 1987; Gekas et al., 2001*).
Klinefelter's syndrome (KS) is a form of primary testicular failure with testicular hypotrophy and elevated gonadotropin plasma levels, and it represents the most common

form of male hypogonadism. The prevalence of KS among infertile men is very high, up to 5% in severe oligozoospermia and 10% in azoospermia (*De Braekeleer & Dao, 1991*). The syndrome usually causes the arrest of spermatogenesis at the primary spermatocyte stage, but occasionally later stages of sperm development are observed. There are two forms of Klinefelter syndrome: nonmosaic, 47,XXY; and mosaic, 47, XXY/ 46, XY. Although previously believed to be sterile, it has been estimated that 25% of nonmosaic Klinefelter syndrome patients have sperm in their ejaculate (*Ferlin et al., 2007*). Men with the mosaic form of the disease may have residual spermatogenesis in their seminiferous tubules (*Foresta et al., 2005*). Klinefelter syndrome patients may try to achieve pregnancy using ICSI, but they risk producing offspring with chromosomal abnormalities (*Reubinoff et al., 1998*).

The karyotype 47,XYY is the second most frequent full aneuploidy of sex chromosomes. The spermatogenesis in XYY individuals range from severe oligozoospermia to normozoospermia (*Skakkebaek et al., 1973; Sharara et al., 1999*).

46,XX chromosomal abnormality is observed mainly in azoospermic males, with frequency of 0.9% (*Mau-Holzmann, 2005*). The phenotype is similar to Klinefelter syndrome, but with normal height and unimpaired intelligence. The *SRY* gene is present in most of the cases (*SRY*+ XX males); in these cases males are invariably infertile, and azoospermia results from testicular atrophy. The other category are *SRY*− XXmales, which assumes a mutation in an autosomal or X-linked gene involved in the sex determining cascade which should substitute the SRY, permitting testicular determination in absence of SRY.

1.1.2 Y chromosome microdeletions

1.1.2.1 Deletions of AZFa, AZFb and AZFc regions

Y chromosome microdeletions represent the etiological factor of 10-15% of idiopathic azoospermia and severe oligozoospermia (*Foresta et al., 2000; Ma et al., 2000*). In 1976, Tiepolo and Zuffardi provided the first evidence that the long arm of the Y chromosome is required for fertility in men, when they karyotyped 1170 men and found that six azoospermic men were missing most of the long arm of Y chromosome (*Tiepolo & Zuffardi, 1976*). Subsequently, this cluster on Yq11 became known as the azoospermia factor or AZF. The use of polymerase chain reaction (PCR) of sequence tagged sites (STS) has made possible the detection of small, interstitial deletions invisible by karyotyping (*Vollrath et al., 1992*). In 1996, the AZF region was subdivided into 25 deletion intervals (D1-D25) and the existence of three non-overlapping subregions, designated AZFa, AZFb and AZFc (*Figure 1A*), was proposed (*Vogt, 1996*). Subsequent DNA sequencing approaches revealed eight large palindromic regions containing an array of different ampliconic sequences (*Kuroda-Kawaguchi et al., 2001*) and demonstrated that these regions harbour a total of 12 different genes/gene families, most of which are exclusively expressed in testises (*Kuroda-Kawaguchi et al., 2001; Tilford et al., 2001, Scaletsky et al., 2003*). An overlap of 1.5Mb between distal AZFb and proximal AZFc was also demonstrated (*Repping et al., 2002*). Ampliconic sequences make up almost all of the AZFc sequence and 50% of the AZFb sequence (*Figure 1B*).

The frequency of AZF deletions in infertile men ranges in worldwide surveys from 5 to 20% (*Vogt, 1998; Krausz et al., 2003*). Y microdeletions are found almost exclusively in patients with azoospermia or severe oligozoospermia (*Simoni et al., 1998*). The prevalence of Y microdeletions among the infertile males from the Republic of Macedonia is 6.4%, among patients with azoospermia 16.7% and among those with severe oligozoospermia 2.8% (*Plaseski et al., 2003*). Deletions most frequently involve AZFc region, less frequently the

AZFb region, and only rarely the AZFa region. The most frequent deletions among Macedonian males are AZFc deletions, while AZFa deletions have not been detected (*Plaseski et al., 2006; Plaseski et al., 2008*).

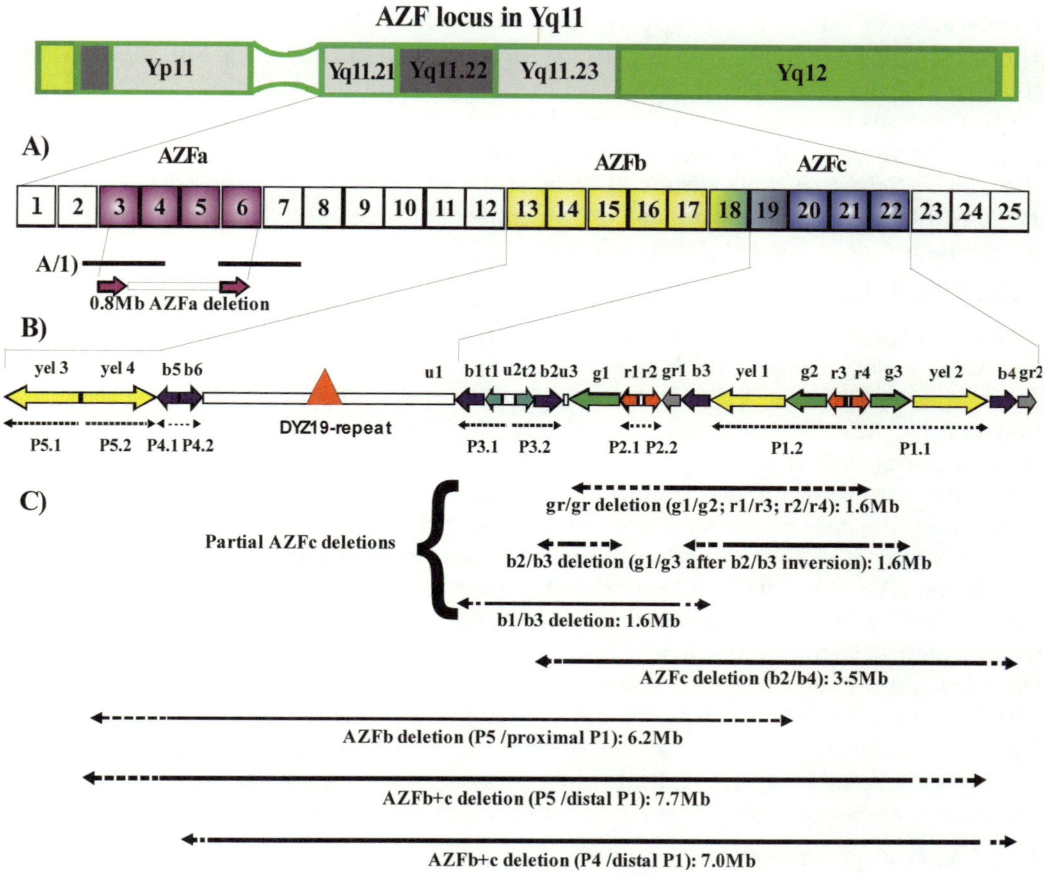

Fig. 1. Schematic view of the AZF locus in Yq1. **A)** Deletion map of AZF locus: 25 intervals (D1-D25) and three AZF regions (AZFa, AZFb and AZFc). **A/1)** Complete AZFa deletion, caused by recombination of two homologous HERV 15Yq1/q2 blocks; **B)** Structural organization of the different amplicons in the AZFb and AZFc regions belonging to five palindromic structures (P1-P5); **C)** Partial and complete AZFc, AZFb and AZFb+c deletions caused by recombination between different amplicons.

Distant homologous recombination between specific palindromic sequences is believed to be the mechanism for majority Yq deletions (Figure 1C) (*Kamp et al., 2000; Repping et al., 2002; Repping et al., 2003*), although deletions based on mechanism of nonhomologous recombination were also identified (*Costa et al., 2008*). The AZFa deletions are located in proximal Yq and are caused by recombination that take place between retroviral homologous sequences. These deletions account for less then 1% of all microdeletions of the Y chromosome reported to be associated with spermatogenic failure. Clinically, AZFa deletions are associated with complete absence of germ cells in the testes (*Vogt, 2005*). Complete deletions of AZFb have a size of 6.23 Mb and extend within a 1.5 Mb of the proximal portion of AZFc. Deletions removing simultaneously part of the AZFb and AZFc regions result from homologous recombination, in which the proximal breakpoints are located in the P5 palindrome and the distal breakpoints mapped in either proximal P1 or distal P1 (*Repping et al., 2002*). Clinically, complete AZFb deletions are associated with meiotic arrest or Sertoly cell-only syndrome (*Ferlin et al., 2003*).

The most common AZFc deletion (b2/b4 deletion) eliminates a 3.5 Mb segment that contains 21 genes and is present in about 1 in 4.000 men worldwide (*Kuroda-Kawaguchi et al., 2001*). Deletions involving the AZFc region account for up to 90% of all Yq deletions with phenotypes varying from azoospermia to severe oligozoospermia (*Reijo et al., 1995, Simoni et al., 1997, Najmabadi et al., 1996)* and occasionally to milder oligozoospermia (*Oliva et al., 1998*). Although natural transmission of Y microdeletions has been reported, majority of the cases arise as a *de novo* event (*Edwards & Bishop , 1997*).

1.1.2.2 Partial AZFc deletions

Partial deletions within the AZFc region (gr/gr and b2/b3) that remove smaller portions of the AZFc region (1.6 and 1.8 Mb) are much more common and are present at various frequencies in different Y haplogroups (*Repping et al., 2003; Vogt, 2005*). Partial and polymorphic AZF deletions have been also reported in the AZFa (*Kamp et al., 2000*) and AZFb regions (*Ferlin et al., 2003*).

While the association of the complete AZFc deletion with spermatogenic failure is well established, the role of partial AZFc deletions and duplications on spermatogenesis and male infertility is still controversial. With the exception of one study among Han-Chinese population (*Wu et al., 2007*), all other studies reported no association between the b2/b3 deletion and impaired spermatogenesis. The results of the gr/gr deletion are more inconsistent; it is considered a new genetic risk factor by a number of research groups (*Kuroda-Kawaguchi et al., 2001; de Llanos et al., 2005; Ferlin et al., 2005; Gianchini et al., 2005, Gianchini et al., 2008*), but not by the others (*Machev et al., 2004; Hucklenbroich et al., 2005; Ravel et al., 2006; Carvalho et al., 2006; Lardone et al., 2007a; Lin et al., 2007*). These contradictory results may in part be due to the methodological differences and differences in the controls (fertile controls, general population, or normozoospermic men).

1.1.2.3 AZFc duplications

In addition to deletions, different duplications at the AZFc region have been reported. Duplications can occur on a chromosome with partial AZFc deletion and generate a chromosome with four DAZ genes, but lacking some STS markers (*Repping S et al., 2003; Repping S et al., 2004*). Recently, AZFc partial duplication has been shown to be a risk factor for male infertility in Taiwan (*Lin et al., 2007*). A higher incidence of increased number of DAZ genes was demonstrated in azoospermic and oligozoospermic men in Slovenia (*Writzl et al., 2005*). Additional studies are needed to determine the role of AZFc partial deletions and duplications in spermatogenesis and male infertility.

1.1.2.4 AZF candidate genes

The AZF regions include genes that are expressed during spermatogenesis and encode proteins necessary for specific stages of spermatogenesis as well as for maintaining the general housekeeping functions of the cells involved (*Lahn & Page, 1997*). The Dead box Y (DBY, recently renamed DDX3Y) encodes a putative RNA helicase. The ubiquitin-specific protease 9Y gene (USP9Y, previously known as DFFRY) encodes a protease with activity specific to ubiquitin that is involved in the regulation of protein metabolism (protein turn-over). Both genes are located at the AZFa region and have homologous genes on the X chromosome. The exact role of the candidate genes in the AZFa region are largely unknown, owing to the extreme rarity of naturally occurring, single-gene-specific mutations. Complete deletions of AZFa region is rare, but is well documented and always associated with Sertoli-cell-only syndrome and consequently azoospermia (*Ferlin et al., 2007*). The translation Initiation Factor 1A Y isoform gene (EIF1AY) and the RNA binding motif (RBM) family are found on AZFb region. EIF1AY encodes an essential translation factor. The PTP-BL-related Y (PRY) family of genes is mapped to AZFb and AZFc regions and encodes proteins proposed to be involved in apoptosis. RBM and deleted-in-azoospermia (DAZ) genes encode RNA-binding proteins that are exclusively expressed in germ cells. In addition to DAZ, chromodomain Y genes (CDY1) are found on the AZFc region and encode a protein involved in DNA remodeling that can acetylate histone H4 in vitro. Among other Y chromosome genes, likely implicated in spermatogenesis but not related to microdeletions, TSPY is a candidate oncogene that, due to its limited expression pattern in germ cells, is thought to function as a proliferation factor during spermatogenesis. The quantities of AZF gene transcripts in testicular tissues of patients with different spermatogenic impairment have been recently examined and an important role of DDX3Y was suggested (*Kleiman et al., 2007; Lardone et al., 2007*).

1.1.3 Androgen receptor CAG repeats

Androgens are essential for male sexual development and for fertility. They act through the AR, which is a transcriptional factor that contains functional domains for DNA binding, ligand binding and transcriptional regulation. The 5' end of exon 1 of the AR gene includes a polymorphic CAG triplet repeat that codes for a polyglutamine tract. The number of CAG repeats in the normal population varies between 10 and 36. Expansion of the polyglutamine tract to >38 repeats in males leads to Kennedy disease [spinal bulbar muscular atrophy (SBMA)] (*LaSpada et al., 1991*). In addition to neurological symptoms, SBMA patients show signs of hypogonadism, such as gynecomastia, impotence, testicular atrophy and reduced fertility.

In vitro studies have demonstrated a negative correlation between CAG repeat size and AR function (*Chamberlain et al., 1994*). The possible association of a long CAG repeat with male infertility in Asian populations was suggested because of a four-fold increase in the risk of impaired spermatogenesis in males who had >28 CAG repeats (*Tut et al., 1997*). Since then, the association of the long CAG repeat number in the AR gene and male infertility has been controversial.

We have also studied the possible effect of long CAG repeat tracts in the AR on infertility among Macedonian men (*Plaseski et al., 2007*). Our results showed that the mean CAG length dos not differ significantly between males with azoospermia, mild oligozoospermia, severe oligozoospermia, normozoospermia, or known causes of infertility and fertile controls. However, we found a significantly higher percentage of CAG repeats >26 ($p = 0.022$), >27 ($p = 0.018$) and >28 ($p = 0.009$) in males with mild oligozoospermia. Thus, our initial results indicated a possible association between CAG repeat length and mild oligozoospermia.

2. Screening for the presence of the most common genetic causes by quantitative fluorescent (QF)-PCR

Screening for chromosomal abnormalities is usually done by cytogenetic analysis and for AZF deletions by PCR analysis of several sequence tagged sites (STSs) in the three AZF regions. Recently, we have described a multiplex QF-PCR method that allows simultaneous detection of the most common genetic causes of male infertility, i.e. sex chromosomal aneuploidies and AZFc and AZFb deletions, and some potential risk factors such as partial AZFc deletions/duplications and AR CAG repeats (*Plaseski et al., 2008*). This 11-plex QF-PCR analysis was shown as a rapid, simple, reliable and inexpensive method that can be used as a first-step genetic analysis in infertile patients. Here, we present a modified system, where we have included additional markers in the AZFa and AZFb region, as well as a marker for determination of the X/ chromosome 3 ratio.

2.1 QF-PCR method

The quantitative fluorescent (QF) polymerase chain reaction (PCR) included 13 markers: amelogenin gene which is present on X and Y chromosomes and allows for the determination of the Y/X ratio (AMEL marker), TAF9B gene that is present on chromosomes X and 3 and permits the determination of x/chr 3 ratio, four polymorphic X-specific short tandem repeat (STR) markers (XHPRT, DXS6803; DXS981 and exon 1 of the AR gene), three non-polymorphic Y-specific markers (SRY gene, sY86 in AZFa and sY134 in AZFb region), polymorphic Y-specific STR marker (DYS448), and co-amplification of DAZ/DAZL, MYPT2Y/MYPT2 and CDY2/CDY1 fragments that permit determination of the DAZ, MYPT2Y, CDY1 and CDY2 gene copy number. The details of the primers used in the 13-plex QF-PCR are given in Table 1, while the location of the markers on the Y chromosome is given in Figure 2.

The AMEL marker exploits the 6bp deletion on the X chromosome sequence, enabling amplification of specific X-chromosome (106 bp) and Y-chromosome sequences (112 bp). The TAF9B marker co-amplifies a fragment of the TAF9B gene on X chromosome (144bp) and the one on chromosome 3 (140 bp). The DAZ gene copy number was quantified using primers that co-amplify a fragment of intron 10 from DAZ gene (208 bp) and from the homologous autosomal locus DAZL on chromosome 3 (211 bp or 251 bp). The two MYPT2Y copies in the AZFc region were co-amplified with the MYPT2 gene on chromosome 1, giving fragments of 181 bp and 176 bp respectively. The relative ratio of the two CDY1 genes in the AZFc region and two CDY2 genes in the AZFb region, which share 98% nucleotide identity was scored by two PCR sets which amplify a 6bp nucleotide difference in the 5′ region, producing fragments of 200 bp for CDY1 and 194 bp for CDY2.

One primer in each set was labeled with 6-FAM or HEX fluorescent dye, which allowed the determination of the length of the different STR and STS alleles and for quantification of the relative Amel Y/Amel X, TAF9B-X/TAF9B-chr. 3, DAZ/DAZL, MYPT2Y/MYPT2 and CDY2/CDY1 ratios on ABIPrism 3130 Genetic Analyzer using a GeneMapper Software v.4.0 (Applied Biosystems, Foster City, CA, USA).

The PCR reaction mixture contained PCR buffer (Applied Biosystems), 50-100 ng genomic DNA, 200 μM each of the four dNTP's (dATP, dCTP, dGTP and dTTP), 2-8 pmol each of the primers, and 1.5U TaqGold polymerase (Applied Biosystems) in a total volume of 15μl. The PCR was performed under the following conditions: initial denaturation step at 95^{0}C for 5 minutes, followed by 28 cycles of 1 minute denaturation at 95^{0}C, 1 minute annealing at 58^{0}C and 1.5 minutes elongation at 72^{0}C; and final elongation at 72^{0}C for 30 minutes.

2.2 QF-PCR results

The normal results of the 13 markers included in the QF-PCR analysis in males without sex chromosome aneuploidies and AZF rearrangements are shown in Table 2 and Figure 3. The

Marker	Chromosome location		Sequence of the primers (5'-3')	Label	Repeat element	Allele size range in bp (expected)	Allele size range in bp (obtained)	Concen-tration (pmol)	Reference
AMEL	Xp22.1-p22.31 Yp11.2-p22.1	(F) (R)	CCC TGG GCT CTG TAA AGA ATA GTG ATC AGA GCT TAA ACT GGG AAG CTG	6-FAM	/	106 112	103 109	2	*Sullivan et al., 1993*
DXS6803	X chr	(F) (R)	GAA ATG TGC TTT GAC AGG AA CAA AAA GGG ACA TAT GCT ACT T	HEX	tetra	/	105-125	6	*Cirigliano et al, 2001*
TAF9B	TAF9B - X chr TAF9B - chr 3	(F) (R)	TTT GAC AGG TAG TTT TGG GTC A TGG TTT TGC CTA GGT CCA GT	6-FAM	/	144 140	147 143	4	*this study*
MYPT2	MYPT2Y - Y (AZFc) MYPT2 - chr 1	(F) (R)	CTC ACT ACA TGA CAT TCA GG GTT TCT TCC CAG TAT CTA GTA CAG TGC	6-FAM	/	181 176	180 175	2	*Machev et al., 2004*
CDY	CDY 1 - Y (AZFc) CDY 2 - Y (AZFb)	(F) (R)	GTT TCT TCC ACT GTA GAA ATT CAC CTC C GAA GTT TGC ATA GTG GAC AGC	6-FAM	/	200 194	203 197	4	*Machev et al., 2004*
DAZ	DAZ - Y (AZFc) DAZL - chr 3	(F) (R)	TTA AGT ACT ACT GTA GAC AC GTT TCT TGT ATA ATG TAG AAG AGT AGA GC	HEX	/	208 211/251*	211 214/254*	6	*Machev et al., 2004*
SRY	Yp11.2-p22.1	(F) (R)	AGT AAA GGC AAC GTC CAG GAT TTC CGA CGA GGT CGA TAC TTA	HEX	/	248	243	4	*Ogilvie et al., 2005*
DXS981	Xq13.1	(F) (R)	CTC CTT GTG GCC TTC CTT AAA TG TTC TCT CCA CTT TTC AGA GTC A	6-FAM	tetra	/	233-257	4	*Edwards et al., 1991*
XHPRT	Xq26.1	(F) (R)	ATG CCA CAG ATA ATA CAC ATC CCC CTC TCC AGA ATA GTT AGA TGT AGG	6-FAM	tetra	/	268-292	4	*Edwards et al., 1992*
AR	Xq11.12	(F) (R)	TCC AGA ATC TGT TCC AGA GCG TGC GCT GTG AAG GTT GCT GTT CCT CA	HEX	tri	/	247-309	8	*Plaseski et al., 2007*
sY134	Y (AZFb)	(F) (R)	GTC TGC CTC ACC ATA AAA CG ACC ACT GCC AAA ACT TTC AA	HEX	/	301	303	4	*Simoni et al., 1999*
sY86	Y (AZFa)	(F) (R)	GTG ACA CAC AGA CTA TGC TTC ACA CAC AGA GGG ACA ACC CT	6-FAM	/	326	317	4	*Simoni et al., 1999*
DYS448	Yq11.2	(F) (R)	CAA GGA TCC AAA TAA AGA ACA GAG A GGT TAT TTC TTG ATT CCC TGT G	6-FAM	hexa	/	346-376	6	*Ogilvie et al., 2005*

* in app. 25% of individuals a 40bp insertion polymorphism in DAZL intron 10 is present (*Machev et al., 2004*)

Table 1. Details of the primers used in the QF-PCR for the detection of the most common causes of male infertility

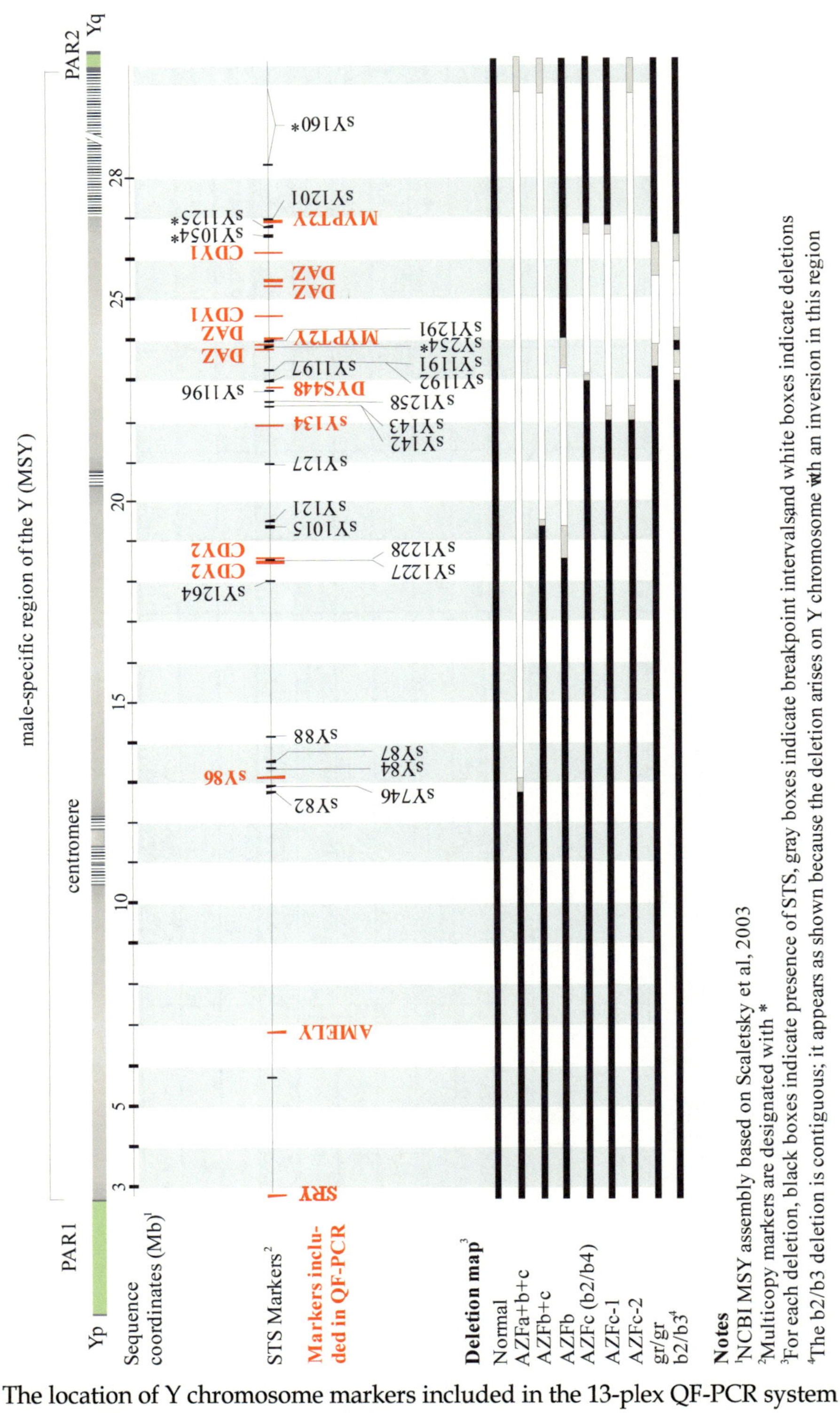

Fig. 2. The location of Y chromosome markers included in the 13-plex QF-PCR system and schematic presentation of AZF deletions detected among Macedonian males

Marker	Normal result	Sex chromosomal aneuploidies			AZF deletions						Partial AZFc deletions			AZFc duplications	
		XXY	XX	XYY	b2/b4	AZFc-1	AZFc-2	AZFb	AZFb+c	AZFa+b+c	gr/gr	b2/b3	gr/gr + b2/b4dup	gr/gr & b2/b4	b2/b3
AMEL Y/X ratio	1 (1/1)	0,5	no Y	2	normal	normal	normal	normal	<1	<1	normal	normal	normal	normal	normal
DAZ/DAZL (Y/chr 3) ratio	2 (4/2)	normal	no DAZ	4 (8/2)	no DAZ	no DAZ	no DAZ	no DAZ	no DAZ	no DAZ	1 (2/2)	1 (2/2)	2 (4/2)	>3 (>6/2)	>3 (>6/2)
MYPT2Y/MYPT2 (Y/chr 1) ratio	1 (2/2)	normal	no MYPT2Y	2 (4/2)	0,5 (1/2)	0,5 (1/2)	no MYPT2Y	normal	no MYPT2Y	no MYPT2Y	0,5 (1/2)	normal	0,5 (1/2)	>1,5 (>3/2)	normal
TAF9B (X/chr 3) ratio	0,5 (1/2)	1 (2/2)	1 (2/2)	normal	normal	normal	normal	normal	normal	normal	normal	normal	normal	normal	normal
CDY2/CDY1 - II (AZFb/AZFc) ratio	1 (2/2)	normal	no CDY1 no CDY2	normal	no CDY1	no CDY1	no CDY1	0,5 (1/2)	no CDY1 no CDY2	no CDY1 no CDY2	2 (2/1)	2 (2/1)	1 (2/2)	<0,5 (2/>4)	<0,5 (2/>4)
DXS6803/DXS 981/ XHPRT/ AR	1 allele of each STR marker	1 or 2 alleles[2]	1 or 2 alleles[2]	normal	normal	normal	normal	normal	normal	normal	normal	normal	normal	normal	normal
SRY	248 bp fragment	normal	normal[3]	normal	normal	normal	normal	normal	normal	normal	normal	normal	normal	normal	normal
sY134	303 bp fragment	normal	no fragment	normal	normal	normal	normal	no fragment	no fragment	no fragment	normal	normal	normal	normal	normal
sY86	317 bp fragment	normal	no fragment	normal	normal	normal	normal	normal	normal	no fragment	normal	normal	normal	normal	normal
DYS 448	1 allele	normal	no fragment	normal	normal	no fragment	no fragment	no fragment	no fragment	no fragment	normal	normal	normal	normal	normal

[1] the ratio is slightly higher in heterozygotes and homozygotes for DAZL polymorphism
[2] one allele in homozygotes and two alleles in heterozygotes for particular marker
[3] normal in SRY+ XX males; no fragment in SRY- XX males

Table 2. Results of the 11-plex QF-PCR in normal males and males with sex chromosomal aneuploidies, AZF deletions, partial AZFc deletions and b2/b4 duplication

normal results in a male DNA samples are presented by a Amel Y/X ratio of 1, due to the presence of one X and one Y chromosome, DAZ/DAZL ratio of 2, due to the presence of 4 DAZ genes in the AZFc region of Y chromosome and two DAZL genes, one on each chromosome 3. Around 30% of the samples showed the presence of a 40bp insertion polymorphism in the DAZL gene in a heterozygous or homozygous state. The DAZ/DAZL ratio was higher in the heterozygotes and homozygotes than in the individuals without this polymorphism due to the area of the 254bp peak being smaller than the 214bp peak. The normal MYPT2/MYPT2Y ratio is around 1 due to the presence of two copies of the gene in the AZFc region of the Y chromosome and one copy on each of the chromosomes 1, while the normal TAF9B-X/TAF9B-chr 3 ratio is 0,5 due to the presence of two copies of the gene on the chromosomes 3 and one copy on the chromosome X in males.

The four STR markers on chromosome X, as well as the one in the AZFb region on chromosome Y generate one PCR fragment due to the presence of one allele of each of the investigated markers. The non-plymorphic markers on the Y chromosome: SRY, sY134 (in the AZFb region) and sY86 (in the AZFa region) gave PCR fragments of 248 bp, 303 bp and 317 bp in males without chromosome aneuploidies and/or AZF rearrangements.

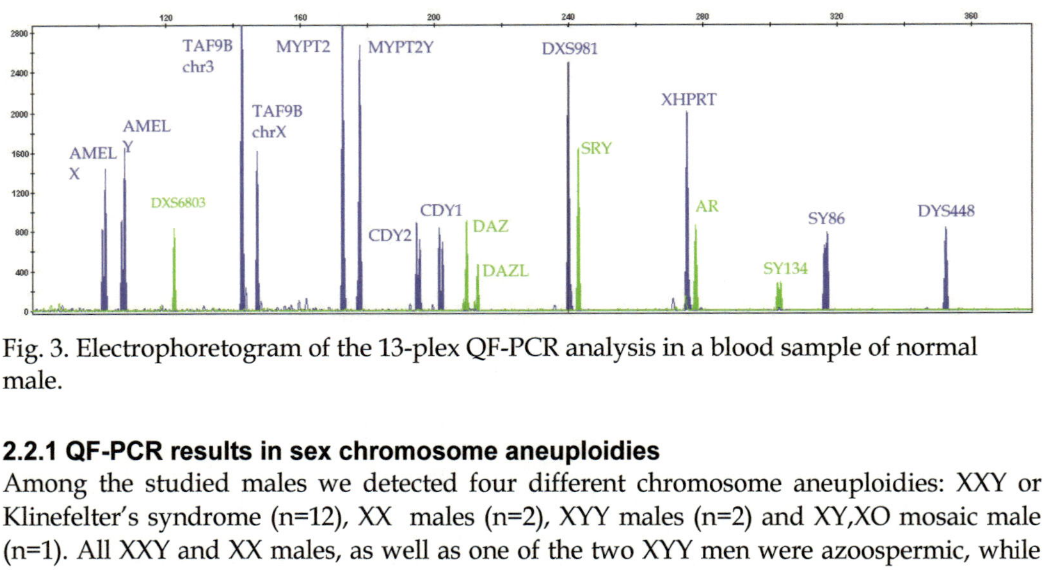

Fig. 3. Electrophoretogram of the 13-plex QF-PCR analysis in a blood sample of normal male.

2.2.1 QF-PCR results in sex chromosome aneuploidies

Among the studied males we detected four different chromosome aneuploidies: XXY or Klinefelter's syndrome (n=12), XX males (n=2), XYY males (n=2) and XY,XO mosaic male (n=1). All XXY and XX males, as well as one of the two XYY men were azoospermic, while the second XYY male and the XY,XO mosaic male presented with severe oligozoospermia. The electrophoreograms of the individuals with sex chromosome aneuploidies are shown in Figures 4-7 and the Y/X, DAZ/DAZL, MYPT2Y/MYPT2 and CDY2/CDY1 ratios are given in Table 2. All detected cases of chromosome aneuploidies were confirmed by cytogenetic analysis.

Klinefelter's syndrome (XXY) was detected by an abnormal Y/X ratio (~0.5), TAF9B-X/TAF9B-chr 3 ratio of ~1 and presence of two alleles from some of the STR markers on the X chromosome in a ratio of approximately 1:1 (Figure 4).

The two XX males were characterized by the absence of the Y fragment from the AMEL Y/X marker, DAZ, MYPT2Y, CDY1 and CDY2 fragments and TAF9B-X/TAF9B-chr 3 ratio of ~1 (Figure 5). In both XX males the SRY fragment was present, sY134, sY86 and DYS 448 fragments were absent and at least one of the four STR markers on the X chromosome showed two alleles. Rarely, in XX males the SRY gene is not present in which case the PCR fragment from the SRY gene would be missing and 11-plex QF-PCR pattern would be same as in DNA from normal females.

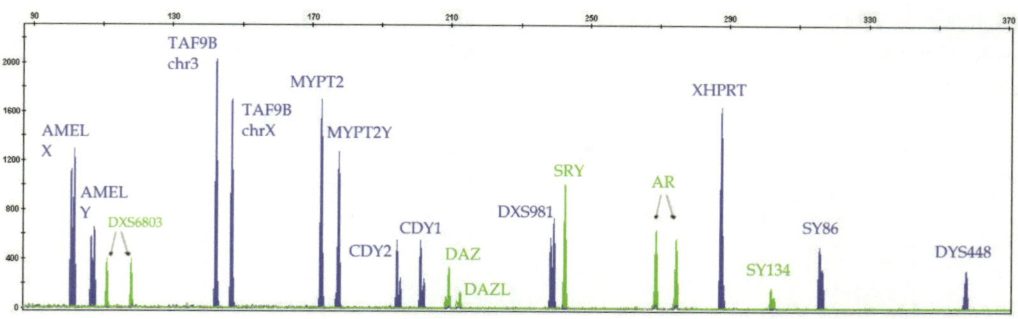

Fig. 4. Electrophoretogram of the 13-plex QF-PCR analysis in a men with Klinefelter's syndrome (XXY).

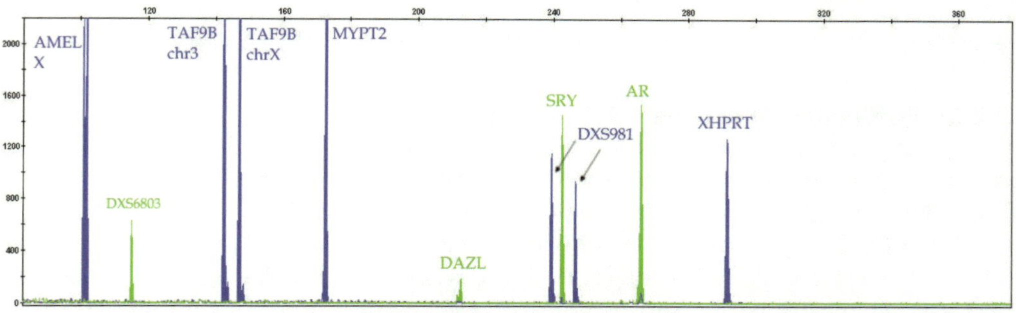

Fig. 5. Electrophoretogram of the 13-plex QF-PCR analysis in a men with XX male syndrome.

The XYY individuals showed also a specific pattern, characterized by abnormal Y/X (~2), DAZ/DAZL (~4) and MYPT2Y/MYPT2 (~2) ratios, while the TAF9B-X/TAF9B-chr 3 and CDY2/CDY1 ratios were within the normal range (Figure 6).

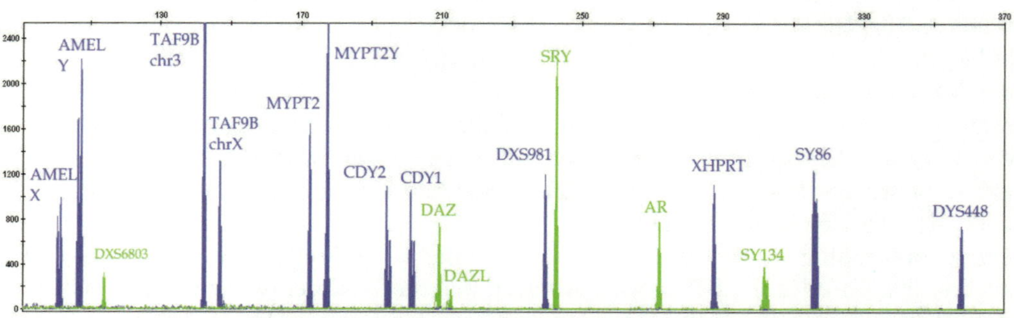

Fig. 6. Electrophoretogram of the 13-plex QF-PCR analysis in a men with XYY syndrome.

The 13-plex QF-PCR of XY,XO mosaic male showed abnormal Y/X (0,35) and MYPT2Y/MYPT2 (0,25) and DAZ/DAZL (0,59) ratios, while the CDY2/CDY1 and TAF9B-X/TAF9B-chr 3 ratios were normal (Figure 7). This result suggested that the Y chromosome is lost in approximately half of the white blood cells in this patient. The result was confirmed on a DNA isolated from a fresh blood sample and by cytogenetic analysis as well. Analysis of DNA extracted from the buccal swab of this patient showed a normal result. Unfortunately we were not able to analyze DNA isolated from the spermatozoa of this patient.

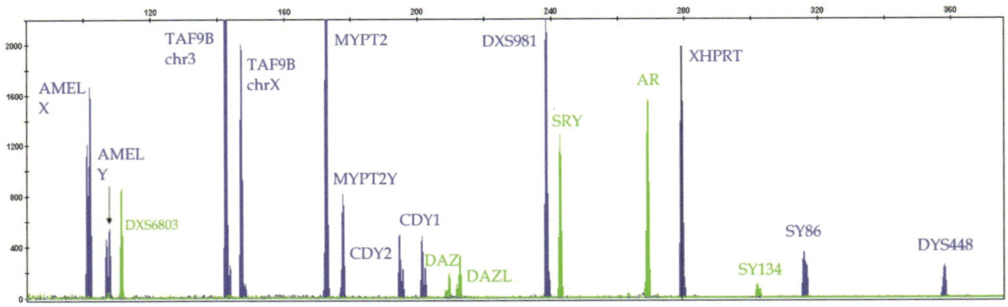

Fig. 7. Electrophoretogram of the 13-plex QF-PCR analysis in a XY/X0 mosaic male.

2.2.2 QF-PCR results in complete AZF deletions

During our previous work we have detected eight different AZF deletions, including the two partial AZFc deletions, gr/gr and b2/b3 deletions (*Plaseski et al., 2006, Plaseski et al., 2008*). Schematic presentation of the deletions is shown in Figure 2.

The 13-plex QF-PCR patterns obtained in the patients with different AZF deletions are given in Table 2. We were able to distinguish all six types of AZF deletions that we detected previously amongst infertile patients (*Plaseski et al., 2006*). In the six patients with b2/b4 deletions the DAZ fragment and the CDY1 fragments were missing, while the MYPT2Y/MYPT2 ratio was decreased suggesting the absence of one of the two MYPT2Y copies on the Y chromosome. All other fragments showed a normal pattern.

The initial screening for AZF deletions following the guidelines for the detection of Y microdeletions showed presence of AZFc deletions in two other patients (*Plaseski et al., 2006*). The analysis with additional STS markers showed that in these two patients the 5′ border of the deletion is identical and lies between sY 134 and sY 142 markers. The 3′ border differs and is identical to the 3′ border of the b2/b4 deletion in one of the two patients, while in the other it extends distal from the AZFc region (Figure 2). These two patients showed an identical pattern for all markers except for MYPT2Y/MYPT2 (Table 2). In one the MYPT2Y fragment was missing (Figure 8), while in the other it was present, but the ratio of MYPT2Y/MYPT2 was decreased to about half suggesting deletion of one MYPT2Y copy. In both patients markers sY134 in the AZFb region and sY86 in AZFa region were present, while the DYS 448 marker was absent.

During our routine screening for Y microdeletions we detected one patient with AZFb deletion. The additional Y STS markers showed that the 5′ border of this deletion is between sY 1228 and sY 1015, while the 3′ border extends in the 5′ part of the AZFc region between sY1291 and sY1191 (Figure 2). This deletion also gave a specific pattern with the 13-plex QF

PCR characterized by the absence of the DYS 448 and sY134 fragments and ratios of DAZ/DAZL and CDY2/CDY1 markers reduced to half (Table 2), suggesting that two of the four DAZ genes in the AZFc regions and one of the two CDY2 genes in the AZFb region were missing.

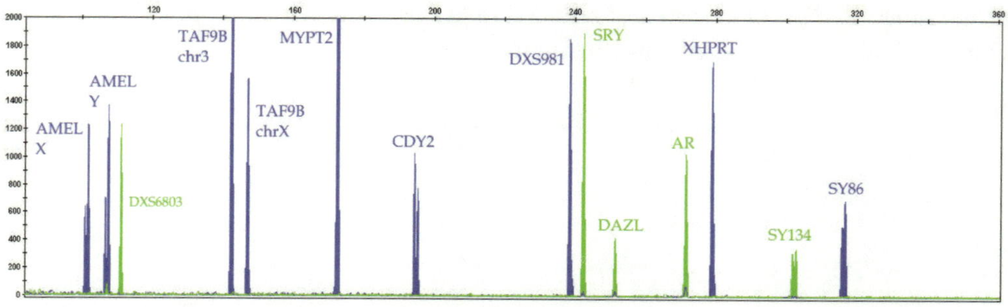

Fig. 8. Electrophoretogram of the 13-plex QF-PCR analysis in a men with AZFc-2 deletion.

The patient with AZFb+c deletion also showed a specific pattern with the 13-plex QF-PCR, which was the same as AZFc-1 deletion in all but sY134 marker that was missing and Y/X AMEL marker which showed a reduced ratio of 0.23, due to the presence of XY/X0 mosaicism (Table 2 and Figure 9). The XY/XO mosaicism was confirmed by cytogenetic analysis.
The QF-PCR result of the AZFa+b+c deletion showed absence of all markers in the AZF a, b and c regions (DAZ, MYPT2Y, CDY1, CDY2, sY134, sY86 and DYS448) (Figure 10). The patient with AZFa+b+c deletion also showed an abnormal Y/X ratio (0,42), suggesting that the Y chromosome was lost in half of the cells in this patient.

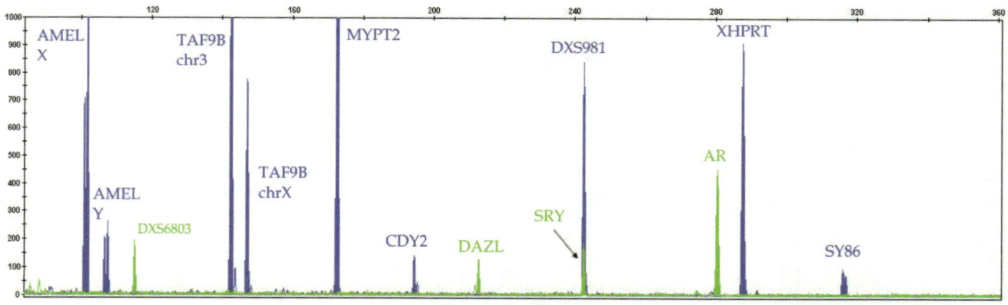

Fig. 9. Electrophoretogram of the 13-plex QF-PCR analysis in a men with AZFb+c deletion.

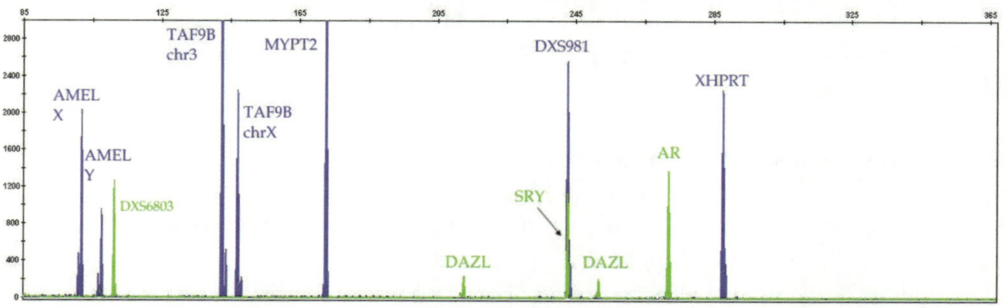

Fig. 10. Electrophoretogram of the 13-plex QF-PCR analysis in a men with AZFa+b+c deletion.

2.2.3 QF-PCR results in partial AZFc deletions

The 13-plex QF-PCR permitted detection of partial AZFc deletions and duplications (Table 2). Both partial AZFc deletions (gr/gr and b2/b3) showed abnormal DAZ/DAZL (~1) and CDY2/CDY1 ratios (~2), but differ in the MYPT2Y/MYPT2 ratios which are within the normal range in b2/b3 deletion and reduced in gr/gr deletion (~0.5). The QF-PCR analysis in men with gr/gr deletion is shown in Figure 11.

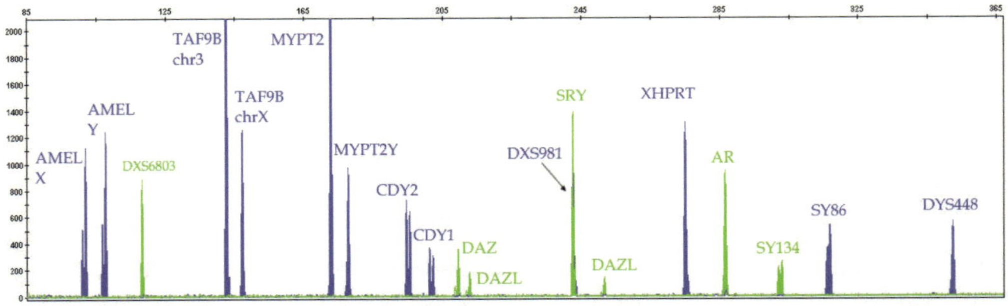

Fig. 11. Electrophoretogram of the 13-plex QF-PCR analysis in a men with gr/gr deletion.

Three of the previously detected patients with gr/gr deletions, showed normal or increased DAZ/DAZL levels, normal, increased or decreased CDY2/CDY1 levels, while the MYPT2Y/MYPT2 ratio was reduced to half, similar to that in the other gr/gr deletions (Figure 12). This rearrangement has probably arisen from gr/gr deletion followed by duplication. All three males with both b2/b4 duplication and gr/gr deletion differ from normal individuals in the MYPT2Y/MYPT2 ratio which is reduced to half.

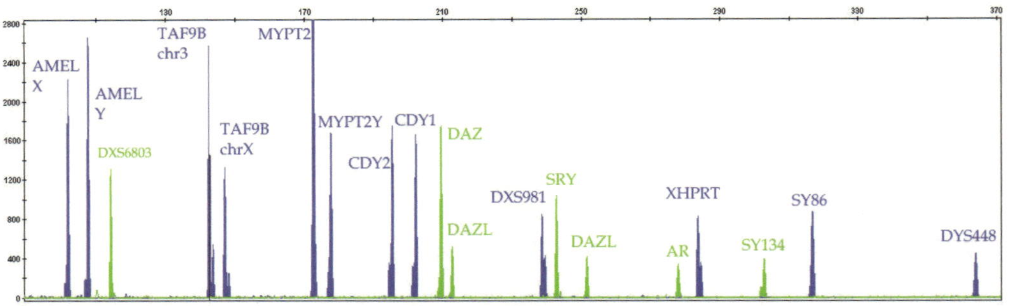

Fig. 12. Electrophoretogram of the 13-plex QF-PCR analysis in a men with b2/b4 duplication and gr/gr deletion.

2.2.4 QF-PCR results in AZFc duplications

The 13-plex QF-PCR detected also the duplications mediated by the amplicons in the AZFc region. Samples with gr/gr or b2/b4 duplications were characterized by increased DAZ/DAZL (>3) and MYPT2Y/MYPT2 (>1.5) ratios and decreased CDY2/CDY1 ratios (<0.5) (Table 2). Samples with partial AZFc duplication on chromosomes with b2/b3 inversion (b2/b3 duplications), showed increased DAZ/DAZL (>3), normal MYPT2Y/MYPT2 and decreased CDY2/CDY1 ratios (<0.5) (Figure 13).

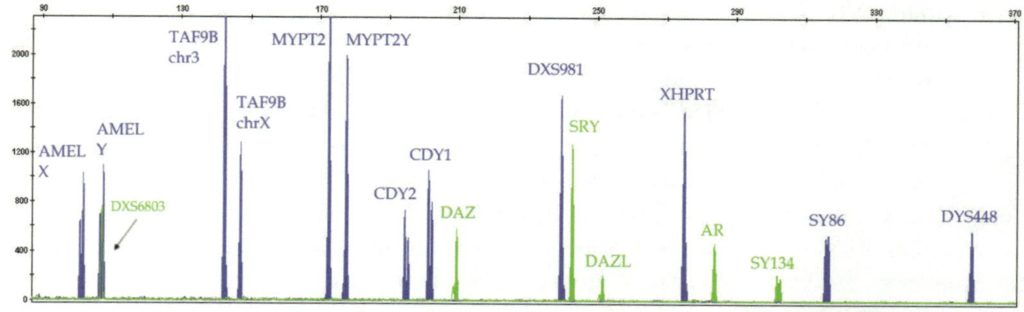

Fig. 12. Electrophoretogram of the 13-plex QF-PCR analysis in a men with b2/b3 duplication.

2.2.5 Detection of the number of AR CAG repeats

An additional advantage of our QF-PCR system is that it can also assess the number of the AR CAG repeats, since one of the STR markers on the X chromosome in the 13-plex QF-PCR involves the CAG repeats in the exon 1 of the AR gene. The PCR amplification using oligonucleotide primers surrounding the CAG repeat region in the exon 1 of the AR gene generated fragments with a size ranging from 247 to 309 bp, corresponding to the 13 to 34 CAG tandem repeats. The number of CAG repeats predicted by the GeneMapper software v.4.0. (Applied BioSystems) was previously compared with the actual CAG repeats determined by direct dideoxy terminator cycle sequencing using the BigDye Terminator Sequencing Kit v1.0 (Applied BioSystems) in several male DNA samples with 14, 19, 21, 25 and 29 CAG repeats.

3. Conclusion

In conclusion, we have developed a rapid, simple, reliable and inexpensive multiplex QF-PCR method, that can be used as a first-step genetic analysis in infertile/subfertile men to detect the most common genetic causes of male infertility (sex chromosomal aneuploidies and AZF deletions) and to study some potential risk factors (AZFc partial deletions and duplications and AR CAG repeats).

4. Acknowledgements

This study was supported in part by grants CRP/MAC09-01 from ICGEB-Trieste and 14-1656/1-10 from the Ministry of Education and Science of the R. Macedonia (both to D. Plaseska-Karanfilska).

5. References

Carvalho CM, Zuccherato LW, Bastos-Rodrigues L, Santos FR, Pena SD (2006) No association found between gr/gr deletions and infertility in Brazilian males. *Mol Hum Reprod* 12:269-273.

Chamberlain NL, Driver ED, Miesfeld RL (1994) The length and location of CAG trinucleotide repeats in the androgen receptor N-terminal domain affect transactivation function. *Nucleic Acids Res* 22:3181-3186.

Cirigliano V, Lewin P, Szpiro-Tapies S, Fuster C, Adinolfi M (2001) Assessment of new markers for the rapid detection of aneuploidies by quantitative fluorescent PCR (QF-PCR). *Ann Hum Genet* 65:421-427.

Costa P, Goncalves R, Ferras C, Fernandes S, Fernandes AT, Sousa M, Barros A (2008) Identification of new breakpoints in AZFb and AZFc. *Mol Hum Reprod* 14:251-8.

De Braekeleer M, Dao TN (1991) Cytogenetic studies in male infertility: a review. *Hum Reprod* 6:245–250.

de Llanos M, Ballesca JL, Gazquez C, Margarit E, Oliva R (2005) High frequency of gr/gr chromosome Y deletions in consecutive oligospermic ICSI candidates. *Hum Reprod* 20:216-220.

Edwards A, Civitello A, Hammond HA, Caskey CT (1991) DNA typing and genetic mapping with trimeric and tetrameric tandem repeats. *Am J Hum Genet* 49:746-756.

Edwards A, Hammond HA, Jin L, Caskey CT, Chakraborty R (1992) Genetic variation at five trimeric and tetrameric tandem repeat loci in four human population groups. *Genomics* 12:241-53.

Edwards RG & Bishop CE (1997) On the origin and frequency of Y chromosome deletions responsible for severe male infertility. *Mol Hum Reprod* 3: 549-54.

Ferlin A, Moro E, Rossi A, Dallapiccola B, Foresta C (2003) The human Y chromosome's azoospermia factor b (AZFb) region: sequence, structure, and deletion analysis in infertile men. *J Med Genet*; 40: 18-24.

Ferlin A, Arredi B, Foresta C (2006) Genetic causes of male infertility. *Reprod Toxicol* 22:133-141.

Ferlin A, Tessari A, Ganz F, Marchina E, Barlati S, Garolla A, Engl B, Foresta C (2005) Association of partial AZFc region deletions with spermatogenic impairment and male infertility. *J Med Genet* 42:209-213.

Ferlin A, Raicu F, Gatta V, Zuccarello D, Palka G, Foresta C (2007) Male infertility: role of genetic background. *Reprod Biomed Online* 14:734–45.

Foresta C, Ferlin A, Moro E, Scandellari C (2000) Y chromosome. *Lancet* 355:234-235.

Foresta C, Garolla A, Bartoloni L, Bettella A, Ferlin A (2005) Genetic abnormalities among severely oligospermic men who are candidates for intracytoplasmic sperm injection. *J Clin Endocrinol Metab* 90:152-6.

Gekas J, Thepot F, Turleau C, Siffroi JP, Dadoune JP, Briault S, Rio M, Bourouillou G, Carré-Pigeon F, Wasels R, Benzacken B; Association des Cytogeneticiens de Langue Francaise (2001) Chromosomal factors of infertility in candidate couples for ICSI: an equal risk of constitutional aberrations in women and men. *Hum Reprod* 16:82-90.

Giachini C, Guarducci E, Longepied G, Degl'Innocenti S, Becherini L, Forti G, Mitchell MJ, Krausz C (2005) The gr/gr deletion(s): a new genetic test in male infertility? *J Med Genet* 42:497-502.

Hecht F, Hecht B (1987) Aneuploidy in humans: dimensions, demography, and dangers of abnormal numbers of chromosomes. In: Vig BK and Sandberg AA (eds) *Aneuploidy: Incidence and Etiology*. Alan R. Liss, New York, pp 9-50.

Hucklenbroich K, Gromoll J, Heinrich M, Hohoff C, Nieschlag E, Simoni M (2005) Partial deletions in the AZFc region of the Y chromosome occur in men with impaired as well as normal spermatogenesis. *Hum Reprod* 20:191-197.

Kamp C, Hirschmann P, Voss H, Huellen K, Vogt PH (2000) Two long homologous retroviral sequence blocks in proximal Yq11 cause AZFa microdeletions as a result of intrachromosomal recombination events. *Hum Mol Genet* 9: 2563-72.

Kleiman SE, Bar-Shira Maymon B, Hauser R, Botchan A, Paz G, Yavetz H, Yogev L (2008) Histone H4 acetylation and AZFc involvement in germ cells of specimens of impaired spermatogenesis. *Fertil Steril* 89:1728-36.

Krausz C, Forti G, McElreavey K (2003) The Y chromosome and male fertility and infertility. *Int J Androl* 26: 70-5.

Kuroda-Kawaguchi T, Skaletsky H, Brown LG, Minx PJ, Cordum HS, Waterston RH, Wilson RK, Silber S, Oates R, Rozen S, Page DC (2001) The AZFc region of the Y chromosome features massive palindromes and uniform recurrent deletions in infertile men. *Nat Genet* 29:279-286.

Lahn BT and Page DC (1997) Functional coherence of the human Y chromosome. *Science* 278:675-80.

LaSpada AR, Wilson EM, Lubahn DB, Harding AE, Fishbeck KH (1991) Androgen receptor gene mutations in X-linked spinal and bulbar muscular atrophy. *Nature* 352: 77-79.

Lardone MC, Parodi DA, Ebensperger M, Peñaloza P, Cornejo V, Valdevenito R, Pommer R, Castro A (2007a) AZFc partial deletions in Chilean men with severe spermatogenic failure. *Fertil Steril* 88:1318-1326.

Lardone MC, Parodi DA, Valdevenito R, Ebensperger M, Piottante A, Madariaga M, Smith R, Pommer R, Zambrano N, Castro A (2007b) Quantification of DDX3Y, RBMY1, DAZ and TSPY mRNAs in testes of patients with severe impairment of spermatogenesis. *Mol Hum Reprod* 13:705-12.

Lin YW, Hsu LC, Kuo PL, Huang WJ, Chiang HS, Yeh SD, Hsu TY, Yu YH, Hsiao KN, Cantor RM, Yen PH (2007) Partial duplication at AZFc on the Y chromosome is a risk factor for impaired spermatogenesis in Han Chinese in Taiwan. *Hum Mutat* 28:486-494.

Ma K, Mallidis C, Bhasin S (2000) The role of Y chromosome deletions in male infertility. *Eur J Endocrinol* 142:418-430.

Machev N, Saut N, Longepied G, Terriou P, Navarro A, Levy N, Guichaoua M, Metzler-Guillemain C, Collignon P, Frances AM, Belougne J, Clemente E, Chiaroni J, Chevillard C, Durand C, Ducourneau A, Pech N, McElreavey K, Mattei M-G, Mitchell MJ (2004) Sequence family variant loss from the AZFc interval of the human Y chromosome, but not gene copy loss, is strongly associated with male infertility. *J Med Genet* 41:814-825.

Mau-Holzmann UA. Somatic chromosomal abnormalities in infertile men and women (2005) Cytogenet Genome Res 111:317–336.

Najmabadi H, Huang V, Yen P, Subbarao MN, Bhasin D, Banaag L, Naseeruddin S, de Kretser DM, Baker HW, McLachlan RI, et al. (1996) Substantial prevalence of microdeletions of the Y-chromosome in infertile men with idiopathic azoospermia and oligozoospermia detected using a sequence-tagged site-based mapping strategy. *J Clin Endocrinol Metab* 81: 1347-52.

Ogilvie CM, Donaghue C, Fox SP, Docherty Z, Mann K (2005) Rapid prenatal diagnosis of aneuploidy using quantitative fluorescence-PCR (QF-PCR). J Histochem Cytochem 53:285-288.

Oliva R, Margarit E, Ballesca JL, Carrio A, Sanchez A, Mila M, Jimenez L, Alvarez-Vijande JR, Ballesta F (1998) Prevalence of Y chromosome microdeletions in oligospermic and azoospermic candidates for intracytoplasmic sperm injection. *Fertil Steril* 70: 506-10.

Plaseski T, Dimitrovski C, Kocevska B, Efremov GD, Plaseska-Karanfilska D (2003) The prevalence of Y chromosome microdeletions among infertile males from the Republic of Macedonia. *Balkan J Med Genet* 6:39-44.

Plaseski T, Noveski P, Kocevska B, Dimitrovski C, Efremov GD and Plaseska-Karanfilska D (2006) AZF deletions in infertile men from the Republic of Macedonia. *Prilozi* 27:5-16.

Plaseski T, Noveski P, Trivodalieva S, Efremov GD, Plaseska-Karanfilska D. Detection of sex chromosome aneuploidies and AZF deletions by QF-PCR. *Genet Test* 12:595-605, 2008.

Ravel C, Chantot-Bastaraud S, El Houate B, Mandelbaum J, Siffroi JP, McElreavey K (2006) GR/GR deletions within the azoospermia factor c region on the Y chromosome might not be associated with spermatogenic failure. *Fertil Steril* 85:229-231.

Reijo R, Lee TY, Salo P, Alagappan R, Brown LG, Rosenberg M, Rozen S, Jaffe T, Straus D, Hovatta O et al. (1995) Diverse spermatogenic defects in humans caused by Y chromosome deletions encompassing a novel RNA-binding protein gene. *Nat Genet* 10: 383-93.

Repping S, Skaletsky H, Lange J, Silber S, Van der Veen F, Oates RD, Pages DC, Rozen S (2002) Recombination between palindromes P5 and P1 on the human Y chromosome causes massive deletions and spermatogenic failure. *Am J Hum Genet* 71:906-922.

Repping S, Skaletsky H, Brown L, van Daalen SK, Korver CM, Pyntikova T, Kuroda-Kawaguchi T, de Vries JW, Oates RD, Silber S, van der Veen F, Page DC, Rozen S (2003) Polymorphism for a 1.6-Mb deletion of the human Y chromosome persists through balance between recurrent mutation and haploid selection. *Nat Genet* 35:247-251.

Repping S, van Daalen SK, Korver CM, Brown LG, Marszalek JD, Gianotten J, Oates RD, Silber S, van der Veen F, Page DC, Rozen S (2004) A family of human Y chromosomes has dispersed throughout northern Eurasia despite a 1.8-Mb deletion in the azoospermia factor c region. *Genomics* 83:1046-1052.

Reubinoff BE, Abeliovich D,Werner M, Schenker JG, Safran A, LewinA (1998) A birth in non-mosaic Klinefelter's syndrome after testicular fine needle aspiration, intracytoplasmic sperm injection and preimplantation genetic diagnosis. *Hum Reprod* 13:1887–1892.

Simoni M, Gromoll J, Dworniczak B, Rolf C, Abshagen K, Kamischke A, Carani C, Meschede D, Behre HM, Horst J, Nieschlag E (1997) Screening for deletions of the Y chromosome involving the DAZ (Deleted in AZoospermia) gene in azoospermia and severe oligozoospermia. *Fertil Steril* 67: 542-7.

Simoni M, Kamischke A, Nieschlag E (1998) Current status of the molecular diagnosis of Y-chromosomal microdeletions in the work-up of male infertility. Initiative for international quality control. *Hum Reprod* 13: 1764-8.

Simoni M, Bakker E, Eurlings MC, Matthijs G, Moro E, Muller CR, Vogt PH (1999) Laboratory guidelines for molecular diagnosis of Y-chromosomal microdeletions. *Int J Androl* 22: 292-9.

Sharara FI (1999) Klinefelter's Syndrome. In: *Encyclopaedia of Reproduction*. Academic Press, New York, vol 2, pp 938-941.

Skaletsky H, Kuroda-Kawaguchi T, Minx PJ, Cordum HS, Hillier L, Brown LG, Repping S, Pyntikova T, Ali J, Bieri T, Chinwalla A, Delehaunty A, Delehaunty K, Du H, Fewell G, Fulton L, Fulton R, Graves T, Hou SF, Latrielle P, Leonard S, Mardis E, Maupin R, McPherson J, Miner T, Nash W, Nguyen C, Ozersky P, Pepin K, Rock S, Rohlfing T, Scott K, Schultz B, Strong C, Tin-Wollam A, Yang SP, Waterston RH, Wilson RK, Rozen S, Page DC (2003) The male-specific region of the human Y chromosome is a mosaic of discrete sequence classes. *Nature* 423:825-837.

Skakkebaek NE, Hultén M, Jacobsen P, Mikkelsen M (1973) Quantification of human seminiferous epithelium. II. Histological studies in eight 47,XYY men. *J Reprod Fertil* 32:391-401.

Sullivan KM, Mannucci A, Kimpton CP, Gill P (1993) A rapid and quantitative DNA sex test: fluorescence-based PCR analysis of X-Y homologous gene amelogenin. *Biotechniques* 15:636-638.

Tiepolo L & Zuffardi O (1976) Localization of factors controlling spermatogenesis in the nonfluorescent portion of the human Y chromosome long arm. *Hum Genet* 34: 119-24.

Tilford CA, Kuroda-Kawaguchi T, Skaletsky H, Rozen S, Brown LG, Rosenberg M, McPherson JD, Wylie K, Sekhon M, Kucaba TA et al (2001) A physical map of the human Y chromosome. *Nature* 409:943-945.

Tut TG, Ghadessy FJ, Trifiro MA, Pinsky L, Yong EL (1997) Long polyglutamine tracts in the androgen receptor are associated with reduced transactivation, impaired sperm production, and male infertility. *J Clin Endocrinol Metab* 82: 3777-3782.

Vogt PH, Edelmann A, Kirsch S, Henegariu O, Hirschmann P, Kiesewetter F, Kohn FM, Schill WB, Farah S, Ramos C et al (1996) Human Y chromosome azoospermia factors (AZF) mapped to different subregions in Yq11. *Hum Mol Genet* 5:933-943.

Vogt PH (1998) Human chromosome deletions in Yq11, AZF candidate genes and male infertility: history and update. *Mol Hum Reprod* 4:739-44.

Vogt PH (2005) AZF deletions and Y chromosomal haplogroups: history and update based on sequence. *Hum Reprod Update* 11:319-336.

Vollrath D, Foote S, Hilton A, Brown LG, Beer-Romero P, Bogan JS, Page DC (1992) The human Y chromosome: a 43-interval map based on naturally occurring deletions. *Science* 258: 52-9.

Writzl K, Zorn B, Peterlin B (2005) Copy number of DAZ genes in infertile men. *Fertil Steril* 84:1522-1525.

Wu B, Lu NX, Xia YK, Gu AH, Lu CC, Wang W, Song L, Wang SL, Shen HB, Wang XR (2007) A frequent Y chromosome b2/b3 subdeletion shows strong association with male infertility in Han-Chinese population. *Hum Reprod* 22:1107-1113.

13

High-Throughput Screening for Highly Functional RNA-*Trans*-Splicing Molecules: Correction of Plectin in Epidermolysis Bullosa Simplex

Verena Wally, Ulrich Koller and Johann W. Bauer
Division of Molecular Dermatology and EB House Austria, Department of Dermatology, Paracelsus Medical University
Austria

1. Introduction

Epidermolysis bullosa (EB) is a very heterogeneous hereditary disease of the skin and mucous membranes, characterized by erosions and blistering after minor traumatization. Up to now at least 12 genes are known to underlie EB, which render structural and mechanical stability of the skin (Fine et al., 2008). The characteristic blister formation occurs on the level of the basement membrane zone and the basal keratinocytes, depending on the gene, which is mutated. In EB simplex (EBS) the split formation in the skin occurs due to cytolysis of the basal keratinocytes, in junctional EB (JEB) within the lamina lucida and in dystrophic EB (DEB) on the dermal aspect of the basement membrane zone. Due to the clinical and genetic heterogeneity of this disease the development of a gene therapy is challenging, since every type of EB has to be targeted separately. Furthermore, the different subtypes differ in their mode of inheritance. Especially for basal EB simplex, where mutations in the keratin 5 (*K5*), keratin 14 (*K14*) and plectin (*PLEC*) genes may cause the clinical phenotype, dominant mutations are frequent. But also in dystrophic EB, where mutations in the collagen VII gene (*COL7A1*) are causative for the disease, dominantly inherited subtypes are known. Another characteristic feature of the involved genes is that many of them are very large and exceed the packaging capacities of commonly used (viral) vectors (e.g. *COL7A1*: ~9,3kb, *PLEC*: ~14.8kb). Functionally, all genes involved in EB have structural significance. Whereas keratin 5 and keratin 14 are major components of the cytoskeleton in basal keratinocytes, plectin is a cytolinker protein, connecting the actin filament network with the microtubules, the intermediate filaments and the hemidesmosomes and desmosomes. Isoforms of plectin are expressed in many cell types and always have "networking" functions. This is the reason why epidermolysis bullosa triggered by mutations in this gene goes along with muscular dystrophy and pyloric atresia. 12 plectin isoforms, differing in their 5′ transcript portion have been identified up to now, most of them differing in their first exon. However, the structure and mode of function is comparable between all isoforms (Rezniczek et al., 2003). Structurally, plectin consists of two globular domains, flanking a central rod domain. The 5′ globular domain is encoded by exons 1 to 30 and is over 4kb in length, whereas the rod is encoded by one single 3.38kb exon. Plectin peptides form homodimers with a central coiled-coil of alpha helices and two globular domains. Within the globular domains the binding sites for its various binding partners are situated. Therefore, mutations in the rod cause mainly EBS with muscular dystrophy, whereas EBS with pylorus atresia is caused by mutations outside exon 31 (Natsuga et al., 2010). In this chapter we describe a *trans*-splicing based gene therapeutic approach on the example of epidermolysis bullosa simplex, caused by mutations in the *PLEC* gene. Based on the first proof-of-principle publication from 2008 we developed a screening method to correct patient fibroblasts with a high efficiency and specificity, rendering this approach a potential candidate for future *in vivo* studies.

2. Gene therapy in EB

For many devastating diseases gene therapy is the only hope for a curative intervention. Many efforts have been made in a spectrum of gene therapeutic strategies, resulting in a small range of gene therapeutic approaches available *in vitro*, each having its advantages and limitations.

A very straight-forward approach is gene supplementation therapy, in which a wildtype cDNA copy of a given mutated gene is brought into a cell to revert the phenotype. This gene complementation approach results in the rescue of the phenotype by providing the functional protein. Full-length cDNA therapy can be used for most recessively inherited diseases, where the transgene does not exceed the size of the packaging capacity of the vector of choice. In EB, cDNA therapy was already used for collagen 17 (*COL17A1*), laminin beta 3 (*LAMB3*) (Dellambra et al., 2000; Dellambra et al., 1998), integrin beta 4 (*ITGB4*) (Dellambra et al., 2001) and collagen 7 (*COL7A1*) (Siprashvili et al., 2010). In 2006, De Luca and his group applied *ex vivo* gene therapy for a patient suffering from recessive dystrophic EB for the first time (Mavilio et al., 2006). Patient's epidermal stem cells were transduced with a *LAMB3* expressing retrovirus. Expanded skin sheets were transplanted onto the anterior parts of the patient's legs, showing complete epidermal regeneration after eight weeks. Molecular analysis confirmed the correct integration of the *LAMB3* chain in the laminin-332 protein, rendering integrity to the transplanted skin section.

Even though great achievements were made also for other genes, cDNA therapy has limitations. In the case of the *LAMB3* approach described above, some case specific characteristics facilitated the success of this application. These were the autosomal recessive mode of inheritance, the limited size of the *LAMB3* coding region, the residual 5% gene expression of the endogenous *LAMB3* alleles (avoiding immune rejection) and the nature of LAMB3 in making part in a trimer, thereby avoiding an excess of the functional protein, as the amount of available laminin-332 is limited by laminin alpha 3 and laminin gamma 2. This last point is crucial as also overexpression of the transgene can have major impact on the therapeutic outcome.

For other genes the starting situation is different. Mutated genes can be very large or dominantly inherited, or they need strict expression control due to their negative interference when overexpressed. Quite contrary, it was found that low levels of functional protein can be sufficient to render a normal phenotype. For this reason cDNA therapy is often complemented with knockdown approaches like RNA interference (RNAi) or antisense oligonucleotides (ASOs) to knock down the mutated gene and minimizing an excess of the transcript.

But not only complementary, but also standing alone such alternative strategies were developed, many of them acting on RNA level. Therapy on RNA level has the advantage that cell targeting does not have to be as strict, since the interfering process can only take place in cells actively expressing the targeted gene. This also regulates the amount of interference, thus avoiding the overexpression of the respective gene. A widely applied approach is the use of interfering RNAs (RNAi). There, specifically designed short-hairpin RNAs (shRNAs) or short interfering RNAs (siRNA) are introduced into cells of interest. After processing, specific 21bp RNA fragments are incorporated in an RNA induced silencing complex (RISC), specifically hybridizing to an allele harbouring a mutation. This leads to the cleavage of the target mRNA (Siomi and Siomi, 2009).

For keratin 14, RNAi was used for characterization studies of EBS (Werner et al., 2004; Russell et al., 2009). However, the drawback of RNAi is that even though theoretically any gene and any mutation can be targeted, the risk of haploinsufficiency has to be considered. To meet this problem, rescue approaches are conducted by introducing the wildtype cDNA, leading to the limitations discussed above.

Another approach on RNA level is the use of ribozymes. Ribozymes are RNA molecules, which can specifically cleave themselves, a DNA or RNA molecule at a specific site, mediating degradation or ligation of yonder. The mostly used ribozymes are hammerhead ribozymes and group-I-intron self-splicing ribozymes. Both have recognition sites specifically hybridizing to a target mRNA, mediating cleavage or splicing. Group-I-self splicing ribozymes can be altered to introduce a desired cDNA portion to be *trans*-spliced 3′ of the endogenous target site. Besides the fact that recognition sites of ribozymes are rather short (~ 30nt for group-I-self splicing introns) and therefore increasing the probability of hybridizing unspecifically or off-target, only downstream gene portions can be replaced. For 5′ mRNA stretches this approach is not applicable. Regarding EB, McLean I and Terron A engineered three ribozymes mediating specific cleavage of EBS underlying keratin 14 (McLean & Terron, 2002). Cleavage of more than 90% of endogenous keratin 14 in cultured keratinocytes was achieved upon transfection. However, no differentiation between wildtype and mutated alleles was possible, resulting in a nearly complete loss of *K14* mRNA, necessitating rescue by ribozyme resistant wildtype keratin 14. Given the limitations of the above mentioned approaches we assume that Spliceosome Mediated RNA *Trans*-splicing (SMaRT) is a promising tool for gene therapy.

2.1 Spliceosome Mediated RNA *Trans*-Splicing

Spliceosome Mediated RNA *Trans*-Splicing (SMaRT) is a gene therapeutic approach, taking advantage of the cell's spliceosome to recombine two distinct pre-mRNAs to result in one mature mRNA. Pre-mRNA splicing is a naturally occurring process during mRNA maturation, which was first seen in trypanosomes, nematodes and recently also in humans (Murphy et al., 1986; Flouriot et al., 2002; Davis et al., 1995). During *trans*-splicing, the spliceosome ligates a 5′ exon from one pre-mRNA with a 3′ exon from another pre-mRNA, thereby producing an "alternative" mature mRNA, composed of exons derived from two different precursors. For SMaRT, this process is utilized to replace a disease causing gene portion by its wildtype copy. With this technology, any coding region of interest can be *trans*-spliced to any targeted, endogenous pre-mRNA (Puttaraju et al., 1999). Depending on the gene portion to be replaced, 5′ exon replacement, 3′ exon replacement and internal exon replacement (IER) are distinct (Figure 1).

Commonly, SMaRT is applied as a therapeutic tool, replacing gene portions harbouring a disease relevant mutation. Such settings were reported for epidermolysis bullosa (*COL7A1, KRT14, PLEC*) (Murauer et al., 2010; Wally et al., 2010; Wally et al., 2008), Duchenne muscular dystrophy (Lorain et al., 2010), cystic fibrosis (Liu et al., 2002; Song et al., 2009), frontotemporal dementia with parkinsonism (Rodriguez-Martin et al., 2009), severe combined immunodeficiency (Zayed et al., 2007), spinal muscular atrophy (Coady et al., 2007), sickle cell anemia and ß-thalassemia (Kierlin-Duncan and Sullenger, 2007). First *in vivo* assays showed the functionality of SMaRT in a mouse model of spinal muscular atrophy (Coady et al., 2008; Coady and Lorson, 2010). However, SMaRT has also been shown to be functional for a number of other approaches like *in vivo* imaging (Walls et al., 2008), antibody and therapeutic protein production (Wang et al., 2009; Iwasaki et al., 2009) and suicide therapy in squamous cell carcinoma (Gruber et al., 2011).

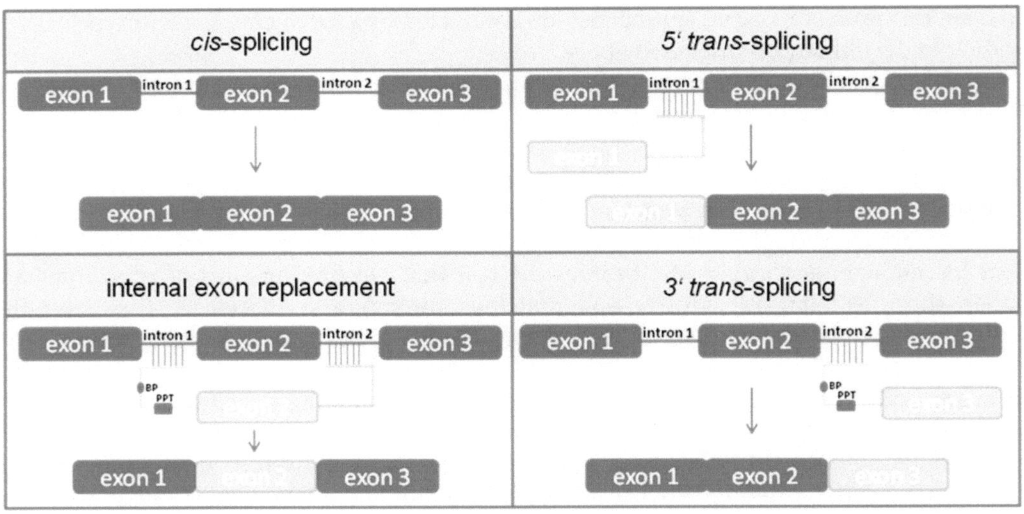

Fig. 1. RNA *trans*-splicing can be performed to replace one or more (a) 5′, (b) 3′ or (c) internal exons.

Technically, SMaRT is triggered by RNA-*trans*-splicing molecules (RTMs), which are specifically engineered for targeting a selected endogenous mRNA. Depending on the type of *trans*-splicing to be applied (5′, 3′ or IER), RTMs have to comprise certain features facilitating the *trans*-splicing process to take place. These are (a) The coding region to be replaced or integrated, (b) a hybridization/binding domain (BD), (c) a spacer region for sterical reasons and (d) splicing elements like a branch point (BP), polypyrimidine tract (PPT) and functional splice sites (SS). For 5′ *trans*-splicing the RTM comprises the 5′ (wildtype) coding sequence to be replaced, a spacer region and a binding domain. The binding domain hybridizes to the targeted intron, facilitating the generation of a mature mRNA mediated by the cell's spliceosome, comprising the 5′ exons from the RTM and the 3′ exons from the endogenous target. For 3′ *trans*-splicing a PPT and a BP have to be included for spliceosome assembly (for 5′ *trans*-splicing PPT and BP are provided by the endogenous target intron). Internal exon replacement is a combination of 5′ and 3′ *trans*-splicing (Figure 1).

Recent studies have shown that the binding domain is crucial for the efficiency, functionality and specificity of the replacement process. The binding domain is cloned reverse and complementary and usually targets the intron adjacent to the most central exon to be replaced. Recent studies showed that slight variations in the sequence can render an RTM from a highly functional to a non-functional or very weak RTM. The mechanisms to consider when rationally designing a binding domain are not yet clearly understood.

3. SMaRT for EBS-MD

Correction of *PLEC* by spliceosome mediated RNA *trans*-splicing was first demonstrated 2008 (Wally et al., 2008). In brief, a rationally designed RTM was engineered, targeting intron 9 to replace the upstream coding sequence including exon 9 of the endogenous *PLEC* mRNA. EBS-MD patient fibroblasts, harbouring a 3bp insertion in exon 9 (1287ins3) (Bauer et al., 2001) were transduced with the RTM and *trans*-splicing was monitored on RNA level, protein level and by immunofluorescence microscopy. An increase of full-length plectin protein by 58,7% was detected in transfected fibroblasts, whereas untreated fibroblasts showed hardly any expression. Even though the whole amount of plectin was still less than in wildtype fibroblasts, characteristic cytoplasmatic plectin-specific staining was detected by immunofluorescence microscopy. On RNA level, semi-quantitative real-time PCR (SQRT-PCR) revealed an increase of 83,42% of plectin mRNA expression. The rationally designed RTM used in this study was designed to cover the 3′ exon 9/intron 10 junction of the plectin pre-mRNA. Even though these results were promising, potential improvement by the variation of the binding domain was likely to be achieved. We therefore established a method to identify highly efficient binding domains for any gene of interest from a large pool of RTMs with randomly generated binding domains. From these libraries highly potent RTMs can be isolated and much information about the design of yonder can be obtained.

4. Principles of a fluorescence based RTM screen

The studies mentioned above showed that the binding domain is crucial for the efficiency and specificity of the *trans*-splicing process. Even minor variations in binding position, length and composition of the BDs result in significantly different efficiencies of the *trans*-splicing process. Rational design and evaluation of RTM binding domains can be an arduous process as there are no convincing criteria for the design of the binding domain. To simplify the process of RTM design we have developed a screening system that can be used to select the most efficient RTMs from a library containing a diversity of RTMs with complementary binding domains (BDs) for a certain target region of a pre-mRNA of interest. Using this method we can test a high number of RTMs for the efficiency of randomly generated binding domains. Binding domains are obtained by sonication or restriction digest of the targeted exonic and/or intronic region of the gene of interest. The resulting fragments have a length between 50 and 400bp (depending on the target region of choice) and are cloned into a fluorescence based RTM backbone. This random cloning results in the inclusion of one or more binding domains in a sense or antisense orientation, thereby resulting in about 50% of RTMs with a binding domain in a correct orientation for target hybridization, which is complementary. The vector backbone consists of a fluorescence reporter gene (e.g. dsRed) as transfection control and a 5′ or 3′ portion of a second fluorescence reporter gene (e.g. acGFP) respectively, mimicking the target gene portion to be *trans*-spliced to, therefore being the *trans*-splicing reporter. The generated RTM libraries are co-transfected with a corresponding target vector, harbouring the targeted full-length exonic and/or intronic region and the respective 5′ or 3′ reporter gene portion. Crucial is the inclusion of functional splice sites at the junctions of the split fluorescence reporter to facilitate *trans*-splicing. Functional *trans*-splicing upon co-transfection results in cells double positive for both reporter genes. The ratio between the transfection control reporter and the *trans*-splicing reporter gives information about the quality of the RTM. Cells transfected by highly functional RTMs show a proportional transfection control expression (dsRed) in relation to the *trans*-splicing reporter (acGFP), whereas RTMs with low *trans*-splicing efficiencies show a high amount of cells expressing exclusively the transfection control and less cells expressing the *trans*-splicing product (i.e. acGFP) as well.

4.1 RTM library construction for plectin and screening for highly functional molecules

For plectin we cloned two 5′ *trans*-splicing libraries. *Trans*-splicing of the RTM to the target results in the restoration of the open reading frame of acGFP, leading to the expression of the full-length protein in RTM and target co-transfected cells. Based on the previously described correction of *PLEC* by 5′ *trans*-splicing (Wally et al., 2008) we selected the target region exon/intron 9 (199bp in length) of *PLEC*, using the acGFP split reporter and dsRed as reporter for RTM transfection.

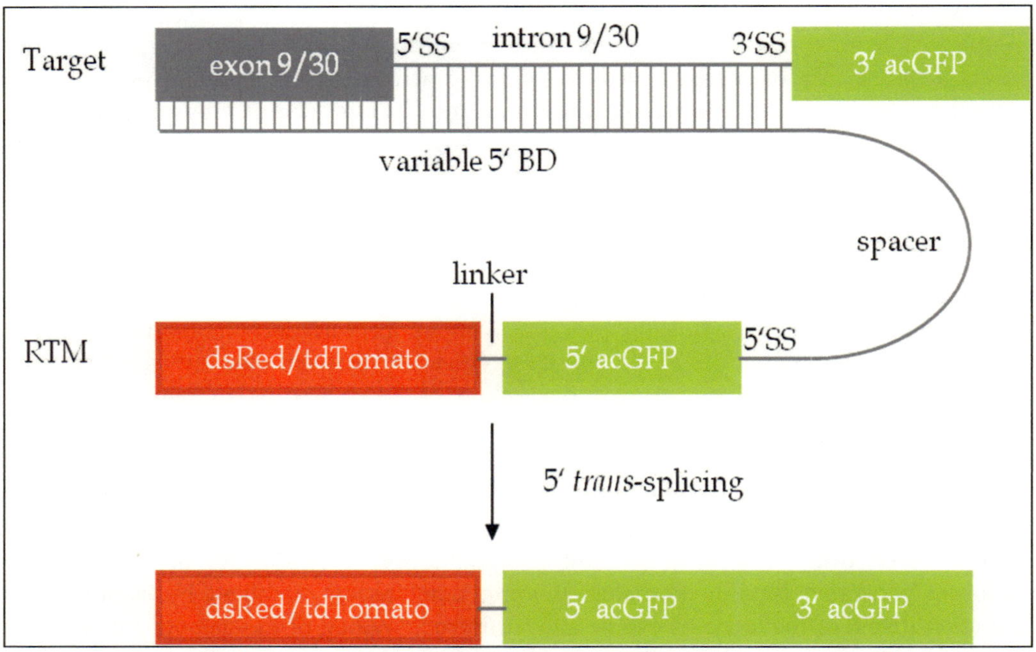

Fig. 2. Schematic depiction of the fluorescence based RTM screening system for the plectin gene.

To widen the spectrum of mutations included in the upstream coding region of *PLEC*, we constructed another library and its respective target molecule for exon/intron 30 (998bp in length) in parallel.

The RTM backbone for the exon/intron 30 specific BD library includes the more intense tdTomato instead of dsRed as RTM transfection control. The RTM screening system requires cells expressing an RTM and a plectin specific target molecule. Interaction between the RTM and target pre-mRNAs by RNA *trans*-splicing leads to the fusion of both split parts of acGFP, thus restoring the full-length coding sequence and expression of acGFP. The target molecule harbors the 3′ acGFP part flanked by a 3′ splice site (SS) and the genomic region of *PLEC* (exon/intron 9 or 30). The RTM contains the 5′ portion of acGFP linked in frame with the reporter gene tdTomato (for exon/intron 30) or dsRed (exon/intron 9) respectively. The 5′ acGFP part is flanked by a functional 5′SS, a short spacer sequence and a binding domain randomly created by fragmenting the *PLEC* target region (Figure 2).

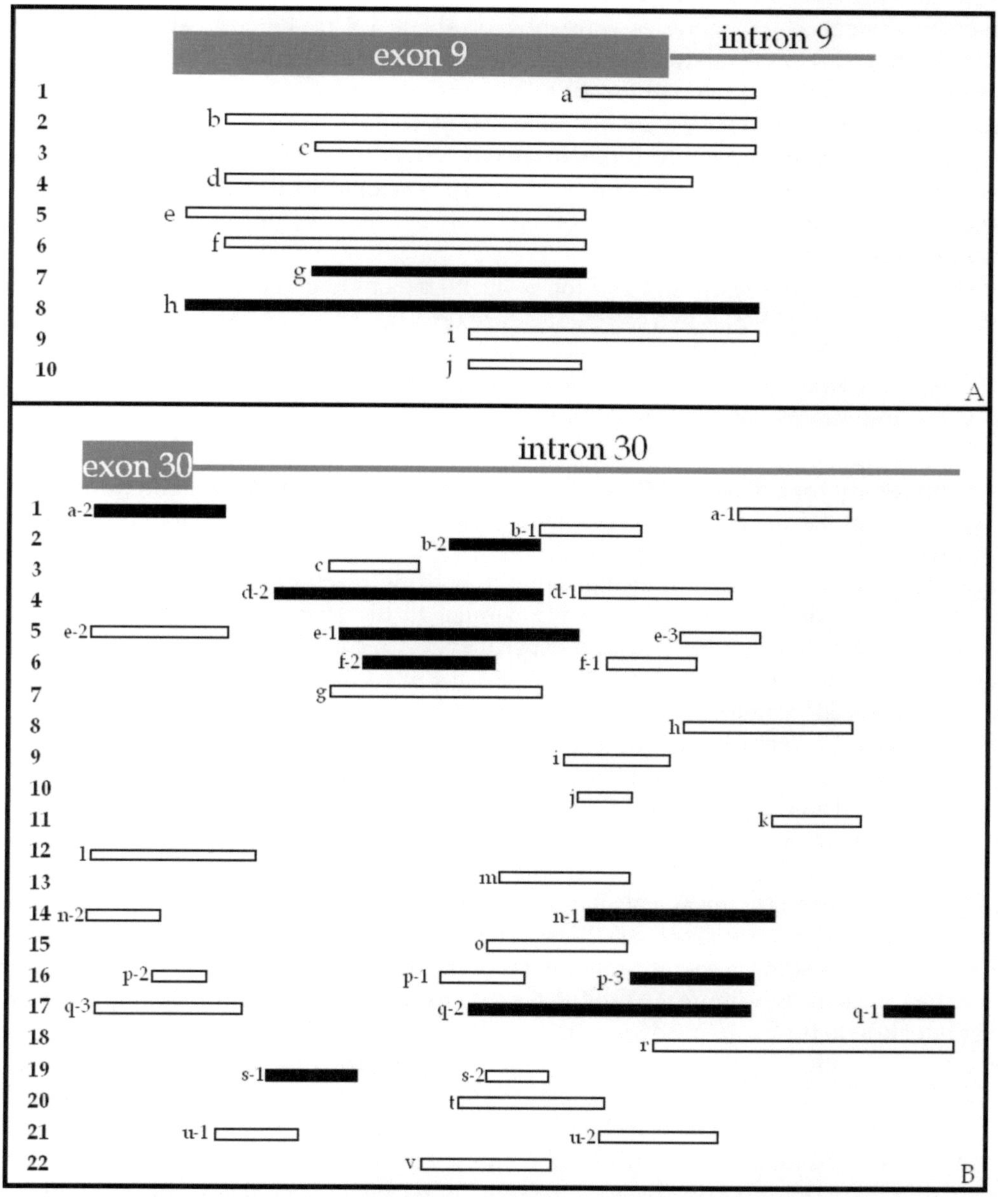

Fig. 3. Composition of the binding domains of all RTMs tested for exon/intron 9 (A) and exon/intron 30 (B).

The 5′ *trans*-splicing arm of the RTM backbone, downstream of the 5′ portion of acGFP, contains a donor (5′) splice site, a short spacer region and a random binding domain created by fragmentation of the respective *PLEC* target region. A high diversity of RTMs with different binding properties to the targeted exon/intron regions was constructed either by sonication (exon/intron 30) or CviJI* digestion (exon/intron 9) of the PCR amplified target region. CviJI* produces blunt end DNA fragments, cleaving between a G and a C of the sequence 5′-PuGCPy-3′. The randomized CviJI* digested, as well as the blunt end repaired sonicated fragments were cloned into the RTM backbone. To show the robustness of the screening system, 5′ BD libraries consisting of about 10^2 to 10^4 individual clones were constructed and several randomly picked clones were sequenced to select those with the correct (complementary) orientation. 10 RTMs from the exon/intron 9 library (Figure 3A) and 22 RTMs from the exon/intron 30 library (Figure 3B) harboring one or more parallel and/or complementary binding domains were tested for their *trans*-splicing efficiency, quantifying GFP expression by semi-quantitative real time PCR (SQRT-PCR) on mRNA level (for exon/intron 30 specific RTMs) and by flow cytometry on protein level (exon/intron 9 and 30 specific RTMs).

For all RTMs (1-10 for ex/in9 and 1-22 for ex/in 30) the binding domains were characterized and mapped (Figure 3). BDs in a complementary orientation (white bars) as well as BDs in a parallel orientation (black bars) were identified. Some RTMs had more than one BD included. BDs were named a to j and a to v respectively. Numbers next to the alphabetic characters indicate their order from 5′ to 3′.

4.1.1 Screening for efficient 5' RTMs targeting exon/intron 9 of the plectin gene

Ten individual RTMs from a 5′ BD library were selected to show the potential and robustness of the RTM screening system. Eight RTMs contain complementary BDs to the target region exon/intron 9, inducing the *trans*-splicing reaction between target and RTM pre-mRNAs. RTMs 7 and 8 harbor a BD parallel to the target region and are therefore included as negative controls in the experiments. Co-transfection of target expression plasmids along with either one of the ten RTMs resulted in a diverse expression profile of dsRed and acGFP (Figure 4). Weak RTMs (1, 7-10) show only low expression levels of dsRED - acGFP protein in comparison to the highly efficient RTMs 2-6. RTMs 7 and 8, harboring parallel BDs, produce a background expression of acGFP in less than 1% of all analyzed cells. The most efficient RTMs 2-6 show functional acGFP expression in 44-67% of all treated cells with a geometric mean of acGFP expression ranging from 6 (RTM 3) to 8 (RTM 6) (Figure 4B). These values reflect the average acGFP expression of all analyzed GFP positive cells. Geometric mean calculations after flow cytometric analysis were performed using the FlowJo software (Treestar). Flow cytometric analysis of RTM 6, 7 and 9 transfected HEK293AD cells show a significant difference in the amount of acGFP expression and fluorescence intensity (Figure 4A). RTM 6 contains a complementary BD, binding exon 9 only, but close to the exon/intron junction, maybe influencing the 5′ splice site on the target molecule. This might be the reason why RTM 6 is significantly more efficient in comparison to RTM 7 or RTM 9, harboring a parallel (RTM 7) or a short antisense BD (RTM 9). No acGFP expression was detected in HEK293AD cells transfected with either target or RTM alone. As the binding position of RTMs 2-6 on the target molecule is similar, there was not much difference in reporter gene expression. Masking almost the whole exon 9 with complementary BDs seems to increase the *trans*-splicing efficiency significantly. RTMs 1, 9 and 10 contain either short BDs specific for a short stretch of the target exon (RTM 10) or for a short portion containing the 5′ exon/intron boundary (RTM 1 and 9). These RTMs induced acGFP expression in less than 14% of transfected cells. Additionally, the intensity of acGFP expression was much lower (Figure 4).

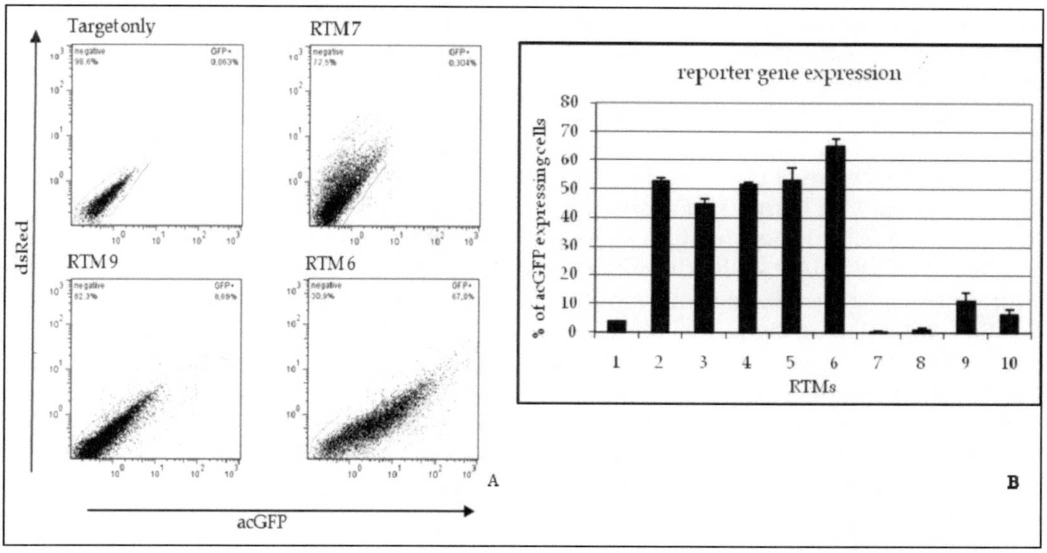

Fig. 4. Exon/intron 9: Expression of the fluorescence reporter genes acGFP and dsRed and the percentage of acGFP positive cells.

4.1.2 Screening for efficient 5′ RTMs targeting exon / intron 30 of the plectin gene

The same experiments as described for exon/intron 9 were conducted for exon/intron 30. This intron was chosen to cover a maximum 5′ *PLEC* gene portion and thereby including more known mutations. Again, flow cytometric analysis was performed with HEK293AD cells co-transfected with RTM and target plasmids. For each RTM two independent co-transfections were performed. Two days after co-transfection, the subset of acGFP expressing cells and the expression level of acGFP was quantified by flow cytometry. The number of acGFP positive cells and the relative amount of acGFP expressed reflect the functionality of RTMs and their respective binding domains. Between 5.10^3-2.10^4 HEK293AD cells were analyzed for each transfection.

After transfecting each of the 22 RTMs, harboring at least one complementary binding domain, together with the target molecule into HEK293AD cells, flow cytometry was performed. The geometric mean of acGFP expression ranged from 1.3 to 3.2 according to the RTM introduced into the target cells. The highly efficient RTMs 12, 13 and 17 showed acGFP expression in over 20% of all transfected cells and had a calculated geometric mean of over 2.6. RTMs with a weak *trans*-splicing efficiency (e.g. RTMs 1, 4, 11) showed a high amount of cells expressing the RTM transfection control gene tdTomato only and less cells expressing acGFP as well (Figure 5B). By setting the highly efficient RTMs 5, 12 and 17 in relation to the weak RTM 22, significant differences in their reporter gene expression were observed (Figure 5A). RTMs 5, 12 and 17 produced significantly higher levels of acGFP. RTM 22 generated only a background expression of acGFP in about 1% of analyzed HEK293AD cells.

Besides flow cytometry, all 22 RTMs with BDs ranging from 57 to 355 nucleotides, complementary to essentially all regions of the exon 30/intron 30 target (Figure 3B), were individually tested for *trans*-splicing induced restoration of acGFP expression by SQRT-PCR. A *PLEC* specific 5′ *trans*-splicing RTM is able to recombine with a target pre-mRNA by a specific 5′ *trans*-splicing reaction. Thus the exon on the target molecule is replaced by the 5′ part of acGFP, leading to the expression of the reporter molecule acGFP in RTM treated cells. *Trans*-splicing between the RTM and target molecule was detected by semi-quantitative real-time PCR (SQRT-PCR). For that, an acGFP specific primer pair was used to quantify the amount of full-length acGFP transcripts present in HEK293AD cells co-transfected with the target molecule plasmid harboring exon/intron 30 of *PLEC* along with either one of the 22 RTMs (Figure 6). This demonstrates that the acceptor (3′) and donor (5′) splice sites on the target molecule and the RTM were recognized by the endogenous splicing machinery and that both acGFP parts were connected by 5′ RNA *trans*-splicing, leading to full-length acGFP expression. By analyzing the amount of expressed acGFP transcripts in co-transfected HEK293AD cells, the influence of different RTM binding domains on *trans*-splicing efficiency can be shown on mRNA level. As a reference gene, GAPDH was used. For the evaluation of the results all RTMs were referred to the weakest RTM 11 (set to 1), producing a low level of acGFP. As shown in Figure 6, RTMs 5, 12 and 17, accomplishing the exon/intron boundary of the target molecule by their complementary BDs, showed a high *trans*-splicing efficiency. RTM 12 achieved an up to 90 fold expression of acGFP transcripts in comparison to RTM 11. Masking the 5′ splice site on the target molecule may direct the ratio of the splicing reactions from *cis* to *trans*, since the binding of splicing factors might be disturbed.

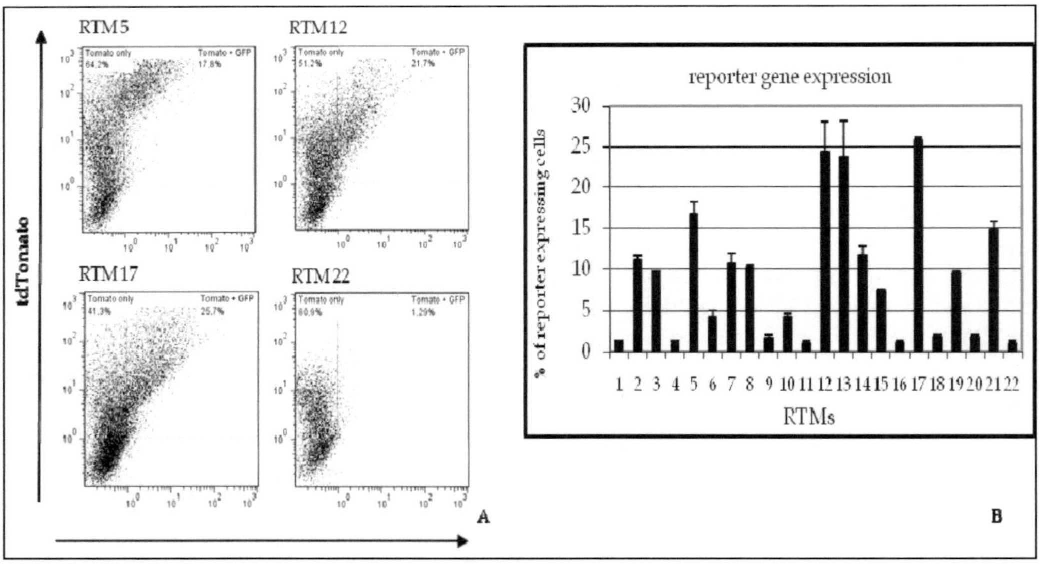

Fig. 5. Exon/intron 30: Expression of the fluorescence reporters acGFP : tdTomato was analyzed using flow cytometry (A) Four RTMs with different BDs show varying ratios of acGFP : tdTomato (B) The percentage of acGFP positive cells is summarized for all RTMs tested.

The data created by flow cytometric analysis (Figure 5) correlates with those obtained from semi-quantitative real-time PCR (SQRT-PCR). RTMs 5, 12 and 17, hybridizing to the exon/intron junction of the target molecule showed high *trans*-splicing efficiencies on mRNA (SQRT-PCR) and protein (flow cytometry) level, indicating the reliability of the RTM screening system. Since the highly efficient RTMs 5, 12 and 17 have similar complementary binding domains (exon/intron junction of the target molecule), this region seems to be the ideal binding position for efficient RNA *trans*-splicing in the case of the *PLEC* gene region exon/intron 30. The blockage of the exon/intron boundary of the target molecule, accomplished by these RTMs, may interfere with recognition of the exon 30 5′ splice site and facilitate *trans*-splicing.

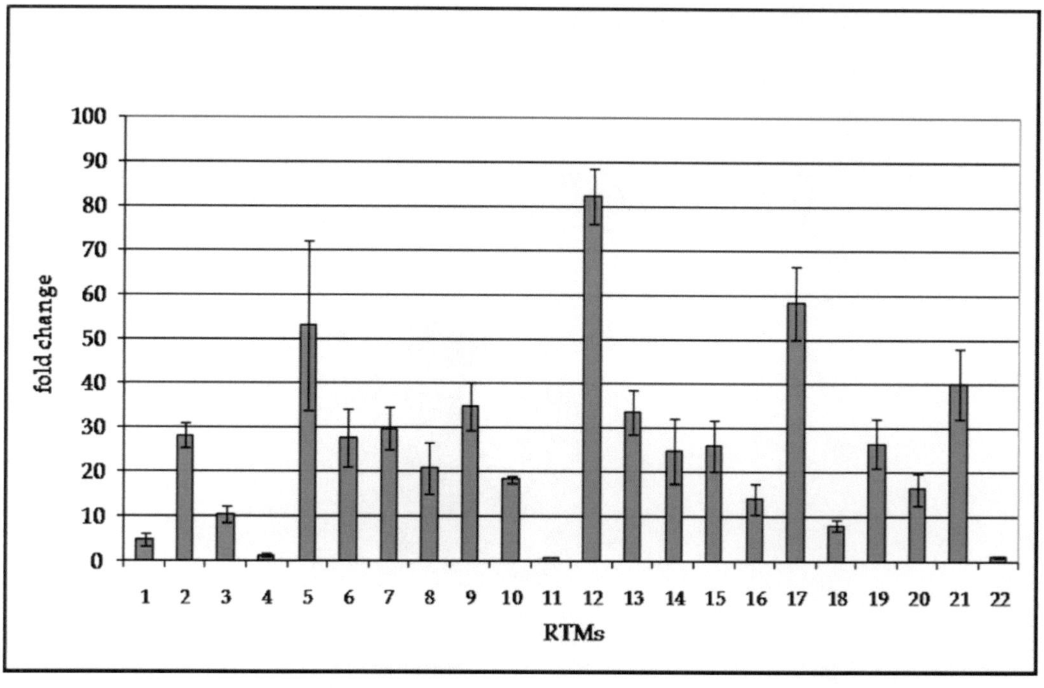

Fig. 6. Exon/intron 30: acGFP expression on mRNA level.

4.2 *Trans*-splicing with endogenous *PLEC* transcripts

One day after transfection of single RTMs into HEK293AD cells, endogenous *trans*-splicing was detected by RT-PCR. Specific *trans*-splicing between the RTM and the endogenous target pre-mRNA of *PLEC* resulted in the fusion of the 5′ portion of acGFP to exon 10 or 31 of *PLEC*. The fusion mRNA was amplified by including an acGFP specific forward primer and an exon 10 or 31 specific reverse primer into the polymerase chain reaction. After gel electrophoresis the 5′acGFP-exon 10/31 *PLEC* fusion PCR product was visible on an agarose gel at a size of 413bp and 542bp respectively (Figure 7). The DNA band was gel purified and sequenced. All RTMs introduced into HEK293AD cells (RTMs specific for exon/intron 9: 1-6, RTMs specific for exon/intron 30: 7, 12, 13), induced endogenous 5′ *trans*-splicing.

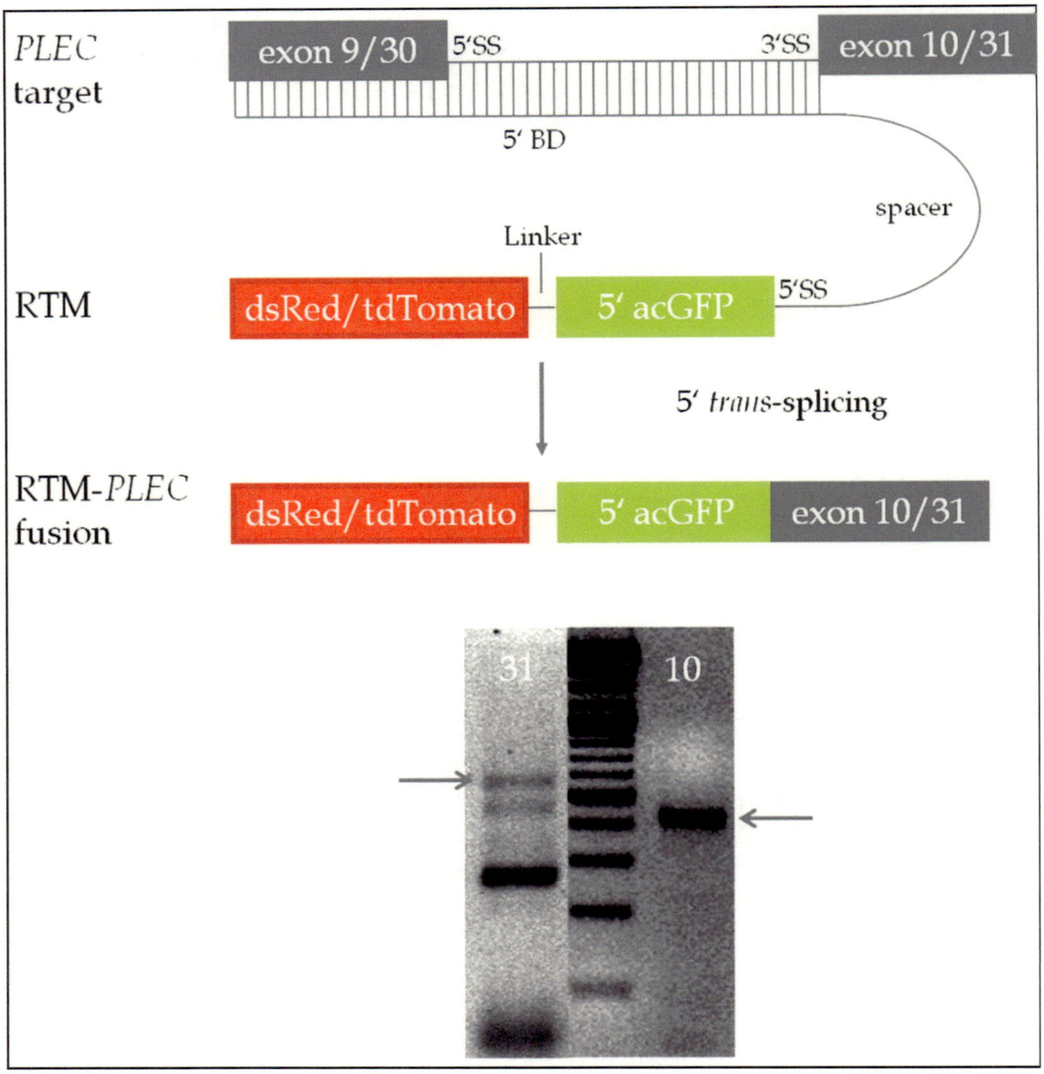

Fig. 7. Single transfection of selected RTMs (exon/intron 9 or 30 RTM screen) into HEK293AD cells resulted in the fusion of the 5′ portion of acGFP of the RTM to the respective endogenous target exon of *PLEC* (exon 10 or exon 31) on pre-mRNA level.

5. Discussion

During the last years it was shown that SMaRT is a functional tool for the correction of disease causing mutations of many genes on mRNA level. Several approaches in different settings (i.e. reporter gene based, endogenous *trans*-splicing, *in vivo* application) have corroborated this assumption (Dallinger et al., 2003; Coady and Lorson, 2010; Wally et al., 2010). Also the applicability of SMaRT beyond mRNA repair was shown, using it for *in vivo* imaging and antibody and protein production. For the latter, therapeutic protein encoding sequences were *trans*-spliced to the highly abundant albumin mRNA, resulting in the expression of the therapeutic molecule (Wang et al., 2009). For epidermolysis bullosa, SMaRT was applied for a number of underlying genes, including *PLEC* (Wally et al., 2008), *COL7A1* (Murauer et al., 2010), *K14* (Wally et al., 2010) and *COL17A1* (our unpublished results). Whereas for *PLEC* and *COL7A1* the binding domains of the RNA-*trans*-splicing molecules (RTMs) were designed empirically, based on preliminary data, the binding domains for *K14* and *COL17A1* resulted from the evaluation of a number of randomly cloned BDs. Using a fluorescence based screening system, we saw that binding domains are crucial for the efficiency and specificity of the *trans*-splicing process. In this reporter-based assay, BDs were tested independently from the influence of gene characteristics and variations in splicing domains. This facilitated a direct comparison of the BDs, revealing a high impact of (a) localization within the targeted exon/intron, (b) composition and (c) length. Comparing obtained data, hints on principles for BD design were extracted. These are: (a) highly functional BDs have a length between 90 and 170bp, (b) masking of the competitive exon/intron junction is mostly beneficial, (c) targeting of a large intron results in more potential and diverse *trans*-splicing results since more binding sites are available. Furthermore, these facts underlay a hierarchy, with length ranging before splice site masking. Best BDs identified in the exon/intron 30 screen had a length of around 140 - 170bp AND masked the respective target splice site. An optimal target intron is not always available, restricting optimization in this aspect. However, screening for BDs also revealed exceptions from the rule. For example binding domains from RTMs 5 and 6 for exon/intron 9 exclusively bind within the exon. Even though we know that also splicing domains and spacer sequences influence *trans*-splicing success, regarding the BDs, it is not yet clearly understood what further influences *trans*-splicing efficiency and specificity. The first published BD for *PLEC* (Wally et al., 2008) masked the target splice site to be used for *trans*-splicing, resulting in reasonable *trans*-splicing rates. However, we still recommend using the fluorescence based screening system, as this is rather facile as soon as vector backbones are cloned. Backbones can be used for any gene of interest and any targeted intron. Within the *K14* gene, the applicability of SMaRT for dominant diseases was shown. The concomitant knock-down of the mutated and the increase of the wildtype allele multiply the effect of correction. Even though endogenous efficiencies are not high level, *trans*-splicing rates can be enough to revert a disease phenotype. Werner et al. showed in an *in vitro* model that dominance is limited and depends on the ratio of wildtype versus mutated *K14* molecules (Werner et al., 2004). Also, for dominant *COL7A1* mutations, overexpression of the wildtype protein can rescue the RDEB phenotype (Fritsch et al., 2009). Finally, Cao et al. showed that dominance is dependent on a certain ratio of wildtype to mutant alleles; in their *in vivo* mouse model a neomycin-resistance gene inserted in intron 1 of *K14* led to a 50% reduction of the mutated *K14* expression, resulting in phenotypically normal pups which showed no blistering (Cao et al., 2001). In view of this ameliorative effect, therapeutic approaches able to reduce the expression of a mutant gene product by 50% could be sufficient. Functional assays with RTM treated patient cells showed a transition of migratory behaviour and invasiveness versus wildtype in respective tests.

An improvement of the screen will be the sorting of analysed cells, resulting in a faster and more restricted identification of highly functional RTMs. Isolation of cells showing a certain ratio of the two fluorescence reporters expressed will increase the number of potential binding domains characterized. Single cell expansion and plasmid extraction will provide highly potential BDs to integrate into an endogenous setting of spliceosome mediated RNA *trans*-splicing.

The development of an RTM selection system has a high impact on *trans*-splicing efficiency and specificity. Further improvements can be made regarding codon usage, nuclear retention signals, promoter selection and mode of delivery. Inclusion of nuclear retention signals might have great influence on the *trans*-splicing efficiency, but also regarding minimization of side effects and background expression of unspliced RTMs. Codon optimization and the use of weaker promoters and enhancers can be used to increase the safety of retrovirally introduced RTMs (Baum and Schambach, 2011; Fath et al., 2011).

Currently, a limiting fact is the lack of mouse models meeting the exigencies of a SMaRT approach. Many mouse models are generated by the inclusion of intron-free genes, making them unfeasible *trans*-splicing experiments. However, mouse models are becoming easier available and creatable. This will pave the way to *in vivo* studies as the basis for clinical trials.

6. Prospects and visions

Bringing spliceosome mediated RNA *trans*-splicing toward clinics is the aim of presumably all conducted studies for mRNA correction. This technology also gives hope to patients suffering from EB subtypes which cannot be treated by commonly used approaches like full-length cDNA based therapy. Patients regarding this have alterations in very large genes like *PLEC, COL7A1* and *COL17A1*, and also those harbouring mutations in dominantly inherited genes, like *K14* and *K5*. The next step will be to show *in vivo*, that *trans*-splicing can convert a disease phenotype to wildtype. The generation of viable, intron-posessing mouse models is a task that is being gone about currently. Looking further, *ex vivo* gene therapy is the currently most favoured approach for epidermolysis bullosa patients. Transplantation of skin sheets derived from autologous epidermal stem cells that were transduced with a respective corrective molecule is the current state of the art. This approach was successfully conducted for full-length cDNA therapy in junctional epidermolysis bullosa in 2006 (Mavilio et al., 2006). There, a 50cm^2 area was replaced on the patient legs. Even five years after transplantation the transplanted areas have not shown any blisters at all and are indistinguishable from healthy skin (De Luca, personal communication).

However, systemic application of SMaRT is the technology to go for, which is not available yet. Delivery of (any) gene therapeutic advice is a problem common to all approaches. Increasing the safety of lenti- and retroviral vectors is being pushed forward with good results. Also the use of transposons like sleeping beauty (Hackett et al., 2010) and piggyBack (Yusa et al., 2011) are promising tools. Finally, targeting is another challenge to be overcome. However, in this case SMaRT has the advantage of being functional only in cells expressing the target gene, therefore minimizing off-target effects in other cell types.

7. References

Bauer JW, Rouan F, Kofler B, Rezniczek GA, Kornacker I, Muss W, Hametner R, Klausegger A, Huber A, Pohla-Gubo G, Wiche G, Uitto J, and Hintner H. (2001). A compound heterozygous one amino-acid insertion/nonsense mutation in the plectin gene causes epidermolysis bullosa simplex with plectin deficiency. *American Journal of Pathology,* Vol.158, No.2, pp. 617-625, ISSN 00029440

Baum C and Schambach A. (2011). Promoter Competition for Gene Therapy of SCID-X1. *Human Gene Therapy,* Vol.22, No.3, pp. 255-256, ISSN 1043-0342

Cao TY, Longley MA, Wang XJ, and Roop DR. (2001). An inducible mouse model for epidermolysis bullosa simplex: Implications for gene therapy. *Journal of Cell Biology,* Vol.152, No.3, pp. 651-656, ISSN 0021-9525

Coady TH, Baughan TD, Shababi M, Passini MA, and Lorson CL. (2008). Development of a single vector system that enhances trans-splicing of SMN2 transcripts. *PLoS ONE,* Vol.3, No.10, pp. e3468, ISSN 1932-6203

Coady TH and Lorson CL. (2010). Trans-Splicing-Mediated Improvement in a Severe Mouse Model of Spinal Muscular Atrophy. *Journal of Neuroscience,* Vol.30, No.1, pp. 126-130, ISSN 0270-6474

Coady TH, Shababi M, Tullis GE, and Lorson CL. (2007). Restoration of SMN function: Delivery of a trans-splicing RNA re-directs SMN2 pre-mRNA splicing. *Molecular Therapy,* Vol.15, No.8, pp. 1471-1478, ISSN 1525-0016

Dallinger G, Puttaraju M, Mitchell LG, Yancey KB, Yee C, Klausegger A, Hintner H, and Bauer JW. (2003). Development of spliceosome-mediated RNA trans-splicing (SMaRT (TM)) for the correction of inherited skin diseases. *Experimental Dermatology, Vol.*12, No.1, pp. 37-46, ISSN 0906-6705

Davis RE, Hardwick C, Tavernier P, Hodgson S, and Singh H. (1995). RNA trans-splicing in flatworms. Analysis of trans-spliced mRNAs and genes in the human parasite, Schistosoma mansoni. *Journal of Biological Chemistry,*Vol. 270, No.37, pp. 21813-21819, ISSN 0021-9258

Dellambra E, Pellegrini G, Guerra L, Ferrari G, Zambruno G, Mavilio F, and De Luca M. (2000). Toward epidermal stem cell-mediated ex vivo gene therapy of junctional epidermolysis bullosa. *Human Gene Therapy,* Vol.11, No.16, pp. 2283-2287, ISSN 1043-0342

Dellambra E, Prislei S, Salvati AL, Madeddu ML, Golisano O, Siviero E, Bondanza S, Cicuzza S, Orecchia A, Giancotti FG, Zambruno G, and De Luca M. (2001). Gene correction of integrin beta(4)-dependent pyloric atresia-functional epidermolysis bullosa keratinocytes establishes a role for beta(4) tyrosines 1422 and 1440 in hemidesmosome assembly. *Journal of Biological Chemistry,* Vol. 276, No.44, pp. 41336-41342, ISSN 0021-9258

Dellambra E, Vailly J, Pellegrini G, Bondanza S, Golisano O, Macchia C, Zambruno G, Meneguzzi G, and De Luca M. (1998). Corrective transduction of human epidermal stem cells in laminin-5-dependent junctional epidermolysis bullosa. *Human Gene Therapy,* Vol.9, No.9, pp. 1359-1370, ISSN 1043-0342

Fath S, Bauer AP, Liss M, Spriestersbach A, Maertens B, Hahn P, Ludwig C, Schafer F, Graf M, and Wagner R. (2011). Multiparameter RNA and Codon Optimization: A Standardized Tool to Assess and Enhance Autologous Mammalian Gene Expression. *PLoS ONE,* Vol.6, No.3, pp. e17596, ISSN 1932-6203

Fine JD, Eady RA, Bauer EA, Bauer JW, Bruckner-Tuderman L, Heagerty A, Hintner H, Hovnanian A, Jonkman MF, Leigh I, McGrath JA, Mellerio JE, Murrell DF, Shimizu H, Uitto J, Vahlquist A, Woodley D, and Zambruno G. (2008). The classification of inherited epidermolysis bullosa (EB): Report of the Third International Consensus Meeting on Diagnosis and Classification of EB. *Journal of the American Academy of Dermatology,*Vol.58, No. 6, pp.931-950, ISSN 0190-9622

Flouriot G, Brand H, Seraphin B, and Gannon F. (2002). Natural trans-spliced mRNAs are generated from the human estrogen receptor-alpha (hER alpha) gene. *Journal of Biological Chemistry,* Vol.277, No.29, pp. 26244-26251, ISSN 0021-9258

Fritsch A, Spassov S, Elfert S, Schlosser A, Gache Y, Meneguzzi G, and Bruckner-Tuderman L. (2009). Dominant negative effects of COL7A1 mutations can be rescued by controlled over-expression of normal collagen VII. *Journal of Biological Chemistry,* Vol.284, No.44, pp. 30248-30256, ISSN 0021-9258

Gruber C, Gratz IK, Murauer EM, Mayr E, Koller U, Bruckner-Tuderman L, Meneguzzi G, Hintner H, and Bauer JW. (2011). Spliceosome-mediated RNA trans-splicing facilitates targeted delivery of suicide genes to cancer cells. *Molecular Cancer Therapeutics,* Vol.10, No.2, pp. 233-241, ISSN 1535-7163

Hackett PB, Largaespada DA, and Cooper LJN. (2010). A Transposon and Transposase System for Human Application. *Molecular Therapy,* Vol.18, No.4, pp. 674-683, ISSN 1525-0016

Iwasaki R, Kiuchi H, Ihara M, Mori T, Kawakami M, and Ueda H. (2009). Trans-splicing as a novel method to rapidly produce antibody fusion proteins. *Biochemical and Biophysical Research Communications,* Vol.384, No.3, pp. 316-321, ISSN 0006-291X

Kierlin-Duncan MN and Sullenger BA. (2007). Using 59-PTMs to repair mutant beta-globin transcripts. *RNA,* Vol.13, No.8, pp. 1317-1327, ISSN 1355-8382

Liu XM, Jiang QS, Mansfield SG, Puttaraju M, Zhang YL, Zhou WH, Cohn JA, Garcia-Blanco MA, Mitchell LG, and Engelhardt JF. (2002). Partial correction of endogenous Delta F508 CFTR in human cystic fibrosis airway epithelia by spliceosome-mediated RNA trans-splicing. *Nature Biotechnology,* Vol.20, No.1, pp. 47-52, ISSN 1087-0156

Lorain S, Peccate C, Le Hir M, and Garcia L. (2010). Exon exchange approach to repair duchenne dystrophin transcripts. *PLoS ONE,* Vol.5, No.5, pp. e10894, ISSN 1932-6203

Mavilio F, Pellegrini G, Ferrari S, Di Nunzio F, Di Iorio E, Recchia A, Maruggi G, Ferrari G, Provasi E, Bonini C, Capurro S, Conti A, Magnoni C, Giannetti A, and De Luca M. (2006). Correction of junctional epidermolysis bullosa by transplantation of genetically modified epidermal stem cells. *Nature Medicine,* Vol.12, No.12, pp. 1397-1402, ISSN 1078-8956

McLean I and Terron A. (May 2002). Ribozyme Gene Therapy Strategies for Keratin Disorders. *Journal of Investigative Dermatology,* Available from Society of Investigative Dermatology

Murauer EM, Gache Y, Gratz IK, Klausegger A, Muss W, Gruber C, Meneguzzi G, Hintner H, and Bauer JW. (2011). Functional Correction of Type VII Collagen Expression in Dystrophic Epidermolysis Bullosa. *Journal of Investigative Dermatology,* Vol.131, No.1, pp. 74-83, ISSN 0022-202X

Murphy WJ, Watkins KP, and Agabian N. (1986). Identification of a novel Y branch structure as an intermediate in trypanosome mRNA processing: evidence for trans splicing. *Cell,* Vol.47, No.4, pp. 517-525, ISSN 0092-8674

Natsuga K, Nishie W, Shinkuma S, Arita K, Nakamura H, Ohyama M, Osaka H, Kambara T, Hirako Y, and Shimizu H. (2010). Plectin Deficiency Leads to Both Muscular Dystrophy and Pyloric Atresia in Epidermolysis Bullosa Simplex. *Human Mutation,* Vol.31, No.10, pp.1687-1698, ISSN 1059-7794

Puttaraju M, Jamison SF, Mansfield SG, Garcia-Blanco MA, and Mitchell LG. (1999). Spliceosome-mediated RNA trans-splicing as a tool for gene therapy. *Nature Biotechnology,* Vol.17, No.3, pp. 246-252, ISSN 0733-222X

Rezniczek GA, Abrahamsberg C, Fuchs P, Spazierer D, and Wiche G. (2003). Plectin 5 '-transcript diversity: short alternative sequences determine stability of gene products, initiation of translation and subcellular localization of isoforms. *Human Molecular Genetics,* Vol.12, No.23, pp. 3181-3194, ISSN 0964-6906

Rodriguez-Martin T, Anthony K, Garcia-Blanco MA, Mansfield SG, Anderton BH, and Gallo JM. (2009). Correction of tau mis-splicing caused by FTDP-17 MAPT mutations by spliceosome-mediated RNA trans-splicing. *Human Molecular Genetics,* Vol.18, No.17, pp. 3266-3273, ISSN 0964-6906

Russell D, Ross H, and Lane EB. (2009). ERK Involvement in Resistance to Apoptosis in Keratinocytes with Mutant Keratin. *Journal of Investigative Dermatology,* Vol.130, No.3, pp. 671-681, ISSN 0022-202X

Siomi H and Siomi MC. (2009). On the road to reading the RNA-interference code. *Nature,* Vol.457, No.7228, pp. 396-404, ISSN 0028-0836

Siprashvili Z, Nguyen NT, Bezchinsky MY, Marinkovich PM, Lane AT, and Khavari PA. (2010). Long-term Type VII Collagen Restoration to Human Epidermolysis Bullosa Skin Tissue. *Human Gene Therapy,* Vol.21, No.10, pp. 1299-1310, ISSN 1043-0342

Song Y, Lou HH, Boyer JL, Limberis MP, Vandenberghe LH, Hackett NR, Leopold PL, Wilson JM, and Crystal RG. (2009). Functional Cystic Fibrosis Transmembrane Conductance Regulator Expression in Cystic Fibrosis Airway Epithelial Cells by AAV6.2-Mediated Segmental Trans-Splicing. *Human Gene Therapy,* Vol.20, No.3, pp. 267-281, ISSN 1043-0342

Walls ZF, Puttaraju M, Temple GF, and Gambhir SS. (2008). A generalizable strategy for imaging pre-mRNA levels in living subjects using spliceosome-mediated RNA trans-splicing. *Journal of Nuclear Medicine,* Vol.49, No.7, pp. 1146-1154, ISSN 0161-5505

Wally V, Brunner M, Lettner T, Wagner M, Koller U, Trost A, Murauer EM, Hainzl S, Hintner H, and Bauer JW. (2010). K14 mRNA reprogramming for dominant epidermolysis bullosa simplex. *Human Molecular Genetics,* Vol.19, No.23, pp. 4715-4725, ISSN 0964-6906

Wally V, Klausegger A, Koller U, Lochmuller H, Krause S, Wiche G, Mitchell LG, Hintner H, and Bauer JW. (2008). 5' trans-splicing repair of the PLEC1 gene. *Journal of Investigative Dermatology,* Vol.128, No.3, pp. 568-574, ISSN 0022-202X

Wang J, Mansfield SG, Cote CA, Jiang PD, Weng K, Amar MJ, Brewer BH, Jr., Remaley AT, McGarrity GJ, Garcia-Blanco MA, and Puttaraju M. (2009). Trans-splicing into highly abundant albumin transcripts for production of therapeutic proteins in vivo. *Molecular Therapy,* Vol.17, No.2, pp. 343-351, ISSN 1525-0016

Werner NS, Windorffer R, Strnad P, Grund C, Leube RE, and Magin TM. (2004). Epidermolysis bullosa simplex-type mutations alter the dynamics of the keratin cytoskeleton and reveal a contribution of actin to the transport of keratin Subunits. *Molecular Biology of the Cell,* Vol.15, No.3, pp.990-1002, ISSN 1059-1524

Yusa K, Zhou LQ, Li MA, Bradley A, and Craig NL. (2011). A hyperactive piggyBac transposase for mammalian applications. *Proceedings of the National Academy of Sciences of the United States of America,* Vol.108, No.4, pp. 1531-1536, ISSN 0027-8424

Zayed H, Xia L, Yerich A, Yant SR, Kay MA, Puttaraju M, McGarrity GJ, Wiest DL, McIvor RS, Tolar J, and Blazar BR. (2007). Correction of DNA protein kinase deficiency by spliceosome-mediated RNA trans-splicing and sleeping beauty transposon delivery. *Molecular Therapy,* Vol.15, No.7, pp. 1273-1279, ISSN 1525-0016

14

Nanomedicine and Drug Delivery Strategies for Treatment of Genetic Diseases

Janet Hsu[1] and Silvia Muro[1,2]
[1]*Fischell Department of Bioengineering*
[2]*Institute for Bioscience and Biotechnology Research*
University of Maryland, College Park
United States of America

1. Introduction

Effective diagnostic and therapeutic intervention of genetic diseases have been particularly pending on technological development. It was not until the last two decades of the past century that molecular biology and recombinant DNA have provided diagnostic and therapeutic tools for these diseases. Since then, our understanding of the biological processes underscoring genetic conditions and the development of technologies enabling their study and treatment have vastly grown, providing scientists and clinicians with means to continue advancing in these directions. Recently, another technology has strongly impacted the fields of molecular biology, medicine, diagnostic and therapeutic development: nanotechnology.

More precisely, nanotechnology focuses on the study and manipulation of matter and processes at the nanometer (10^{-9} m) scale, encompassing the atomic, molecular, and macromolecular scales. In this chapter, we use the term nanotechnology from a more broad perspective, referring to devices fabricated at the sub-micrometer scale, a size compatible with that of large biological macromolecular complexes and cellular organelles, which are often referred to as nano- as well, due to the nanoscale of their architectural and/or functional components. The application of nanotechnology principles and tools to the field of medicine, known as nanomedicine, is also a relatively young field that has vastly expanded within the last couple of decades to render new diagnostic and treatment approaches. However, delivery of active agents assisted by these technologies is still a relatively unexplored strategy in the case of genetic diseases.

This chapter discusses some of the technological advances regarding the application of nanomedicine to the treatment of genetic conditions. Some basic foundation on the design and features of these technologies are provided, including targeting, transport, and delivery capabilities of drug delivery systems. Applications in the context of genetic diseases are also discussed, including treatment of phenotypic symptoms and complications associated to these conditions, and correction therapies, such as treatment with small molecules, non-viral gene therapies, cell therapies, and enzyme replacement therapies.

2. Types and properties of drug delivery tools used in nanomedicine

An area of research where nanotechnology and nanomedicine applications have been particularly prolific pertains to delivery of diagnostic and therapeutic agents. Drug delivery carriers are macromolecular assemblies that can incorporate imaging and therapeutic compounds of distinct nature, such as small chemicals, fluorophores and biosensors, peptides and proteins, and oligonucleotides and genes. They can be designed to improve the solubility of these cargo molecules and their bioavailability, and also to control their circulation, biodistribution in the body, and release rate, altogether enhancing their efficacy (Langer, 1998, Duncan, 2003, Panyam & Labhasetwar, 2003, Moghimi, et al., 2005).

2.1 Nanocarrier design

A broad spectrum of materials (biological, synthetic and semi-synthetic) assembled in a variety of conformational arrays (from linear structures to branched and dendritic counterparts, micelles, hollow capsules, porous or solid particles, etc.) have been designed to help in diagnostic and therapeutic interventions (Langer, 1998, Discher & Eisenberg, 2002). Examples of these include carbon nanostructures, quantum dots, metal particles, liposomes, and formulations based on natural and/or synthetic polymers (Figure 1). The composition and architecture of these systems play an important role in determining their translational capabilities, including their ability to carry cargoes of different chemistries and their loading capacity, stability, biodegradability and overall biocompatibility, and various functional aspects (Moghimi, et al., 2001, El-Sayed, et al., 2005, Stayton, et al., 2005, Torchilin, 2006).

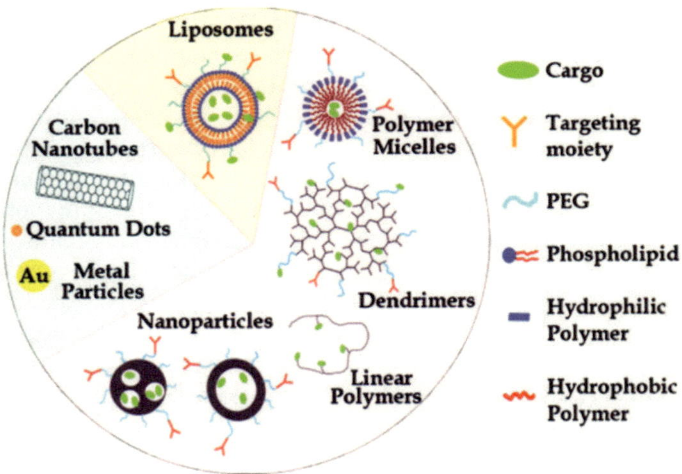

Fig. 1. Composition and architecture of carriers and other assemblies (not drawn to scale) utilized in nanomedicine for diagnosis, imaging, and drug delivery. Yellow, purple, and blue colors correspond to formulations discussed in sections 2.1.1, 2.1.2, and 2.1.3.

2.1.1 Lipid vesicles

Lipid-based micelles (encapsulating vesicles formed by a single phospholipid layer, ranging from ~5 to 100 nm in diameter) and mostly liposomes (vesicles delimited by a phospholipid bilayer, with sizes from 50 nm to several micrometers) have been extensively studied for more than half a century in the context of transport of diagnostic and therapeutic agents (Musacchio & Torchilin, 2011). These vesicles can be constructed with natural lipids, mainly derivatives of phosphatidyletanolamine, phosphatidylcholine, phosphatidylserine, and phosphatidylglycerol, to mimic cellular membranes. Because phospholipids can spontaneously form lipid bilayer-contained capsules in aqueous solution, hydrophilic

molecules can be loaded within the inner volume of the vesicle or attached on the liposome surface, while hydrophobic cargo can be embedded within the bilayer. Targeting moieties with affinity to markers in the body, imaging molecules, and/or polymer coats (discussed below) can be incorporated on the surface in order to enhance their circulation, provide selective targeting, and improve transport (Minko, et al., 2006, Musacchio & Torchilin, 2011).
Yet, liposomes can only bear a relatively low degree of said modifications, rendering them relatively unstable and susceptible for rapid clearance, mainly due to deposition of plasma immunoglobulins and proteins on their surface, favoring uptake by macrophages of the reticuloendothelial system (Moghimi & Szebeni, 2003). New approaches are combining polymers with liposomal formulations to improve these aspects (Musacchio & Torchilin, 2011).

2.1.2 Polymer nanocarriers

Polymers are macromolecules that result from covalent linkage of smaller structural units or repeats referred to as monomers, and can be designed from fully synthetic to biological blocks (Moghimi, et al., 2001). Some examples of synthetic polymers employed in drug delivery include chemically inert and non-toxic materials such as poly(methyl methacrylate), poly(acrylic acid), polyacrylamide, poly(vinyl alcohol), and poly(ethylene glycol), among many others. Biological polymers include (but are not restricted to) natural gums, polysaccharide-, and polypeptide-based formulations (e.g., chitosan, sodium alginate, gelatin, albumin, etc.). Also commonly used due to their biocompatibility and ability to be degraded in the body are polyanhydrides, polyorthoesters, polycaprolactone, polylactides, polyglycolides, and poly(lactide-co-glycolides). These carriers encompass linear polymers, branched polymers and tree-like hyperbranched dendrimers, self-assembled polymersomes (the polymer counterpart of liposomes), and more stable particles, with overall sizes ranging from a few nanometers to several micrometers (Torchilin, 2006). They can endure a degree of modification higher than that of lipososomes, rendering multifunctional formulations that can carry therapeutics, targeting moieties, and imaging agents (Duncan, 2003).
Among them, the polyether poly(ethylene glycol), a polymer of ethylene oxide also known as PEG (Figure 2B in section 2.2.1), is one of the polymers most broadly used in nanomedicine due to its high hydrophilicity and, hence, its ability to solubilize hydrophobic drugs, minimize interaction with the immune system, and prolong the circulation of compounds (Moghimi, et al., 2001, Panyam & Labhasetwar, 2003). PEG can be directly linked to the therapeutic cargo of interest (oligonucleotides or DNA, proteins, small molecules, etc), or it can be coupled to or grafted onto other carriers (Moghimi, et al., 2003).
Poly(lactide-co-glycolide), known as PLGA, is an FDA-approved material that is also commonly used for drug delivery due to its biocompatibility: PLGA is hydrolyzed into lactic and glycolic acids with minimal toxicity (Mundargi, et al., 2008) and the rate of degradation can be adjusted by modification of the particle size and the lactide-to-glycolide ratio for controlled release of the cargo (Panyam & Labhasetwar, 2003). In addition, endo-lysosomal escape of PLGA carriers can be regulated to some extent by modifying these design parameters (Panyam, et al., 2002), which is useful for gaining access to other cell compartments. This is also a property of cationic polymers, such as poly-L-lysine and poly(ethylenimine) (PEI), whose amine groups become protonated at endosomal pH, resulting in osmotic swelling that bursts the endosome (Sonawane, et al., 2003). Although these polymers are useful for transfection in cell cultures, due to toxicity, other experimental formulations more amenable for *in vivo* applications are being explored. This is the case for pH-sensitive poly(acrylic acid) derivative carriers that act as proton sponges within

lysosomes, and temperature-responsive polyelectrolyte hydrogels whose hydration rate varies with temperature, leading to changes in the carrier volume within the endo-lysosomal compartment (Yessine & Leroux, 2004, El-Sayed, et al., 2005, Choi, et al., 2006).
Also natural polymers, such as chitosan, are often exploited for their pH sensitivity and bioadhesive properties. Chitosan is cationic under neutral or basic conditions, favoring adhesion to negatively-charged membranes of cells, and is depolymerized under acidic conditions, resulting in pH controlled drug release (Agnihotri, et al., 2004). Since chitosan is mucoadhesive and favors permeabilization through the gastrointestinal epithelial layer, this polymer is particularly useful to deliver agents by the oral route (Agnihotri, et al., 2004). Polymer dendrimers are also suitable for transport across the intestine due to their small size and ability to enhance permeability of the epithelial layer (Kitchens, et al., 2005).

2.1.3 Carbon nanostructures, metal particles and quantum dots

In addition to liposomes and (synthetic or natural) polymer carriers, carbon nanostructures, quantum dots, and metal particles are becoming more commonly used in nanomedicine. These materials are often employed in the design of biosensors for diagnostic applications, and also some derivatives have been studied in the context of drug delivery.
Carbon nanostructures (~1-3 nm diameter, (Chen, et al., 2003)), such as single- or multi-walled carbon nanotubes, carbon nanospheres, extended carbon nanocube networks, etc., possess interesting physical properties suitable for applications in nanotechnology, electronics, and optics. They are highly stable and versatile in terms of their structural conformation, charge, strength, flexibility, etc. (Cheung, et al., 2010). This material can also be functionalized with drugs and/or biomolecules for diagnostic and therapeutic purposes.
Quantum dots (QDs) are semiconductors fabricated from a combination of metals and non-metals (Choi & Frangioni, 2010). These nanoparticles (~2-10 nm diameter) have unique photophysical properties, e.g., upon excitation they emit fluorescence that is brighter and more stable than that of traditional fluorophores, and their size can be varied to achieve excitation and emission at different wavelengths. They can be detected with high sensitivity, which along with their stability, provides an ideal ground for the design of *ex vivo* screening technologies, such as the case of effective diagnosis of genetic diseases (Bailey, et al., 2009).
Metal nanoparticles are also used in biosensors due to their charge, high sensitivity, and output stability. Gold is often used for imaging and biosensing due to its biocompatibility and unique optical sensitivity (Cai, et al., 2008). Phosphor particles contain rare earth metals and have similar characteristics as QDs, being highly photostable and rendering virtually no autofluorescence, yet their larger size limits their applications (Corstjens, et al., 2005).
While the formulations described above are mostly employed for *ex vivo* diagnostic applications due to toxicity, iron oxide nanoparticles, preferentially 10-100 nm in size (Shubayev, et al., 2009), which can be additionally coupled to polymers, are being explored for imaging and drug delivery. These carriers can be functionalized with various cargoes and have been shown to be relatively suitable for transport of therapeutics (Shubayev, et al., 2009). They present low toxicity, being biocompatible for *in vivo* applications. Iron oxide and, particularly, superparamagnetic iron oxide (SPIO) nanoparticles exhibit magnetic properties, which is used for MRI imaging (Kamaly & Miller, 2010) and also provides an opportunity to control particle transport by external magnets (Nacev, et al., 2010).

2.2 Pharmacokinetics, targeting, and sub-cellular transport of nanocarriers

Development of effective diagnostic techniques and therapeutic delivery methods carry a number of important challenges, many of which may be overcome with the input of nanomedicine approaches. The size scale of nanomedicines and the degree of manipulation to which they can be subjected, make these endeavors seemingly tangible. Drug delivery carriers can be functionalized to improve control of their circulation and biodistribution in the body at the tissue, cellular, and sub-cellular level. This can be achieved by incorporating immune-evading moieties and/or affinity molecules that favor adhesion to either general or specific biological markers, depending on the degree of selectivity required. In addition, when carriers are targeted to cellular receptors involved in endocytic transport or coupled to cell penetrating peptides, or if they are designed to modify the permeability of cellular barriers, they also provide delivery to a variety of intracellular compartments, such as the lysosome, cytosol, nuclei, etc., and can furthermore be transported at some extent across cellular layers, a requirement for a number of clinical goals (Langer, 1998, Moghimi, et al., 2001, Panyam & Labhasetwar, 2003, Sahay, et al., 2010, Sawant & Torchilin, 2010).

2.2.1 Circulation and clearance

When administered *in vivo*, therapeutic agents are often recognized as foreign substances and, consequently, are rapidly cleared from the body (Moghimi, et al., 2001, Yoo, et al., 2010). This is a general obstacle of classical means of drug delivery that also applies to chemicals used as palliative treatment of symptoms associated to genetic diseases, and more specific small molecules used to regulate affected metabolic pathways, inhibitors and activators of the affected molecules, chaperones to improve folding and stability, and recombinant proteins and enzymes used for replacement therapies. Clearance of foreign compounds in the body occurs mainly by the reticuloendothelial system and other elements of the immune system, as well as by renal filtration (Moghimi & Szebeni, 2003). Resident macrophages in the alveoli remove substances administered into the lungs through the respiratory tract, Kupffer's cells in the liver sinusoids remove materials that enter the portal circulation through the gastrointestinal epithelium, materials administered in the systemic circulation are cleared mainly by the spleen and liver, and the lymph nodes remove substances that arrive to the tissue parenchyma by draining them through the lymphatics.

For most applications, including those designed for treatment of genetic conditions, e.g., mostly applicable to small molecule therapies and enzyme replacement therapies, rapid clearance is detrimental as it minimizes the chances of the delivered agent to reach its targets in the body and accumulate there at amounts amenable to render significant efficacy. Avoiding recognition by said clearance systems, e.g., by designing immune evasive strategies leading to lengthening of the life-span of the cargo, can improve the efficiency.

One strategy to control this parameter consists of coupling to poly(ethylene glycol) or PEG, known as PEGylation or stealth technology. PEG helps form a hydrophilic brush around cargoes and/or their carriers, minimizing interactions with plasma opsonins, the complement, professional phagocytes, and lymphocytes which provide specific immunity (Moghimi & Szebeni, 2003) (Figure 2A and 2B). As a consequence, certain physiochemical properties of the cargo (such as hydrophobicity) are altered, allowing the platform to gain solubility and to remain elusive from immune detection. This prolongs the circulation in the bloodstream from a few hours to days, which favors lengthened medicinal effects and less frequent administrations (Moghimi & Szebeni, 2003, Musacchio & Torchilin, 2011).

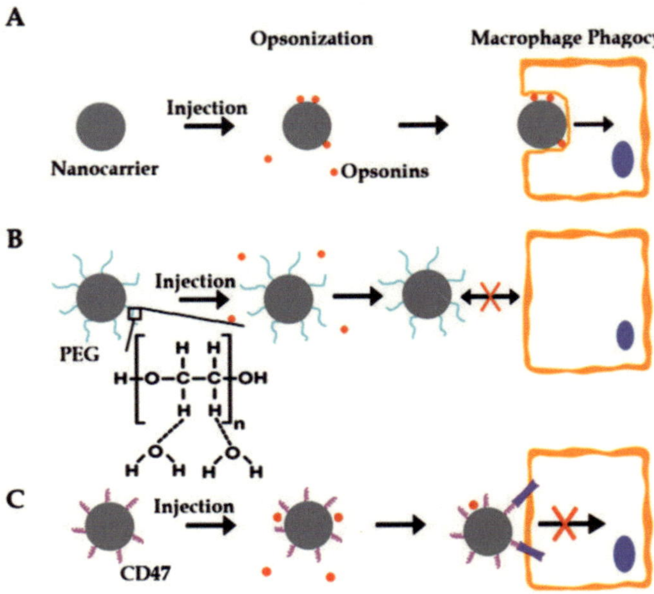

Fig. 2. Strategies to minimize rapid clearance of nanocarriers. (A) Poly(ethylene glycol) or PEG minimizes interaction with plasma proteins and binding to macrophages. (B) CD47 binding to the surface of immune cells inhibits engulfment and phagocytosis.

Other strategy to minimize drug removal takes advantage of the natural mechanism by which red blood cells in the body avoid clearance by elements of the innate immune system. This is the case for CD47 (Figure 2C), a transmembrane protein that acts like a marker of the "self" by binding to its cognate receptor expressed on leukocytes, inhibitory receptor signal regulatory protein alpha (SIRPα). CD47 binding to SIRPα inhibits phagocytosis, in part via regulation of the cytoskeleton and inhibition of engulfing structures. Incorporation of CD47 on drug carrier surfaces reduces attachment to neutrophils and macrophages, therefore prolonging circulation and inhibiting inflammation (Stachelek, et al., 2011).

In addition to controlling the solubility level, half-life in circulation, and immune system recognition, nanocarriers can also improve control of the drug efficacy upon release in the case of therapeutic interventions where administration is local. Localized implantation of bioactive agents embedded within porous matrices and/or hydrogels capable of responding to microenvironment properties can provide controlled release and effects (Tokarev & Minko, 2010). Encapsulation within these formulations can also provide sustained release over prolonged periods of time, as oppose to bulk delivery of a naked therapeutic (Tokarev & Minko, 2010), which can apply to the release of encapsulated drugs and also bioactive substances produced by cells encapsulated within these matrices (discussed in section 3.4).

2.2.2 Targeting

As described above, nanomedicines can improve the bioavailability and pharmacokinetics of diagnostic and therapeutic agents, also protecting them from rapid degradation. In order to maximize their efficacy, carriers can also be designed to help maximize bioadhesion to areas in the body where their action is required, a strategy known as targeting (Figure 3).

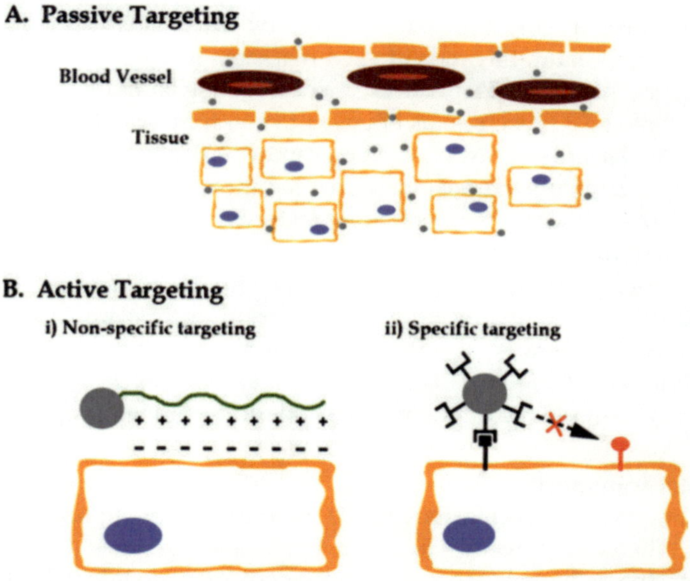

Fig. 3. Passive (A) and active (B) targeting of drug carriers helps localize their cargo within the body, either via non-specific interactions with the target cells (i) or more specific recognition of particular surface markers (ii).

In some cases, general enhanced delivery throughout the body, rather than specific delivery to particular organs, is preferred. This is the case for genetic conditions that affect multi-organ systems due to ubiquitous distribution of the molecular markers or functions affected, such as in many monogenic disorders with both peripheral and central nervous system components. Since most therapeutics do not present intrinsic affinity to cells in the body, coupling them to carriers with affinity properties provides advantages. Hydrophilic and slightly positively-charged polymers provide affinity to the negatively-charged plasma membrane of cells (Panyam & Labhasetwar, 2003, El-Sayed, et al., 2005). Also, these systems can be coupled to affinity moieties that enhance bioadhesion. This is the case for promiscuous affinity peptides such as Tat, antennapedia, and other sequences that gain access to the plasma membrane of cells due to their positively-charged nature (Suk, et al., 2006, Sawant & Torchilin, 2010) (Figure 3Bi), similarly to polymer carriers described above.

In other cases, more specific localization of drug cargoes and imaging agents is necessary for optimal effects, such as the case of diseases with more prominent symptoms in particular organs or cell types (Langer, 1998, Torchilin, 2006, Pardridge, 2010). Moreover, such specific targeting may also reduce potential side effects of the therapeutic in non-intended targets. For instance, carriers injected in the circulation are passively targeted to organs irrigated by the vascular bed immediately downstream the area of administration (first pass phenomenon), such as the case of pulmonary accumulation of carriers administered intravenously. Also, nanocarriers can gain preferential access to organs irrigated by discontinuous blood vessels (Figure 3A), which do not pose a barrier from free diffusion of substances between the circulation and tissue, such as in the liver, an organ considered a main therapeutic target for many monogenic diseases that affect metabolic pathways.

However, delivery of therapeutics to most other sites in the body requires more complex and precise strategies of active targeting. This can be achieved by coupling to affinity moieties that recognize specific markers expressed by the cells which require intervention (Figure 3Bii), including natural ligands of such markers, proteins and peptides, antibodies and their fragments, sugars, and aptamers. Also, targeting to markers that are expressed under certain pathological processes (as opposed to control physiological conditions) helps favoring delivery to disease sites (Muro & Muzykantov, 2005, Bareford & Swaan, 2007).

Whether it is due to targeting via positively-charged moieties or by specific affinity means, targeted delivery of drug carriers offers advantages over direct targeting of therapeutics. Apart from the described advantages posed by increased solubility, circulation time, and release control, carriers bearing multiple copies of an affinity moiety display greater affinity due to this multivalency, compared to drugs that are directly coupled to one copy of the same affinity molecule (Muro, et al., 2006a). As described below, multivalency of targeted carriers also provides tight binding to cell surface receptors, which can favor uptake within the cell, a necessary requirement for many diagnostic and therapeutic applications.

2.2.3 Sub-cellular transport

For most applications the molecular targets for intervention are intracellular (Langer, 1998, Torchilin, 2006). Therefore, targeting to selected cells and tissues is not sufficient to attain significant effects, the delivered cargoes must also gain access to intracellular compartments where their molecular targets are located. Interventions related to RNA interference or delivery of antisense oligonucleotides require transport of these cargoes to the cytosol of the cell, where the target is accessible. This is also the case for delivery of some chaperones, inhibitors or activators, enzymes and other proteins located in the cytosol or sub-cellular organelles such as the mitochondria, peroxisomes, etc., which can be re-directed to these compartments by signal peptides if delivered previously to the cytosol. Gene therapies also require delivery to the cytosol, with subsequent transport to the cell nucleus. In all these cases, cytosolic delivery can be granted mainly by two routes: direct transport of the cargoes and/or their carriers from the extracellular space to the cytosol of cells, or engulfment by the plasma membrane and uptake into vesicular compartments (Muro & Muzykantov, 2005, Suk, et al., 2006, Bareford & Swaan, 2007, Sahay, et al., 2010).

Several strategies have been designed to directly overcome the plasmalemma, gaining access to the cytosol. These include physical means such as electroporation and ultrasound, where a local electric or ultrasound pulse is exerted in the immediate post-administration period, causing transient enhancement of the plasmalemma permeability (Trollet, et al., 2008), and biolistic particle delivery systems, where penetration into cells is gained by means of tungsten or gold particles that are propelled by a "gene gun" across the plasma membrane (O'Brien, et al., 2001). Other methods providing a similar outcome relate to polycationic lipids used to assist cell transfection, which can bind negatively charged proteoglycans at the cell surface and favor cytosolic delivery by porating the plasmalemma (Dincer, et al., 2005, Zuhorn, et al., 2005). Positively-charged cell penetrating peptides (such as RGD and Tat peptides) also bind to the cell surface due to electrostatic interactions and can facilitate cytosolic delivery of cargoes (Magzoub, et al., 2005, Suk, et al., 2006).

As opposed to gaining access to the cell interior by direct penetration into the cytosol, uptake within endocytic vesicles and subsequent selective permeabilization of these compartments for cytosolic release is another major area of research regarding the design of precise nanomedicines (Figure 4A). For instance, drug carriers can be targeted to cell surface receptors involved in endocytosis (Muro & Muzykantov, 2005, Bareford & Swaan, 2007, Pardridge, 2010, Sahay, et al., 2010). This term refers to a group of processes by which cells engulf extracellular material with their plasma membrane, followed by pinching off the resulting vesicles into the cytosol. Uptake by endocytosis is regulated by numerous pathways (clathrin- and caveolar-mediated mechanisms, macropinocytosis, phagocytosis, and other non-classical mechanisms), and most commonly results in transport of the internalized materials to endosomes and lysosomes (Bareford & Swaan, 2007, Sahay, et al., 2010). This strategy is ideal in the case of delivery of therapeutic agents whose action is required at said sub-cellular compartments, such as in the case of carrier-assisted delivery of enzyme replacement for lysosomal storage disorders (Figure 4A right) (Garnacho, et al., 2008, Muro, et al., 2008, Muro, 2010, Hsu, et al., 2011). For those cases where delivery to the cytosol and access to other sub-cellular compartments is required (Figure 4A left), carriers can be coupled to fusogenic peptides derived from bacterial toxins (e.g., hemaglutinnin and GALA peptides), which can induce poration of the endosomal membrane in response to gradual pH lowering in these compartments (Kakudo, et al., 2004). Carriers themselves can also be designed to overcome endosomal membranes, such as in the case of pH-sensitive poly(acid) carriers and temperature-responsive poly(electrolyte) hydrogels (Yessine & Leroux, 2004, Stayton, et al., 2005, Choi, et al., 2006, Oishi, et al., 2006).

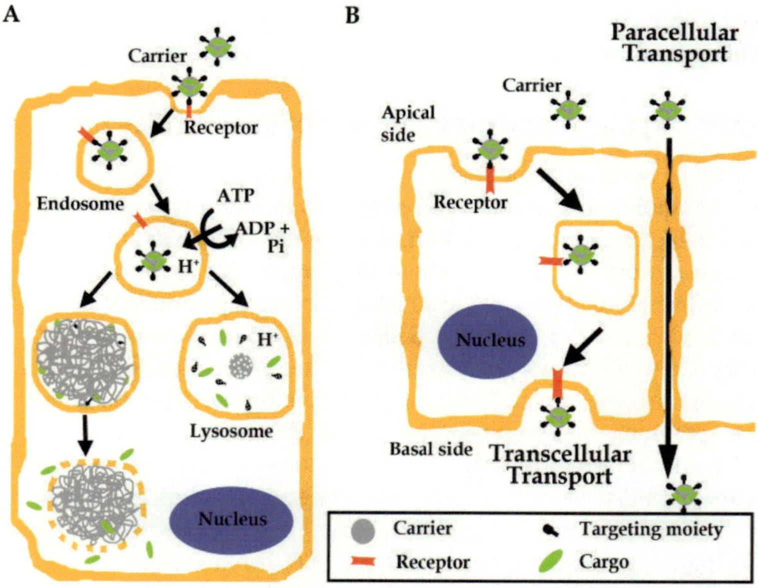

Fig. 4. Sub-cellular delivery of nanocarriers. (A) Endocytosis of carriers can lead to transport to endosomes and lysosomes, where acidic pH and hydrolases can degrade the carrier components and release the therapeutic cargo. Alternatively, pH-sensitive carriers can destabilize the endosome, releasing the cargo to the cytosol. (B) Transport across cellular layers can take place either via paracellular transport between adjacent cells or via transcytosis across the cell body (by vesicular mediated endocytosis and exocytosis).

Finally, effective accumulation within particular tissues requires penetration across cellular barriers. This is most evident in the example of diagnostic and therapeutic agents aimed to exert their activities in the central nervous systems (Pardridge, 2010), and those which need to be transported across the gastrointestinal epithelial layer upon oral administration (Kitchens, et al., 2005, Serra, et al., 2009, Park, et al., 2011). In addition, except for a few cases of vascular beds characterized by discontinuous endothelium where free diffusion is granted, transport of substances from the bloodstream into the irrigated tissues is regulated by the layer of endothelial cells that separate the microvascular wall from the tissue parenchyma and this poses an obstacle to penetration (Pardridge, 2010). Transport of hydrophilic and/or relatively large substances (molecular chaperones, proteins and enzymes, polysaccharides, and oligo- and poly-nucleotides) across endothelial or epithelial barriers is restricted to the transcellular or paracellular routes (Figure 4B). The transcellular route involves internalization of materials on the apical membrane via endocytosis, traffic of endocytic vesicles across the cell body, and exocytosis at the basolateral membrane (transcytosis; Figure 4B left), which occurs mainly via clathrin- and caveolar-mediated pathways (Muro, et al., 2004, Bareford & Swaan, 2007). Due to its safety, this route is preferred for transport into the central nervous system, which can be achieved to some extent by targeting receptors such as the folate, insulin, low density lipoprotein, and transferrin receptors (Hilgenbrink & Low, 2005, Pardridge, 2010, Musacchio & Torchilin, 2011). The paracellular pathway (Figure 4B right) involves transport between adjacent cells via regulation of the junctions that interlock them (Dejana, 2004). This may lead to more uncontrolled, passive transport compared to the transcellular route, hence it is less desired in gaining access into the brain, whereas it seems relatively safe for transport across the gastrointestinal epithelium in oral applications (Kitchens, et al., 2005, Park, et al., 2011).

3. Nanomedicine applications for treatment of genetic diseases

Several properties of nanomedicine designs, mainly pertaining their biocompatible size and high degree of manipulation that allow adaptation to different biomedical applications, have caused this field to be considered a new technological revolution. Nanotechnology has opened new possibilities for *ex vivo* detection methods (e.g., applicable to mutation screening) as well as biomarkers of disease, with several technologies being also applicable for *in vivo* imaging (Cai, et al., 2003, Corstjens, et al., 2005, Bailey, et al., 2009, Cheung, et al., 2010, Choi & Frangioni, 2010). These strategies are considerably more sensitive than traditional methods, permitting detection in smaller samples and/or providing more accurate measurements and tracings of the parameters of interest. From the therapeutic perspective, nanomedicine strategies hold considerable promise to improve control parameters such as the solubility, stability, clearance, biodistribution, sub-cellular transport, controlled release of therapeutic cargoes of diverse nature, improving their efficacy and minimizing potential side effects (Langer, 1998, Moghimi, et al., 2001, Stayton, et al., 2005, Torchilin, 2006).

For the most part, these technologies are still at the experimental stage, particularly those that require *in vivo* administration as opposed to those designed for *ex vivo* diagnosis and detection. However, research has shown a great potential of these platforms for clinical translation in the near future, with some examples being already available in the market, mostly in the case of cancer therapeutics. Although relatively unexplored in the case of genetic deficiencies, the use of nanomedicine principles and strategies for diagnosis and treatment of these conditions is a rapidly growing field with highly promising perspectives.

3.1 Small molecule therapy

Small molecule therapy typically encompasses chemicals used either for palliative care of symptoms or more specifically designed to cope with a particular landmark that regulates disease progression. In many cases, their small size and chemical properties are relatively permissive of diffusion through the body and cells, with relatively good efficacy. However, in other cases they suffer from the obstacles discussed in section 2.2 above, including rapid clearance, inactivation, and sub-optimal access through biological barriers.

For instance, when delivered intravenously rapid loss of therapeutic activity may arise from the direct interaction with blood components and elements of the reticuloendothelial or immune systems. This can be prevented by encapsulating small molecule therapeutics within carriers designed to minimize interaction with said clearance or inactivating systems, prolong their circulation, enhance their accumulation in certain areas of the body, and control their release over long periods of time. Some examples of such applications in the realm of intravenous administration of small molecule therapies for genetic conditions have been reported, such as the case of treatment of hemophilia with coagulation factors encapsulated in biocompatible liposomes, which prolongs the therapeutic window (Yatuv, et al., 2010), or enhanced efficacy of liposomal formulations of antibiotics to treat lung infections in cystic fibrosis (CF) (Mugabe, et al., 2005, Rukholm, et al., 2006). In other cases, interaction with blood components is desired, yet formulation as a nanocarrier still provides therapeutic advantages, such as the case of hexadentate-terminated hydroxypyridinone-based dendrimers, an iron chelating formulation that has been shown to effectively sequester excess iron in haemochromatosis and the thalassaemias (Zhou, et al., 2006).

Regarding penetration in the body, nanomedicine formulations can also help by providing means to modulate viscosity of physiological barriers, such as the sputum in the lungs in the case of inhaled drugs, or enhance the permeability of cellular barriers, such as that encountered by oral drugs in the gastrointestinal epithelium or small molecules that can not cross from the bloodstream into the brain. For instance, the thick lung sputum encountered in CF patients is a major obstacle for effective penetration of classical inhaled therapeutics, hindering access to the underlining epithelial layer. Encapsulation of antibiotics within liposomes modified with amiloride hydrochloride has been shown to force water retention and reduce viscosity of the sputum, resulting in enhanced release and effects (Chougule, et al., 2006). Liposomes modified with the bioadhesive metal, gallium, improved delivery of antibiotics in the CF airways, permitting reduction of the administered dose by an order of magnitude compared to the naked antibiotic (Halwani, et al., 2008). Biodegradable PEGylated PLGA nanoparticles have also been shown to effectively cross the sputum, which has been used to enhance delivery of proteosome inhibitors in CF (Vij, et al., 2010).

With regard to delivery of small molecules by the oral route (preferred to minimize cost and improve patient compliance), encapsulation in enteric-coated capsules is typically required. Classically, bulk capsules protect therapeutics from exposure to the acidic environment in the stomach. Coupling to nanocarriers has shown advantages in this arena, particularly regarding intestinal absorption. This has been shown in the case of oral delivery of anti-diabetic agents by solid lipid particles, which effectively decreased glucose in circulation (Nnamani, et al., 2010) or the case of PLGA nanocarriers encapsulating curcumin for CF, which surpassed the effects of its non-encapsulated counterpart (Cartiera, et al., 2010). Similar results were rendered using chitosan nanocarriers designed for pH-sensitive release and enhanced mucoadhesive potential, resulting in improved absorption of anti-diabetic drugs (Wong, 2010). A combination of classical oral delivery formulations and nanotechnologies, e.g., chitosan nanocarriers encased within enteric-coated capsules for insulin delivery, has shown enhanced results, reflecting the potential of nanomedicine to impact oral delivery of active therapeutics (Cui, et al., 2009, Sonaje, et al., 2010).

Another important cellular barrier encountered by some small molecule therapies is that of the blood-brain interface, which forces more invasive means of local delivery, including direct injection or implantation of the naked therapeutic agent or different scaffolds containing said therapeutic into the brain, e.g., by intracerebral or intraventricular, administration (Menei, et al., 2000, Nakaji-Hirabayashi, et al., 2009, Emerich, et al., 2010). In this regard, prolonged circulation and stability rendered by nanocarriers can enhance the chances of drug diffusion into the brain parenchyma. As discussed in section 2.2.3, carriers targeted to particular transporters of the blood-brain barrier can also improve entry into the central nervous system. Examples illustrating this are those that capitalize on targeting the transferrin receptor, which provides transendothelial transport by a clathirn-mediated mechanism. This has been explored for delivery of nerve growth factor for Huntingon's disease (Kordower, et al., 1994). Nanocarriers have also been used as vehicles to assist in transporting chelating agents into the brain for iron capture and removal in Alzheimer's disease, also with potential in Huntington's and Parkinson's diseases (Liu, et al., 2009).
Similar nanomedicine strategies can improve delivery of other small molecule therapies for genetic diseases, including hormones to control regulatory pathways, antibiotics, growth factors, cofactors, inhibitors or activators that act upstream or downstream of affected pathways, chaperones that favor proper protein folding, and other chemicals.

3.2 Enzyme therapy

The term enzyme therapy describes the administration of exogenous enzymes to replace their defective endogenous counterparts (enzyme replacement therapy or ERT) and can also be extended beyond the treatment of genetic diseases with impaired enzyme production, for instance in cases where administration of additional enzymes that are not encountered endogenously in the human body can help alleviate phenotypic symptoms. Classical examples of the first approach have been applied to the treatment of lysosomal storage disorders (LSDs), mostly caused by genetic defects affecting enzymes involved in lysosomal degradation of varied substrates (Burrow, et al., 2007), neuropathic phenylketonuria (PKU) as a consequence of a defect in phenylalanine hydroxylase (PAH) (Kim, et al., 2004, Harding & Blau, 2010), or prolidase deficiency affecting collagen metabolism (Colonna, et al., 2008b), among many others. The second approach is illustrated in examples pertaining, for instance, administration of alginate lyase to degrade components of infectious biofilms in CF (Lamppa, et al., 2011) or delivery of uricase for gout treatment (Sherman, et al., 2008).
However, effective delivery of enzymes often suffers from the impediments stated above for small molecule therapies, with the added disadvantages that arise from using proteins as therapeutic agents: susceptibility to proteases, high potential for immunogenicity, and even more reduced penetration within tissues and cells in the body. Hence, these therapeutic strategies represent good targets for improvement by nanomedicine approaches.
For instance, several lysosomal ERTs are clinically available, providing a marked phenotypic improvement. However, in many cases, production of antibodies against the administered recombinant enzymes hinders the efficacy of this treatment over time, which represents a major obstacle for treatment of these chronic conditions (Ponder, 2008, Linthorst, et al., 2004). This could be ameliorated by encapsulating or coupling said enzymes within immuno-evasive carriers or polymers, such as those described in section 2.2.1. Some preliminary attempts in this direction include the case of delivery of PEG-modified dextranase, which achieved prolonged activity by bypassing immunorecognition in a mouse model of LSD mimicked by lysosomal accumulation of dextran (Mumtaz & Bachhawat, 1994). Similar strategies of PEGylation have been useful for delivery of uricase for gout

treatment in hyperuricemia (Sherman, et al., 2008), non-mammalian phenylalanine ammonia lyase for treatment of PKU (Ikeda, et al., 2005), or alginate lyase delivery targeted to CF infections (Lamppa, et al., 2011).

In addition to protecting from inactivation and immunogenic responses, by masking the enzymes from the immune and clearance systems, it is expected that these strategies involving incorporation of PEG in the formulation will also provide prolonged circulation, hence enhancing the chances to reach tissues and cell targets in the body, a capacity otherwise considerably restricted for large molecules such as these enzymes. Encapsulation within or coupling to liposomes and polymer carriers, as well as the incorporation of active targeting moieties, may help these aspects. Some examples of these applications were explored in the late 70's, such as in the case of enhanced delivery of glucocerebrosidase deficient in Gaucher disease upon encapsulation within liposomes (Dale, et al., 1979), or liposomes coupled to aggregated immunoglobulins or apolipoproteins for enhanced enzyme targeting to polymorphonucleocytes for treatment of Batten disease (Weissmann, et al., 1975, Steger & Desnick, 1977). Yet, not many subsequent works have risen from these seminal studies, adapting the rapid evolving arena of nanomedicine to formulations for treatment of genetic conditions, and both fields have developed independently. A recent attempt to bridge this gap studied enhancement of delivery of acid sphingomyelinase or α-galactosidase (deficient in types A-B Niemann-Pick disease or Fabry disease, respectively) to peripheral organs and the brain, which was achieved by coupling said enzymes to polymer nanocarriers targeted to intercellular adhesion molecule-1 (ICAM-1), a molecule present in multiple tissues and cell types in the body, whose expression is highly upregulated in many pathological conditions (Garnacho, et al., 2008, Muro, 2010, Hsu, et al., 2011).

This type of strategy can not only assists with targeting of enzymes through the body, but it can also provide access to intracellular compartments where their action is required, improving efficacy. This can be achieved by either exploiting targeting to receptors involved in endocytic transport and/or carriers capable of transporting materials across the plasma membrane or the membranous envelop of intracellular compartments (described in section 2.2.3). This is the case for prolidase delivery by chitosan nanoparticles, which enhance absorptive endocytosis of the enzyme into cells, with subsequent pH-triggered release to the cytosol (Colonna, et al., 2008a), or enhanced delivery of acid sphingomyelinase or α-galactosidase to lysosomal compartments by ICAM-1-targeted nanocarriers (Muro, et al., 2006b, Garnacho, et al., 2008, Hsu, et al., 2011). In the latter example, ICAM-1 targeting provides a means for switching the entry pathway of lysosomal enzymes within cells from clathrin-mediated endocytosis, typically induced by binding of mannose or mannose-6-phosphate residues present on the naked lysosomal enzymes to the corresponding cell receptors, to cell adhesion molecule (CAM)-mediated endocytosis induced by ICAM-1 targeting. This provides an advantage for those cases when the pathology itself tends to alter the expression or function of cell receptors, such as the case of the mannose-6-phosphate receptor in some LSDs (Dhami & Schuchman, 2004, Cardone, et al., 2008). Finally, transport across cellular barriers, greatly impaired for many enzyme therapies, could be improved by formulating said enzymes as their nanocarrier counterparts, as those described in section 2.2.3, enabling these treatment strategies to reach the central nervous system or to be converted into oral delivery modalities.

3.3 Gene therapy

In a broad definition, gene therapy encompasses the modulation of the expression of genes affected in genetic conditions, which can be achieved at the level of providing codifying gene sequences that can enable the transcription and translation of functional proteins otherwise affected by these defects, or other regulatory sequences that can up-regulate or down-regulate said expression at any stage during transcription or translation. This is inclusive of, but not limited to, delivery of cDNA to replace the codifying sequence of the affected gene, or delivery of oligonucleotides for correction of mRNA transcripts by mRNA insertion/deletion, small interference RNA (siRNA) for silencing, etc.

This strategy capitalizes on viral vectors, given that many viruses can actively bind to cell surface receptors, enter cells by endocytosis, and gain access to the cytosol and the nucleus, in certain cases, by escaping the endo-lysosomal vesicles in which they are contained (Campbell & Hope, 2005). These viruses have evolved mechanisms capable of "sensing" the lowering pH within endosomes and lysosomes, e.g., by protonation of amphiphilic molecules, which can then destabilize and porate the endo-lysosomal membrane (Campbell & Hope, 2005). Delivery of said nucleic acid-based therapeutics has been shown to be markedly effective when using viral vectors, which is attributable to their innate ability to effectively deliver double-stranded or single-stranded DNA or RNA molecules within cells.

Most strategies attempted include somatic gene transfer in animal models using adenovirus, adeno-associated virus, herpesvirus and, more recently, retrovirus and lentivirus vectors capable of integrating the exogenous gene sequences into the host genome for prolonged expression (Wilson, 2004, Sands & Davidson, 2006). Other strategies consist of transforming cells *ex vivo* by viral vectors to express functional proteins, with subsequent local implantation of the transformed cells in the body (Ohashi, et al., 2000, Karolewski & Wolfe, 2006). However, while these strategies are highly promising, their current translational application is still limited due to cargo size limitations and mainly safety concerns that involve immunogenicity and potential for random insertions in the host genome.

In this regard, nanomedicine offers an opportunity to develop complementary approaches to traditional gene therapy. For instance, PEGylation strategies can improve the masking from the immune system, such as the case of PEGylated DNA/nanoparticles shown to provide effective intraocular transfection for retinitis pigmentosa while avoiding immune recognition (Cai, et al., 2008), or PEGylation of adenoviruses to confer protection against neutralizing antibodies (O'Riordan, et al., 1999), which may enable subsequent administrations. Similarly, encapsulation of the viral vectors themselves within polymer materials can also minimize immunogenicity, illustrated by successful gene transduction using adenoviruses encapsulated into PLGA microspheres (Turner, et al., 2007).

Encapsulation or complexation of nucleic acid material within liposomes or polymer carriers (lipoplexes or polyplexes) is also being optimized in order to avoid utilization of protein-rich viral capsids (arguably highly immunogenic) and viral genetic elements. Properties such as immune evasion, improved penetration through viscous fluids, targeting to particular cellular markers, and membrane permeabilization (those of the plasmalemma or intracellular compartments), discussed in section 2.2, are being built in these systems, to enable them to achieve delivery of nucleic acid materials. For instance, addition of albumin to polyplexes improves penetration through the sputum and provides transfection in CF (Di Gioia, et al., 2008). Bioadhesive and pH-responsive properties of chitosan nanoparticles, along with its lack of toxicity, can also benefit delivery of gene therapies (Agnihotri, et al., 2004), including oral gene delivery applications such that of coagulation factor VIII in a hemophilia mouse model (Dhadwar, et al., 2010) or glucagon-liked peptide 1 (GLP-1) to reduce blood glucose in diabetes (Jean, et al., 2011).

As discussed for other therapeutic applications, these nanomedicine strategies can be targeted to particular receptors encountered in cells where transfection is needed. As an example, this has been shown in the case of lipoplexes encoding for low-density lipoprotein receptor (LDLR) and targeted to the tranferrin receptor to provide expression of LDLR for treatment of familial hypercholesterolemia (Shichiri, et al., 2003). The same targeting strategy has been used for expression of glial-derived neurotrophic growth factor (GDNF) to reduce neurotoxicity in Parkinson's disease (Zhang, et al., 2006).

Coupling to cell penetrating peptides and/or carrier scaffolds amenable for escaping from endocytic compartments (discussed in section 2.2.3), reminiscent of viral escape from these vesicles, improves the efficacy of transfection. Examples illustrating these strategies are those of facilitated transfection by PEGylated PEI encasing oligonucleotides for Duschenne muscular dystrophy, hemophilia, and CF (Lee, et al., 2004, Carrabino, et al., 2005, Dif, et al., 2006, Sirsi, et al., 2008), lipoplexes coupled to arginine-glycine-aspartic acid (RGD) peptides that can bind to integrins (Scott, et al., 2001), or direct coupling of DNA to cell penetrating peptides, such as in the case of gene therapy for Fabry disease (Lavigne, et al., 2008).

3.4 Cell therapy

Cell therapy has been largely utilized as a therapeutic generating system, where cells from healthy subjects or cells from the patient properly modified are implanted in the body to provide sustained production of a molecule of interest that is innately defective in the diseased patient. Hence, the cell itself can be considered the vehicle of delivery and sustained effects can be achieved. This is beneficial in the case of certain proteins, hormones, and small molecules (such as neurotrophic factors) that display short circulatory longevity and are easily subjected to proteases, shortening their therapeutic effects.

By directly producing these molecules at the required site, cell therapy provides a means to bypass secondary strategies to stabilize said molecules or the necessity for enabling crossing of physiological barriers. This is the case for implantation of alginate microparticles carrying recombinant fibroblasts for sustained systemic release of α-glucuronidase for mucopolysaccharidosis VII (Ross, et al., 2000a). Local implantation of the encapsulated cells into the brain lateral ventricles circumvents the blood-brain barrier and results in considerable delivery of the secreted enzyme (Ross, et al., 2000b). Similarly, implantation of encapsulated, genetically modified fibroblasts capable of producing ciliary neurotrophic factor (CNTF), a neuroprotective agent, in the brain or within vitreous humor of the eye have been explored in the context of treatment for Huntington's disease and retinitis pigmentosa (Emerich, et al., 1996, Tao, et al., 2002, Bloch, et al., 2004).

In most of these applications, encapsulation of cells to be implanted within polymer matrices is advantageous, if not required, in order to create a protective physical barrier to the immune system while permitting sustained release of the therapeutic by the implanted cells. Such scaffolds can avoid unwanted cell escape and neoplastic growth, yet allow oxygen and nutrients to access the matrix to maintain cell viability, while permitting therapeutics to be secreted to the surrounding environment. In this regard, nanotechnology has permitted nano-scale manipulation of these materials to achieve controlled diffusion, limiting immune response while supporting sustained release of the therapeutic molecules. An example of this strategy capitalizes on the use of alginate poly(L-lysine) hydrogels, an immune elusive and non-toxic polymer, (Koch, et al., 2003) with a nanoporous architecture, suitable to allow minimal yet sufficient nutrient exchange (Desai, et al., 2004).

Reduced access to elements of the immune system may also provide an avenue for use of allografts or xenografts, as in the case of long term implantation into rats of bovine islet cells encapsulated within alginate poly(L-lysine) microcapsules (Lanza, et al., 1999). Similarly, this property can be exploited to achieve more sustained therapeutic effects, such as those obtained in the case of genetically modified endothelial cells in treatment of hemophilia A, effective for ~150 days (Lin, et al., 2002), modified myoblasts to secrete erythropoietin, hence reducing the need of constant blood transfusions and hormone injections for treatment of the thalassemias (Dalle, et al., 1999), or encapsulated fibroblasts that release GDNF for Parkinson's disease, which was effective for up to 2 years (Zurn, et al., 2001).

4. Conclusion

During the last 2-3 decades, the development of nanotechnologies for medical applications has provided important new avenues to improve diagnosis and treatment of human maladies. Said nanomedicines display a considerable degree of control of parameters such as increased solubility of various cargoes, evasion from the immune system, controlled circulation, improved stability, enhanced biodistribution in the body, modulatable transport into and/or across cells, and controlled release at the final destination. These approaches can be applied to the development of sensors and imaging agents with improved detection and diagnostic sensitivity, and also delivery of therapeutic strategies pertaining to small molecule, enzyme, gene, and cell therapies. Several nanoconstructs with varied chemical nature, architectural design, and functional properties have been successfully translated into the clinics, mainly for applications other than treatment of genetic conditions. Although, their application in this field has been only modestly explored, these systems rather represent general platforms, offering a unique opportunity to develop alternative and complementary therapeutic interventions applicable to the treatment of genetic diseases.

5. Acknowledgments

The authors would like to acknowledge the financial support from the Nanobiotechnology Program of the Maryland Department of Business and Economic Development, the University of Maryland Minta Martin Foundation, grant 09BGIA2450014 from the American Heart Association, and grant R01HL098416 from the National Institutes of Health (SM).

6. References

Agnihotri, S. A., Mallikarjuna, N. N. & Aminabhavi, T. M. (2004). Recent advances on chitosan-based micro- and nanoparticles in drug delivery. *J Control Release*, Vol.100, No.1, (Nov 5), pp. 5-28, 0168-3659 (Print), 0168-3659 (Linking)

Bailey, V. J., Puleo, C. M., Ho, Y. P., Yeh, H. C. & Wang, T. H. (2009). Quantum dots in molecular detection of disease. *Conf Proc IEEE Eng Med Biol Soc*, Vol.2009, pp. 4089-4092, 1557-170X (Print), 1557-170X (Linking)

Bareford, L. M. & Swaan, P. W. (2007). Endocytic mechanisms for targeted drug delivery. *Adv Drug Deliv Rev*, Vol.59, No.8, (Aug 10), pp. 748-758, 0169-409X (Print), 0169-409X (Linking)

Bloch, J., Bachoud-Levi, A. C., Deglon, N., Lefaucheur, J. P., Winkel, L., Palfi, S., Nguyen, J. P., Bourdet, C., Gaura, V., Remy, P., Brugieres, P., Boisse, M. F., Baudic, S., Cesaro, P., Hantraye, P., Aebischer, P. & Peschanski, M. (2004). Neuroprotective gene therapy for Huntington's disease, using polymer-encapsulated cells engineered to secrete human ciliary neurotrophic factor: results of a phase I study. *Hum Gene Ther*, Vol.15, No.10, (Oct), pp. 968-975, 1043-0342 (Print), 1043-0342 (Linking)

Burrow, T. A., Hopkin, R. J., Leslie, N. D., Tinkle, B. T. & Grabowski, G. A. (2007). Enzyme reconstitution/replacement therapy for lysosomal storage diseases. *Curr Opin Pediatr*, Vol.19, No.6, (Dec), pp. 628-635, 1040-8703 (Print), 1040-8703 (Linking)

Cai, H., Zhu, N., Jiang, Y., He, P. & Fang, Y. (2003). Cu@Au alloy nanoparticle as oligonucleotides labels for electrochemical stripping detection of DNA hybridization. *Biosens Bioelectron*, Vol.18, No.11, (Oct 1), pp. 1311-1319, 0956-5663 (Print), 0956-5663 (Linking)

Cai, X., Conley, S. & Naash, M. (2008). Nanoparticle applications in ocular gene therapy. *Vision Res*, Vol.48, No.3, (Feb), pp. 319-324, 0042-6989 (Print), 0042-6989 (Linking)

Campbell, E. M. & Hope, T. J. (2005). Gene therapy progress and prospects: viral trafficking during infection. *Gene Ther*, Vol.12, No.18, (Sep), pp. 1353-1359,

Cardone, M., Porto, C., Tarallo, A., Vicinanza, M., Rossi, B., Polishchuk, E., Donaudy, F., Andria, G., De Matteis, M. A. & Parenti, G. (2008). Abnormal mannose-6-phosphate receptor trafficking impairs recombinant alpha-glucosidase uptake in Pompe disease fibroblasts. *Pathogenetics*, Vol.1, No.1, pp. 6, 1755-8417 (Electronic)

Carrabino, S., Di Gioia, S., Copreni, E. & Conese, M. (2005). Serum albumin enhances polyethylenimine-mediated gene delivery to human respiratory epithelial cells. *J Gene Med*, Vol.7, No.12, (Dec), pp. 1555-1564, 1099-498X (Print), 1099-498X (Linking)

Cartiera, M. S., Ferreira, E. C., Caputo, C., Egan, M. E., Caplan, M. J. & Saltzman, W. M. (2010). Partial correction of cystic fibrosis defects with PLGA nanoparticles encapsulating curcumin. *Mol Pharm*, Vol.7, No.1, (Feb 1), pp. 86-93, 1543-8392 (Electronic), 1543-8384 (Linking)

Chen, R. J., Bangsaruntip, S., Drouvalakis, K. A., Kam, N. W., Shim, M., Li, Y., Kim, W., Utz, P. J. & Dai, H. (2003). Noncovalent functionalization of carbon nanotubes for highly specific electronic biosensors. *Proc Natl Acad Sci U S A*, Vol.100, No.9, (Apr 29), pp. 4984-4989, 0027-8424 (Print), 0027-8424 (Linking)

Cheung, W., Pontoriero, F., Taratula, O., Chen, A. M. & He, H. (2010). DNA and carbon nanotubes as medicine. *Adv Drug Deliv Rev*, Vol.62, No.6, (Apr 30), pp. 633-649, 1872-8294 (Electronic), 0169-409X (Linking)

Choi, H. S. & Frangioni, J. V. (2010). Nanoparticles for biomedical imaging: fundamentals of clinical translation. *Mol Imaging*, Vol.9, No.6, (Dec), pp. 291-310, 1536-0121 (Electronic), 1535-3508 (Linking)

Choi, S. H., Lee, S. H. & Park, T. G. (2006). Temperature-Sensitive Pluronic/Poly(ethylenimine) Nanocapsules for Thermally Triggered Disruption of Intracellular Endosomal Compartment. *Biomacromolecules*, Vol.7, No.6, (Jun), pp. 1864-1870,

Chougule, M. B., Padhi, B. K. & Misra, A. (2006). Nano-liposomal dry powder inhaler of Amiloride Hydrochloride. *J Nanosci Nanotechnol*, Vol.6, No.9-10, (Sep-Oct), pp. 3001-3009, 1533-4880 (Print), 1533-4880 (Linking)

Colonna, C., Conti, B., Perugini, P., Pavanetto, F., Modena, T., Dorati, R., Iadarola, P. & Genta, I. (2008a). Ex vivo evaluation of prolidase loaded chitosan nanoparticles for the enzyme replacement therapy. *Eur J Pharm Biopharm*, Vol.70, No.1, (Sep), pp. 58-65, 0939-6411 (Print), 0939-6411 (Linking)

Colonna, C., Conti, B., Perugini, P., Pavanetto, F., Modena, T., Dorati, R., Iadarola, P. & Genta, I. (2008b). Site-directed PEGylation as successful approach to improve the enzyme replacement in the case of prolidase. *Int J Pharm*, Vol.358, No.1-2, (Jun 24), pp. 230-237, 0378-5173 (Print), 0378-5173 (Linking)

Corstjens, P. L., Li, S., Zuiderwijk, M., Kardos, K., Abrams, W. R., Niedbala, R. S. & Tanke, H. J. (2005). Infrared up-converting phosphors for bioassays. *IEE Proc Nanobiotechnol*, Vol.152, No.2, (Apr), pp. 64-72, 1478-1581 (Print), 1478-1581 (Linking)

Cui, F., Qian, F., Zhao, Z., Yin, L., Tang, C. & Yin, C. (2009). Preparation, characterization, and oral delivery of insulin loaded carboxylated chitosan grafted poly(methyl methacrylate) nanoparticles. *Biomacromolecules*, Vol.10, No.5, (May 11), pp. 1253-1258, 1526-4602 (Electronic). 1525-7797 (Linking)

Dale, G. L., Kuhl, W. & Beutler, E. (1979). Incorporation of glucocerebrosidase into Gaucher's disease monocytes in vitro. *Proc Natl Acad Sci U S A*, Vol.76, No.1, (Jan), pp. 473-475, 0027-8424 (Print), 0027-8424 (Linking)

Dalle, B., Payen, E., Regulier, E., Deglon, N., Rouyer-Fessard, P., Beuzard, Y. & Aebischer, P. (1999). Improvement of mouse beta-thalassemia upon erythropoietin delivery by encapsulated myoblasts. *Gene Ther*, Vol.6, No.2, (Feb), pp. 157-161, 0969-7128 (Print), 0969-7128 (Linking)

Dejana, E. (2004). Endothelial cell-cell junctions: happy together. *Nat Rev Mol Cell Biol*, Vol.5, No.4, (Apr), pp. 261-270,

Desai, T. A., West, T., Cohen, M., Boiarski, T. & Rampersaud, A. (2004). Nanoporous microsystems for islet cell replacement. *Adv Drug Deliv Rev*, Vol.56, No.11, (Sep 22), pp. 1661-1673, 0169-409X (Print), 0169-409X (Linking)

Dhadwar, S. S., Kiernan, J., Wen, J. & Hortelano, G. (2010). Repeated oral administration of chitosan/DNA nanoparticles delivers functional FVIII with the absence of antibodies in hemophilia A mice. *J Thromb Haemost*, Vol.8, No.12, (Dec), pp. 2743-2750, 1538-7836 (Electronic), 1538-7836 (Linking)

Dhami, R. & Schuchman, E. H. (2004). Mannose 6-phosphate receptor-mediated uptake is defective in acid sphingomyelinase-deficient macrophages: implications for Niemann-Pick disease enzyme replacement therapy. *J Biol Chem*, Vol.279, No.2, (Jan 9), pp. 1526-1532,

Di Gioia, S., Rejman, J., Carrabino, S., De Fino, I., Rudolph, C., Doherty, A., Hyndman, L., Di Cicco, M., Copreni, E., Bragonzi, A., Colombo, C., Boyd, A. C. & Conese, M. (2008). Role of biophysical parameters on ex vivo and in vivo gene transfer to the airway epithelium by polyethylenimine/albumin complexes. *Biomacromolecules*, Vol.9, No.3, (Mar), pp. 859-866, 1526-4602 (Electronic), 1525-7797 (Linking)

Dif, F., Djediat, C., Alegria, O., Demeneix, B. & Levi, G. (2006). Transfection of multiple pulmonary cell types following intravenous injection of PEI-DNA in normal and CFTR mutant mice. *J Gene Med*, Vol.8, No.1, (Jan), pp. 82-89, 1099-498X (Print), 1099-498X (Linking)

Dincer, S., Turk, M. & Piskin, E. (2005). Intelligent polymers as nonviral vectors. *Gene Ther*, Vol.12 Suppl 1, (Oct), pp. S139-145,

Discher, D. E. & Eisenberg, A. (2002). Polymer vesicles. *Science*, Vol.297, No.5583, (Aug 9), pp. 967-973,

Duncan, R. (2003). The dawning era of polymer therapeutics. *Nat Rev Drug Discov*, Vol.2, No.5, (May), pp. 347-360,

El-Sayed, M. E., Hoffman, A. S. & Stayton, P. S. (2005). Smart polymeric carriers for enhanced intracellular delivery of therapeutic macromolecules. *Expert Opin Biol Ther*, Vol.5, No.1, (Jan), pp. 23-32,

Emerich, D. F., Lindner, M. D., Winn, S. R., Chen, E. Y., Frydel, B. R. & Kordower, J. H. (1996). Implants of encapsulated human CNTF-producing fibroblasts prevent behavioral deficits and striatal degeneration in a rodent model of Huntington's disease. *J Neurosci*, Vol.16, No.16, (Aug 15), pp. 5168-5181, 0270-6474 (Print), 0270-6474 (Linking)

Emerich, D. F., Mooney, D. J., Storrie, H., Babu, R. S. & Kordower, J. H. (2010). Injectable hydrogels providing sustained delivery of vascular endothelial growth factor are neuroprotective in a rat model of Huntington's disease. *Neurotox Res*, Vol.17, No.1, (Jan), pp. 66-74, 1476-3524 (Electronic), 1029-8428 (Linking)

Garnacho, C., Dhami, R., Simone, E., Dziubla, T., Leferovich, J., Schuchman, E. H., Muzykantov, V. & Muro, S. (2008). Delivery of acid sphingomyelinase in normal and niemann-pick disease mice using intercellular adhesion molecule-1-targeted polymer nanocarriers. *J Pharmacol Exp Ther*, Vol.325, No.2, (May), pp. 400-408, 1521-0103 (Electronic), 0022-3565 (Linking)

Halwani, M., Yebio, B., Suntres, Z. E., Alipour, M., Azghani, A. O. & Omri, A. (2008). Co-encapsulation of gallium with gentamicin in liposomes enhances antimicrobial activity of gentamicin against Pseudomonas aeruginosa. *J Antimicrob Chemother*, Vol.62, No.6, (Dec), pp. 1291-1297, 1460-2091 (Electronic), 0305-7453 (Linking)

Harding, C. O. & Blau, N. (2010). Advances and challenges in phenylketonuria. *J Inherit Metab Dis*, Vol.33, No.6, (Dec), pp. 645-648, 1573-2665 (Electronic), 0141-8955 (Linking)

Hilgenbrink, A. R. & Low, P. S. (2005). Folate receptor-mediated drug targeting: from therapeutics to diagnostics. *J Pharm Sci*, Vol.94, No.10, (Oct), pp. 2135-2146, 0022-3549 (Print)

Hsu, J., Serrano, D., Bhowmick, T., Kumar, K., Shen, Y., Kuo, Y. C., Garnacho, C. & Muro, S. (2011). Enhanced endothelial delivery and biochemical effects of alpha-galactosidase by ICAM-1-targeted nanocarriers for Fabry disease. *J Control Release*, Vol.149, No.3, (Feb 10), pp. 323-331, 1873-4995 (Electronic), 0168-3659 (Linking)

Ikeda, K., Schiltz, E., Fujii, T., Takahashi, M., Mitsui, K., Kodera, Y., Matsushima, A., Inada, Y., Schulz, G. E. & Nishimura, H. (2005). Phenylalanine ammonia-lyase modified with polyethylene glycol: potential therapeutic agent for phenylketonuria. *Amino Acids*, Vol.29, No.3, (Nov), pp. 283-287, 0939-4451 (Print), 0939-4451 (Linking)

Jean, M., Alameh, M., Buschmann, M. D. & Merzouki, A. (2011). Effective and safe gene-based delivery of GLP-1 using chitosan/plasmid-DNA therapeutic nanocomplexes in an animal model of type 2 diabetes. *Gene Ther*, (Mar 17), pp. 1476-5462 (Electronic), 0969-7128 (Linking)

Kakudo, T., Chaki, S., Futaki, S., Nakase, I., Akaji, K., Kawakami, T., Maruyama, K., Kamiya, H. & Harashima, H. (2004). Transferrin-modified liposomes equipped with a pH-sensitive fusogenic peptide: an artificial viral-like delivery system. *Biochemistry*, Vol.43, No.19, (May 18), pp. 5618-5628,

Kamaly, N. & Miller, A. D. (2010). Paramagnetic liposome nanoparticles for cellular and tumour imaging. *Int J Mol Sci*, Vol.11, No.4, pp. 1759-1776, 1422-0067 (Electronic), 1422-0067 (Linking)

Karolewski, B. A. & Wolfe, J. H. (2006). Genetic correction of the fetal brain increases the lifespan of mice with the severe multisystemic disease mucopolysaccharidosis type VII. *Mol Ther*, Vol.14, No.1, (Jul), pp. 14-24, 1525-0016 (Print)

Kim, W., Erlandsen, H., Surendran, S., Stevens, R. C., Gamez, A., Michols-Matalon, K., Tyring, S. K. & Matalon, R. (2004). Trends in enzyme therapy for phenylketonuria. *Mol Ther*, Vol.10, No.2, (Aug), pp. 220-224, 1525-0016 (Print), 1525-0016 (Linking)

Kitchens, K. M., El-Sayed, M. E. & Ghandehari, H. (2005). Transepithelial and endothelial transport of poly (amidoamine) dendrimers. *Adv Drug Deliv Rev*, Vol.57, No.15, (Dec 14), pp. 2163-2176, 0169-409X (Print)

Koch, S., Schwinger, C., Kressler, J., Heinzen, C. & Rainov, N. G. (2003). Alginate encapsulation of genetically engineered mammalian cells: comparison of production devices, methods and microcapsule characteristics. *J Microencapsul*, Vol.20, No.3, (May-Jun), pp. 303-316, 0265-2048 (Print), 0265-2048 (Linking)

Kordower, J. H., Charles, V., Bayer, R., Bartus, R. T., Putney, S., Walus, L. R. & Friden, P. M. (1994). Intravenous administration of a transferrin receptor antibody-nerve growth factor conjugate prevents the degeneration of cholinergic striatal neurons in a model of Huntington disease. *Proc Natl Acad Sci U S A*, Vol.91, No.19, (Sep 13), pp. 9077-9080, 0027-8424 (Print), 0027-8424 (Linking)

Lamppa, J. W., Ackerman, M. E., Lai, J. I., Scanlon, T. C. & Griswold, K. E. (2011). Genetically engineered alginate lyase-PEG conjugates exhibit enhanced catalytic function and reduced immunoreactivity. *PLoS One*, Vol.6, No.2, pp. e17042, 1932-6203 (Electronic), 1932-6203 (Linking)

Langer, R. (1998). Drug delivery and targeting. *Nature*, Vol.392, No.6679 Suppl, (Apr 30), pp. 5-10,

Lanza, R. P., Jackson, R., Sullivan, A., Ringeling, J., McGrath, C., Kuhtreiber, W. & Chick, W. L. (1999). Xenotransplantation of cells using biodegradable microcapsules. *Transplantation*, Vol.67, No.8, (Apr 27), pp. 1105-1111, 0041-1337 (Print), 0041-1337 (Linking)

Lavigne, M. D., Yates, L., Coxhead, P. & Gorecki, D. C. (2008). Nuclear-targeted chimeric vector enhancing nonviral gene transfer into skeletal muscle of Fabry mice in vivo.

FASEB J, Vol.22, No.6, (Jun), pp. 2097-2107, 1530-6860 (Electronic), 0892-6638 (Linking)

Lee, J. S., Lee, M. & Kim, S. W. (2004). A new potent hFIX plasmid for hemophilia B gene therapy. *Pharm Res*, Vol.21, No.7, (Jul), pp. 1229-1232, 0724-8741 (Print), 0724-8741 (Linking)

Lin, Y., Chang, L., Solovey, A., Healey, J. F., Lollar, P. & Hebbel, R. P. (2002). Use of blood outgrowth endothelial cells for gene therapy for hemophilia A. *Blood*, Vol.99, No.2, (Jan 15), pp. 457-462, 0006-4971 (Print), 0006-4971 (Linking)

Linthorst, G. E., Hollak, C. E., Donker-Koopman, W. E., Strijland, A. & Aerts, J. M. (2004). Enzyme therapy for Fabry disease: neutralizing antibodies toward agalsidase alpha and beta. *Kidney Int*, Vol.66, No.4, (Oct), pp. 1589-1595, 0085-2538 (Print)

Liu, G., Men, P., Perry, G. & Smith, M. A. (2009). Metal chelators coupled with nanoparticles as potential therapeutic agents for Alzheimer's disease. *J Nanoneurosci*, Vol.1, No.1, (Jun 1), pp. 42-55, 1939-0653 (Electronic)

Magzoub, M., Pramanik, A. & Graslund, A. (2005). Modeling the endosomal escape of cell-penetrating peptides: transmembrane pH gradient driven translocation across phospholipid bilayers. *Biochemistry*, Vol.44, No.45, (Nov 15), pp. 14890-14897,

Menei, P., Pean, J. M., Nerriere-Daguin, V., Jollivet, C., Brachet, P. & Benoit, J. P. (2000). Intracerebral implantation of NGF-releasing biodegradable microspheres protects striatum against excitotoxic damage. *Exp Neurol*, Vol.161, No.1, (Jan), pp. 259-272, 0014-4886 (Print), 0014-4886 (Linking)

Minko, T., Pakunlu, R. I., Wang, Y., Khandare, J. J. & Saad, M. (2006). New generation of liposomal drugs for cancer. *Anticancer Agents Med Chem*, Vol.6, No.6, (Nov), pp. 537-552, 1871-5206 (Print), 1871-5206 (Linking)

Moghimi, S. M., Hunter, A. C. & Murray, J. C. (2001). Long-circulating and target-specific nanoparticles: theory to practice. *Pharmacol Rev*, Vol.53, No.2, (Jun), pp. 283-318,

Moghimi, S. M., Hunter, A. C. & Murray, J. C. (2005). Nanomedicine: current status and future prospects. *FASEB J*, Vol.19, No.3, (Mar), pp. 311-330, 1530-6860 (Electronic), 0892-6638 (Linking)

Moghimi, S. M. & Szebeni, J. (2003). Stealth liposomes and long circulating nanoparticles: critical issues in pharmacokinetics, opsonization and protein-binding properties. *Prog Lipid Res*, Vol.42, No.6, (Nov), pp. 463-478,

Mugabe, C., Azghani, A. O. & Omri, A. (2005). Liposome-mediated gentamicin delivery: development and activity against resistant strains of Pseudomonas aeruginosa isolated from cystic fibrosis patients. *J Antimicrob Chemother*, Vol.55, No.2, (Feb), pp. 269-271, 0305-7453 (Print), 0305-7453 (Linking)

Mumtaz, S. & Bachhawat, B. K. (1994). Enhanced intracellular stability and efficacy of PEG modified dextranase in the treatment of a model storage disorder. *Biochim Biophys Acta*, Vol.1199, No.2, (Mar 2), pp. 175-182,

Mundargi, R. C., Babu, V. R., Rangaswamy, V., Patel, P. & Aminabhavi, T. M. (2008). Nano/micro technologies for delivering macromolecular therapeutics using poly(D,L-lactide-co-glycolide) and its derivatives. *J Control Release*, Vol.125, No.3, (Feb 11), pp. 193-209, 1873-4995 (Electronic), 0168-3659 (Linking)

Muro, S. (2010). New biotechnological and nanomedicine strategies for treatment of lysosomal storage disorders. *Wiley Interdiscip Rev Nanomed Nanobiotechnol*, Vol.2, No.2, (Mar-Apr), pp. 189-204, 1939-0041 (Electronic), 1939-0041 (Linking)

Muro, S., Dziubla, T., Qiu, W., Leferovich, J., Cui, X., Berk, E. & Muzykantov, V. R. (2006a). Endothelial targeting of high-affinity multivalent polymer nanocarriers directed to intercellular adhesion molecule 1. *J Pharmacol Exp Ther*, Vol.317, No.3, (Jun), pp. 1161-1169,

Muro, S., Garnacho, C., Champion, J. A., Leferovich, J., Gajewski, C., Schuchman, E. H., Mitragotri, S. & Muzykantov, V. R. (2008). Control of endothelial targeting and intracellular delivery of therapeutic enzymes by modulating the size and shape of ICAM-1-targeted carriers. *Mol Ther*, Vol.16, No.8, (Aug), pp. 1450-1458, 1525-0024 (Electronic)

Muro, S., Koval, M. & Muzykantov, V. (2004). Endothelial endocytic pathways: gates for vascular drug delivery. *Curr Vasc Pharmacol*, Vol.2, No.3, (Jul), pp. 281-299,

Muro, S. & Muzykantov, V. R. (2005). Targeting of antioxidant and anti-thrombotic drugs to endothelial cell adhesion molecules. *Curr Pharm Des*, Vol.11, No.18, pp. 2383-2401,

Muro, S., Schuchman, E. H. & Muzykantov, V. R. (2006b). Lysosomal enzyme delivery by ICAM-1-targeted nanocarriers bypassing glycosylation- and clathrin-dependent endocytosis. *Mol Ther*, Vol.13, No.1, (Jan), pp. 135-141,

Musacchio, T. & Torchilin, V. P. (2011). Recent developments in lipid-based pharmaceutical nanocarriers. *Front Biosci*, Vol.16, pp. 1388-1412, 1093-4715 (Electronic), 1093-4715 (Linking)

Nacev, A., Beni, C., Bruno, O. & Shapiro, B. (2010). Magnetic nanoparticle transport within flowing blood and into surrounding tissue. *Nanomedicine (Lond)*, Vol.5, No.9, (Nov), pp. 1459-1466, 1748-6963 (Electronic), 1743-5889 (Linking)

Nakaji-Hirabayashi, T., Kato, K. & Iwata, H. (2009). Hyaluronic acid hydrogel loaded with genetically-engineered brain-derived neurotrophic factor as a neural cell carrier. *Biomaterials*, Vol.30, No.27, (Sep), pp. 4581-4589, 1878-5905 (Electronic), 0142-9612 (Linking)

Nnamani, P. O., Attama, A. A., Ibezim, E. C. & Adikwu, M. U. (2010). SRMS142-based solid lipid microparticles: application in oral delivery of glibenclamide to diabetic rats. *Eur J Pharm Biopharm*, Vol.76, No.1, (Sep), pp. 68-74, 1873-3441 (Electronic), 0939-6411 (Linking)

O'Brien, J. A., Holt, M., Whiteside, G., Lummis, S. C. & Hastings, M. H. (2001). Modifications to the hand-held Gene Gun: improvements for in vitro biolistic transfection of organotypic neuronal tissue. *J Neurosci Methods*, Vol.112, No.1, (Nov 15), pp. 57-64, 0165-0270 (Print), 0165-0270 (Linking)

O'Riordan, C. R., Lachapelle, A., Delgado, C., Parkes, V., Wadsworth, S. C., Smith, A. E. & Francis, G. E. (1999). PEGylation of adenovirus with retention of infectivity and protection from neutralizing antibody in vitro and in vivo. *Hum Gene Ther*, Vol.10, No.8, (May 20), pp. 1349-1358, 1043-0342 (Print), 1043-0342 (Linking)

Ohashi, T., Yokoo, T., Iizuka, S., Kobayashi, H., Sly, W. S. & Eto, Y. (2000). Reduction of lysosomal storage in murine mucopolysaccharidosis type VII by transplantation of normal and genetically modified macrophages. *Blood*, Vol.95, No.11, (Jun 1), pp. 3631-3633, 0006-4971 (Print)

Oishi, M., Kataoka, K. & Nagasaki, Y. (2006). pH-responsive three-layered PEGylated polyplex micelle based on a lactosylated ABC triblock copolymer as a targetable and endosome-disruptive nonviral gene vector. *Bioconjug Chem*, Vol.17, No.3, (May-Jun), pp. 677-688,

Panyam, J. & Labhasetwar, V. (2003). Biodegradable nanoparticles for drug and gene delivery to cells and tissue. *Adv Drug Deliv Rev*, Vol.55, No.3, (Feb 24), pp. 329-347,

Panyam, J., Zhou, W. Z., Prabha, S., Sahoo, S. K. & Labhasetwar, V. (2002). Rapid endo-lysosomal escape of poly(DL-lactide-co-glycolide) nanoparticles: implications for drug and gene delivery. *FASEB J*, Vol.16, No.10, (Aug), pp. 1217-1226,

Pardridge, W. M. (2010). Biopharmaceutical drug targeting to the brain. *J Drug Target*, Vol.18, No.3, (Apr), pp. 157-167, 1029-2330 (Electronic), 1026-7158 (Linking)

Park, K., Kwon, I. C. & Park, K. (2011). Oral protein delivery: Current status and future prospect *Reactive and Functional Polymers*, Vol.71, No.3, (March 2011), pp. 280-287,

Ponder, K. P. (2008). Immune response hinders therapy for lysosomal storage diseases. *J Clin Invest*, Vol.118, No.8, (Aug), pp. 2686-2689, 0021-9738 (Print)

Ross, C. J., Bastedo, L., Maier, S. A., Sands, M. S. & Chang, P. L. (2000a). Treatment of a lysosomal storage disease, mucopolysaccharidosis VII, with microencapsulated recombinant cells. *Hum Gene Ther*, Vol.11, No.15, (Oct 10), pp. 2117-2127, 1043-0342 (Print), 1043-0342 (Linking)

Ross, C. J., Ralph, M. & Chang, P. L. (2000b). Somatic gene therapy for a neurodegenerative disease using microencapsulated recombinant cells. *Exp Neurol*, Vol.166, No.2, (Dec), pp. 276-286, 0014-4886 (Print), 0014-4886 (Linking)

Rukholm, G., Mugabe, C., Azghani, A. O. & Omri, A. (2006). Antibacterial activity of liposomal gentamicin against Pseudomonas aeruginosa: a time-kill study. *Int J Antimicrob Agents*, Vol.27, No.3, (Mar), pp. 247-252, 0924-8579 (Print), 0924-8579 (Linking)

Sahay, G., Alakhova, D. Y. & Kabanov, A. V. (2010). Endocytosis of nanomedicines. *J Control Release*, Vol.145, No.3, (Aug 3), pp. 182-195, 1873-4995 (Electronic), 0168-3659 (Linking)

Sands, M. S. & Davidson, B. L. (2006). Gene therapy for lysosomal storage diseases. *Mol Ther*, Vol.13, No.5, (May), pp. 839-849, 1525-0016 (Print)

Sawant, R. & Torchilin, V. (2010). Intracellular transduction using cell-penetrating peptides. *Mol Biosyst*, Vol.6, No.4, (Apr), pp. 628-640, 1742-2051 (Electronic), 1742-2051 (Linking)

Scott, E. S., Wiseman, J. W., Evans, M. J. & Colledge, W. H. (2001). Enhanced gene delivery to human airway epithelial cells using an integrin-targeting lipoplex. *J Gene Med*, Vol.3, No.2, (Mar-Apr), pp. 125-134, 1099-498X (Print), 1099-498X (Linking)

Serra, L., Domenech, J. & Peppas, N. A. (2009). Engineering design and molecular dynamics of mucoadhesive drug delivery systems as targeting agents. *Eur J Pharm Biopharm*, Vol.71, No.3, (Mar), pp. 519-528, 1873-3441 (Electronic), 0939-6411 (Linking)

Sherman, M. R., Saifer, M. G. & Perez-Ruiz, F. (2008). PEG-uricase in the management of treatment-resistant gout and hyperuricemia. *Adv Drug Deliv Rev*, Vol.60, No.1, (Jan 3), pp. 59-68, 0169-409X (Print), 0169-409X (Linking)

Shichiri, M., Tanaka, A. & Hirata, Y. (2003). Intravenous gene therapy for familial hypercholesterolemia using ligand-facilitated transfer of a liposome:LDL receptor gene complex. *Gene Ther*, Vol.10, No.9, (May), pp. 827-831, 0969-7128 (Print), 0969-7128 (Linking)

Shubayev, V. I., Pisanic, T. R., 2nd & Jin, S. (2009). Magnetic nanoparticles for theragnostics. *Adv Drug Deliv Rev*, Vol.61, No.6, (Jun 21), pp. 467-477, 1872-8294 (Electronic), 0169-409X (Linking)

Sirsi, S. R., Schray, R. C., Guan, X., Lykens, N. M., Williams, J. H., Erney, M. L. & Lutz, G. J. (2008). Functionalized PEG-PEI copolymers complexed to exon-skipping oligonucleotides improve dystrophin expression in mdx mice. *Hum Gene Ther*, Vol.19, No.8, (Aug), pp. 795-806, 1557-7422 (Electronic), 1043-0342 (Linking)

Sonaje, K., Chen, Y. J., Chen, H. L., Wey, S. P., Juang, J. H., Nguyen, H. N., Hsu, C. W., Lin, K. J. & Sung, H. W. (2010). Enteric-coated capsules filled with freeze-dried chitosan/poly(gamma-glutamic acid) nanoparticles for oral insulin delivery. *Biomaterials*, Vol.31, No.12, (Apr), pp. 3384-3394, 1878-5905 (Electronic), 0142-9612 (Linking)

Sonawane, N. D., Szoka, F. C., Jr. & Verkman, A. S. (2003). Chloride accumulation and swelling in endosomes enhances DNA transfer by polyamine-DNA polyplexes. *J Biol Chem*, Vol.278, No.45, (Nov 7), pp. 44826-44831, 0021-9258 (Print), 0021-9258 (Linking)

Stachelek, S. J., Finley, M. J., Alferiev, I. S., Wang, F., Tsai, R. K., Eckells, E. C., Tomczyk, N., Connolly, J. M., Discher, D. E., Eckmann, D. M. & Levy, R. J. (2011). The effect of CD47 modified polymer surfaces on inflammatory cell attachment and activation. *Biomaterials*, Vol.32, No.19, (Jul), pp. 4317-4326, 1878-5905 (Electronic), 0142-9612 (Linking)

Stayton, P. S., El-Sayed, M. E., Murthy, N., Bulmus, V., Lackey, C., Cheung, C. & Hoffman, A. S. (2005). 'Smart' delivery systems for biomolecular therapeutics. *Orthod Craniofac Res*, Vol.8, No.3, (Aug), pp. 219-225,

Steger, L. D. & Desnick, R. J. (1977). Enzyme therapy. VI: Comparative in vivo fates and effects on lysosomal integrity of enzyme entrapped in negatively and positively charged liposomes. *Biochim Biophys Acta*, Vol.464, No.3, (Feb 4), pp. 530-546, 0006-3002 (Print)

Suk, J. S., Suh, J., Choy, K., Lai, S. K., Fu, J. & Hanes, J. (2006). Gene delivery to differentiated neurotypic cells with RGD and HIV Tat peptide functionalized polymeric nanoparticles. *Biomaterials*, (Oct), pp. 5143-5150.

Tao, W., Wen, R., Goddard, M. B., Sherman, S. D., O'Rourke, P. J., Stabila, P. F., Bell, W. J., Dean, B. J., Kauper, K. A., Budz, V. A., Tsiaras, W. G., Acland, G. M., Pearce-Kelling, S., Laties, A. M. & Aguirre, G. D. (2002). Encapsulated cell-based delivery of CNTF reduces photoreceptor degeneration in animal models of retinitis pigmentosa. *Invest Ophthalmol Vis Sci*, Vol.43, No.10, (Oct), pp. 3292-3298, 0146-0404 (Print), 0146-0404 (Linking)

Tokarev, I. & Minko, S. (2010). Stimuli-responsive porous hydrogels at interfaces for molecular filtration, separation, controlled release, and gating in capsules and membranes. *Adv Mater*, Vol.22, No.31, (Aug 17), pp. 3446-3462, 1521-4095 (Electronic), 0935-9648 (Linking)

Torchilin, V. P. (2006). Multifunctional nanocarriers. *Adv Drug Deliv Rev*, Vol.58, No.14, (Dec 1), pp. 1532-1555, 0169-409X (Print)

Trollet, C., Scherman, D. & Bigey, P. (2008). Delivery of DNA into muscle for treating systemic diseases: advantages and challenges. *Methods Mol Biol*, Vol.423, pp. 199-214, 1064-3745 (Print), 1064-3745 (Linking)

Turner, P., Petch, A. & Al-Rubeai, M. (2007). Encapsulation of viral vectors for gene therapy applications. *Biotechnol Prog*, Vol.23, No.2, (Mar-Apr), pp. 423-429, 8756-7938 (Print), 1520-6033 (Linking)

Vij, N., Min, T., Marasigan, R., Belcher, C. N., Mazur, S., Ding, H., Yong, K. T. & Roy, I. (2010). Development of PEGylated PLGA nanoparticle for controlled and sustained drug delivery in cystic fibrosis. *J Nanobiotechnology*, Vol.8, pp. 22, 1477-3155 (Electronic), 1477-3155 (Linking)

Weissmann, G., Bloomgarden, D., Kaplan, R., Cohen, C., Hoffstein, S., Collins, T., Gotlieb, A. & Nagle, D. (1975). A general method for the introduction of enzymes, by means of immunoglobulin-coated liposomes, into lysosomes of deficient cells. *Proc Natl Acad Sci U S A*, Vol.72, No.1, (Jan), pp. 88-92, 0027-8424 (Print)

Wilson, J. M. (2004). Adeno-associated virus and lentivirus pseudotypes for lung-directed gene therapy. *Proc Am Thorac Soc*, Vol.1, No.4, pp. 309-314, 1546-3222 (Print), 1546-3222 (Linking)

Wong, T. W. (2010). Design of oral insulin delivery systems. *J Drug Target*, Vol.18, No.2, (Feb), pp. 79-92, 1029-2330 (Electronic), 1026-7158 (Linking)

Yatuv, R., Robinson, M., Dayan-Tarshish, I. & Baru, M. (2010). The use of PEGylated liposomes in the development of drug delivery applications for the treatment of hemophilia. *Int J Nanomedicine*, Vol.5, pp. 581-591, 1178-2013 (Electronic), 1176-9114 (Linking)

Yessine, M. A. & Leroux, J. C. (2004). Membrane-destabilizing polyanions: interaction with lipid bilayers and endosomal escape of biomacromolecules. *Adv Drug Deliv Rev*, Vol.56, No.7, (Apr 23), pp. 999-1021,

Yoo, J. W., Chambers, E. & Mitragotri, S. (2010). Factors that control the circulation time of nanoparticles in blood: challenges, solutions and future prospects. *Curr Pharm Des*, Vol.16, No.21, (Jul), pp. 2298-2307, 1873-4286 (Electronic), 1381-6128 (Linking)

Zhang, P., Rogelj, S., Nguyen, K. & Wheeler, D. (2006). Design of a highly sensitive and specific nucleotide sensor based on photon upconverting particles. *J Am Chem Soc*, Vol.128, No.38, (Sep 27), pp. 12410-12411, 0002-7863 (Print), 0002-7863 (Linking)

Zhou, T., Neubert, H., Liu, D. Y., Liu, Z. D., Ma, Y. M., Kong, X. L., Luo, W., Mark, S. & Hider, R. C. (2006). Iron binding dendrimers: a novel approach for the treatment of haemochromatosis. *J Med Chem*, Vol.49, No.14, (Jul 13), pp. 4171-4182, 0022-2623 (Print), 0022-2623 (Linking)

Zuhorn, I. S., Bakowsky, U., Polushkin, E., Visser, W. H., Stuart, M. C., Engberts, J. B. & Hoekstra, D. (2005). Nonbilayer phase of lipoplex-membrane mixture determines endosomal escape of genetic cargo and transfection efficiency. *Mol Ther*, Vol.11, No.5, (May), pp. 801-810,

Zurn, A. D., Widmer, H. R. & Aebischer, P. (2001). Sustained delivery of GDNF: towards a treatment for Parkinson's disease. *Brain Res Brain Res Rev*, Vol.36, No.2-3, (Oct), pp. 222-229

15

Consanguinity and Its Effect on Morbidity and Congenital Disorders Among Arabs in Israel

Sharkia Rajech[1,2], Athamny Esmael[1], Khatib Mohamad[3], Sheikh-Muhammad Ahmad[3], Azem Abdussalam[4] and Mahajnah Muhammad[5]

[1]*The Triangle Regional Research and Development Center*

[2]*Beit-Berl Academic College*

[3]*The Galilee Society - The Arabs National Society for Research and Health Services*

[4]*Department of Biochemistry, Faculty of Life Sciences, Tel-Aviv University*

[5]*Child Development and Pediatric Center, Hillel Yaffe Medical Center, Affiliated with the Rappaport Faculty of Medicine, Technion, Haifa*

Israel

1. Introduction

Genetic diseases, especially autosomal recessive diseases, are rare in the general population. However, they become unusually frequent in certain communities worldwide as a result of genetic isolation due to social, geographic or religious factors. When a new mutation is inserted in such a population it spreads rapidly, leading to an increased prevalence of carriers and a large number of affected homozygous individuals. There are high frequencies of genetic diseases and congenital disorders among Arab populations (Tadmouri et al., 2009; Teebi & S.A. Teebi 2005). The high rates of genetic diseases and congenital disorders in the Arab populations can be attributed to several factors including: a) The high rate of traditional consanguineous marriages, which increases the frequency of autosomal recessive diseases; b) a relatively high birth rate of infants with chromosomal disorders related to advanced maternal age such as Down Syndrome and other trisomies; c) a relatively high birth rate of infants with malformations due to new dominant mutations related to advanced paternal age; d) large family sizes, which may increase the number of affected children in families with autosomal recessive conditions; and e) the lack of public health measures directed at the prevention of congenital and genetically determined disorders, and the shortage of genetic services and inadequate health care prior to and during pregnancy (Al-Gazali et al., 2006; Teebi, 2010, as cited in Teebi, 1010). Thus, in Arab populations, several recessive diseases like Cystic Fibrosis, Phenylketonuria, Beta Thalassemia and Wilson disease are very frequent. However, due to the tribal society style life among Arab and consecutive genetic founder effects, the distribution of autosomal recessive disorders among the Arab populations is not uniformly distributed, but shows large geographic differences (Teebi & S.A. Teebi 2005; Zolotogora 2002).

Consanguinity has been recognized as the main social factor related to a high prevalence of genetic and congenital disorders in Arab communities' worldwide (Bener et al., 2007; Bittles

& Hamamy 2010, as cited in Teebi, 2010; Jaber et al., 1992; Sharkia et al., 2010; Zlotogora, 1997). Consanguineous marriage refers to a union contracted between biologically related individuals. In clinical genetics, this includes relationships of second cousins or closer (Bittles & Hamamy 2010, as cited in Teebi, 2010). The phenomenon of consanguineous marriages has been common in different societies worldwide, especially in the Arab rural populations due to socio-cultural factors like maintenance of family structure, and properties or ease of marital arrangements (Alper et al., 2004; Qidwai et al., 2003; Varela et al., 2003). The prevalence of consanguineous marriages in the Arab world is considered to be much higher (35% - 55%) as compared to Western countries (~1%) (Bittles, 2001; Jaber et al. 1998). Recently, different studies of various Arab societies have shown that the consanguinity rates decrease with time (Hamamy et al., 2005; Khlat, 1988; Sharkia et al., 2008). Consanguinity rates in various societies were found to be dependent on multiple factors e.g. religion, educational level, local traditions socio-economic status and demography (Fuster & Colantonio, 2004; Jaber et al., 1996,). The Arab population of Israel reaches about 1.5 million people consisting of about 84 % Muslims, 8 % Christians and 8% Druze (Central Bureau of Statistics, 2010). The Arab community in Israel is characterized by some unique features: most of the population lives in villages or towns which were founded by small numbers of originators and the majority of families have a large number of children. It was also believed that the favorite marriage is the consanguineous one (Jaber et al., 2000). It was found that the frequency of consanguineous marriages in the Arab society in Israel is about 44% (half of which are first cousin marriages) and its incidence is highest in rural areas (Jaber et al., 1994). Consanguinity was recently found to have decreased (Sharkia et al., 2008), in selected Arab communities in Israel but its rate is still high as compared to western communities.

The relationship between consanguineous marriages, inherited genetic diseases and congenital malformation has been studied for many decades. During the 1950s in Japan, a high frequency of infant mortality was associated with consanguinity (Schull, 1958). A study that focused on the consanguinity effects on common adult diseases among the Qatari population revealed a strong correlation between high rates of common adult diseases and consanguineous marriages (Bener et al., 2007). In another study which explored the genetic aspect of beta-Thalassemia among 130 inflicted families from the West Bank and Gaza, 77.3% of the tested couples were found to carry the same mutation. Actually, 77.9% of these couples were from consanguineous marriages (Ayesh et al., 2005). Furthermore, the high rate of infant mortality among the Palestinian population was related to consanguineous marriages (Pedersen, 2002). It was found that consanguineous marriages were a major cause of congenital malformation among the Arab communities in Israel (Jaber et al., 1992). Various forms of congenital malformation of the central nervous system, speech and infertility were found at a higher frequency in those individuals whose parents are family-related, than those with unrelated parents (Bromiker et al., 2004; Zlotogora, 1997). A high proportion of infant mortality due to congenital malformation in the Arab community in Israel is mainly caused by the high frequency of consanguineous marriages (Zlotogora et al., 2003). A report published by Abu-Rabia & Maroun (2005) showed that consanguinity negatively affects children's reading abilities. Recently, it was found that the prevalence of neurological hereditary diseases and mental retardation was associated with consanguinity in selected samples of Arab communities in Israel (Sharkia et al., 2010). From the geneticist's point of view, consanguineous marriage alleviates genetic diagnostics. One main scientifically useful feature of consanguinity is that it facilitates homozygosity mapping of disease related genes. The present study was undertaken to determine the prevalence of various genetic and congenital disorders and their association with parental consanguinity in a selected sample of the Israeli Arab community. Investigation of hereditary disorders is vital for improving health care. This can be achieved by identifying and diagnosing their molecular genetic basis, with a view to developing preventative intervention measures aimed at reducing the occurrence of these inherited genetic disorders.

2. Subjects and methods

2.1 Study population and sample

This research is based on data from the socio-economic survey (SES) conducted by the Galilee Society (GS) and Al Ahali Center in the year 2007. This survey included a sample of 3,173 households. This sample was a stratified multi-stage random sample which was designed in three stages: selection of enumeration areas in one stratification level, selection of thirty responsive households in the chosen enumeration area and selection of two persons, male and female, from persons aged 10 years and above from each household that was chosen in the second stage. The total rate of completed questionnaires in this survey was 81.9% of the households in the field.

This sample was divided into four levels of stratification: Region (North, Center, Haifa and South), Community Classification (urban communities "A" with a population over 15,000 and urban communities "B" with a population between 5,000 and 15,000, rural communities with a population less than 5,000), Locality Type (unrecognized and recognized by the Israeli authorities), and Locality Characteristics (mixed: Arabs and others, unmixed: Arabs only).

The following criteria were used in calculating the sample size: Use of the unemployment indicator (rate of unemployment) as a principal indicator in defining the margin of error which was estimated according to previous data at around 12%, Period of confidence is 95%, The ultimate margin of error for the principal indicator (rate of unemployment) is 3% on the stratification level.

Therefore the size of the stratification level is:

$$n_h = \frac{t^2 S^2 D}{e^2} \qquad h = 1,\ldots 18$$

n_h the number of persons in one stratification level

$S^2 = p(1-p)$

p is the rate of prevalence of the principal feature studied in the survey (unemployment)

t is the confidence factor that expresses the period of confidence

e is the ultimate margin of error in estimating the indicator

D is the effect of sample design of multi-stage stratified samples and is estimated at 1.2.

The result is that the number of persons in one stratification level equals to 564 persons:

$$n_h = \frac{(4)(0.12)(0.88)(1.2)}{(0.03)^2} = 564$$

Since we are covering 18 true levels, the number of persons (N) in the sample in all levels is 10,152 persons

$$N= 564*18 =10152$$

It is important to note that the required number of persons applies to persons in the labor force because the principal feature that was studied (unemployment) is only related to persons in the labor force. Since the sample selection was households, and not persons, therefore we had to choose a number of households which included approximately 10,152 persons in the labor force. According to previous data, the number of persons in the labor force is on average 3.2 persons per household, thus the sample size becomes 3,173 households. Since 30 responsive households were selected from each enumeration area, the required number of enumeration areas was 107.1 and was adjusted to 109 areas, i.e. 3,173 households in order to correlate the enumeration areas with the different levels of stratification.

The target population consisted of all Israeli Arab households that reside inside the green line, and focused on individuals aged 15 years and above during 2007. The study group comprised the full pediatric population (0-18 year old), that was affected with one or more types of disorders caused by congenital, illness or during birth cause. The sample excluded children with disorders caused by accidents or environmental factors. The total number of the study group was 565 affected children.

2.2 Survey questionnaire and data collection

For the current study we used two parts from the general questionnaire that contained:

a. Identification information for the household and the relationship of the household to its head, gender, age, religion and place.
b. Personal status information: included marital status, whether husband and wife are related, and the degree of consanguinity, and the number of births for married women.
c. Health status information: included incidence of chronic diseases, disabilities, kinds of disabilities, and causes of disabilities, availability of supplementary health insurance, and places of treatment.

The response compliance rate was 81.0% of the total households who were visited in the enumeration areas where refusals were recorded.

Questionnaires were completed through face to face interviews. The fieldwork team was recruited from a group of field experienced surveyors. A training course was conducted for these surveyors by the supervisors and the project administrators. The total rate of completed questionnaires in this survey was 82% of the households in the field, which was a total of 107 areas out of 109.

2.3 Consanguinity

Information on consanguinity between the parents was obtained through the interviews. Relationships were grouped into two major categories: consanguineous and non-consanguineous marriages, defined as follows:

Consanguineous marriage: This group included two main levels of relationships:

a. First cousins and closer. These include double-first cousins (in which all grandparents are shared) and first cousins in which the couple are parallel or cross cousins of either paternal or maternal descent;
b. Distant relative marriages, in which the members of the couple were relatives but not with first-degree relations, for example they were first cousin once removed, second cousin, second cousin once removed.

Non-consanguineous marriage: The couple is not related.

2.4 Data analysis

The SPSS program was used for data management and descriptive statistical analysis. The statistical significance of associations between consanguinity and various types of disorders was examined by means of the χ^2 test.

3. Results

Of 3,173 total marriages (households), 1267 (39.9%) were consanguineous and 1906 (60.01%) were non-consanguineous. The various subtypes of consanguinity was observed; 19.7% (N=623) were first-cousin marriage type and a similar incidence was found for distant relative marriage type (N=644, 20.3%). Of the 6,017 total children (siblings) from all the family samples, 565 children were found to have one or more kinds of various types of disorders, comprising an overall prevalence of 93.9 per 1000 children sampled.

The total numbers of affected children of varying degrees separated into those from consanguineous and from non-consanguineous marriages are presented in Table 1. More than half of affected children (56%) were found to be products of parental consanguinity; 68.4% of this prevalence was offspring of first cousins or closer, and 31.6% were offspring of distant relatives. About 44% of the affected children were born to unrelated couples. There was a significant difference in the prevalence between the offspring of consanguineous versus non-consanguineous mating for various types of examined disorders. All reported disorders were more frequent in consanguineous marriages, except for the respiratory disorders which were more frequent in non-consanguineous marriages, indicating that there is a significant association between consanguinity and types of disorders, and that genetic factors are probably the underlying cause.

Type of disorders	Number of affected children	Consanguineous n (%)			Non-consanguineous n (%)	χ^2	p
		Total	FC	DR			
Respiratory	130	56 (21.5)	32 (57.1)	24 (42.9)	74 (78.5)	16.6	0.003
Mental	53	28 (52.8)	19 (67.8)	9 (32.2)	25 (47.2)	14.03	0.002
Physical	160	90 (56.3)	68 (75.5)	22 (24.5)	70 (43.7)	13.25	0.001
Visual	100	66 (66)	47 (71.2)	19 (28.8)	34 (34)	15.2	0.0013
Hearing	77	51 (66.2)	36 (70.5)	15 (29.5)	26 (33.8)	6.06	0.0020
Other Hereditary Disorders	45	25 (55.5)	14 (56)	11 (44)	20 (45.5)	18.41	0.000
Total	**N=565**	**316 (56%)**	**216 (68.4)**	**100 (31.6)**	**249 (44%)**	17.98	0.000

Table 1. Distribution of disorder types among Offspring from Consanguineous and Non-consanguineous Marriages

Table 2 records the numbers and prevalence of disorder types among all the siblings aged 0 to 18 in the presented families. The data shows that approximately 31% (565 cases) of the siblings from all 356 families had one or more kinds of diseases with a prevalence range of 22% to 40%. This indicates that there is an associated familial background. Selected characteristics of affected children with disorders types are presented in Table 3. The prevalence of disorders' types was higher in boys (60%) than in girls (40%), this difference was significant. The detailed age distribution recorded in the table shows that the most (70%) of affected children were in the 10 to 18-year age group.

Types of disorders	Number of families	All siblings aged between 0 and18 years in the families	Number and percentage of affected children (%)
Respiratory	70	420	130 (30)
Mental	33	132	53 (40)
Physical	89	445	160 (35.9)
Visual	92	460	100 (21.7)
Hearing	41	205	77 (37.5)
Other Hereditary disorders	31	155	45 (29)
Total	356	1817	565 (31.9)

Table 2. Number and percentage of affected children from of all children siblings in the families

Age (years)	Affected children with disorders' types						
	Respiratory	Mental	Physical	Visual	Hearing	Other Hereditary disorders	Total Affected children N (%)
< 5	30 (32.6)	9 (9.7)	20 (21.7)	9 (9.7)	19 (20.6)	5 (5.4)	92 (16.2)
5-10	15 (19.7)	7 (9.2)	19 (25)	17 (22.3)	15 (19.7)	3 (3.9)	76 (13.4)
10 -15	19 (17.7)	15 (14.1)	26 (24.2)	28 (26.1)	12 (11.2)	7 (6.5)	107 (19)
>15	66 (22.7)	22 (7.5)	95 (32.7)	46 (5.8)	31 (10.6)	30 (10.3)	290 (51.4)
Gender							P<0.05 sig=0.01
Male	80 (23.5)	33 (9.7)	107 (31.5)	56 (16.5)	38 (11.2)	25 (7.3)	339 (60)
Female	50 (22.1)	20 (8.8)	53 (23.4)	44 (19.4)	39 (17.2)	20 (11.1)	226 (40)
Total	130 (23)	53 (9.3)	160 (28.3)	100 (17.6)	77 (13.6)	45 (7.9)	565 (100)
							P<0.05 sig=0.00

Table 3. Age and Gender of affected Children with disorders' types

Table 4 compares the prevalence of disorders' types among the offspring from three category causes of disorders: illness, congenital and during birth. Most (97%) of the disorders causes among affected children were illness and congenital. The illness cause was recorded in 300 cases (53.2%) and in 251 cases (44.4%) there was a congenital cause. Only 14 cases (2.4%) were caused by "during birth".

Cause of Disorder	Children with types of disorders						
	Respiratory diseases	Mental disorders	Physical disorders	Visual disorders	Hearing disorders	Other Hereditary disorders	Total N (%)
Illness	81 (62.3)	13 (24.5)	101 (63.1)	52 (52)	28 (36.3)	25 (55.5)	300 (53.2)
Congenital	48 (36.9)	37 (69.8)	57 (35.6)	45 (45)	46 (59.7)	18 (40)	251 (44.4)
During birth	1 (0.8)	3 (5.6)	2 (1.2)	3 (3)	3 (3.8)	2 (4.4)	14 (2.4)
Total	130	53	160	100	77	45	565

Table 4. Frequency of disorders' types by cause of disorders

4. Discussion

The highest prevalence of congenital malformations and genetic diseases was reported in the Eastern Mediterranean region, with >65 affected children per 1,000 live births as opposed to 52/1,000 live births in Europe, North America and Australia (Alwan & Modell, 2003). In the selected sample for the present study we found that various types of disorders affected, on average, 93.9 per 1000 children. This finding indicates that morbidity in the studied population is considerably more prevalent than in Eastern Mediterranean regions as well as in western societies.

The phenomenon of consanguineous marriages has been common in the Arab world for many decades and its prevalence is considered to be much higher (35% - 55%) as compared to that (~1%) of Western countries (Bittles, 2001; Jaber et al., 1998; Tadmouri et al., 2009). Nevertheless, despite the previously reported decrease in the rate of consanguineous marriages within selected regions of Israeli Arab communities (Sharkia et al., 2008), the consanguinity rate is still high in this community as the current study indicates. Our study, which is based on data obtained from all regions of the Israeli Arab community, showed that the incidence of consanguinity is relatively high with a rate of about 40%. Approximately 50% of all these consanguineous marriages are of the first-cousin and closer marriage type. These findings can be explained by the preference of consanguineous marriages in Arab populations that are related to socio-cultural factors. It has been reported that consanguineous marriages have a negative effect on reproductive health factors in general. Consanguinity is still the most common risk factor for a high frequency of autosomal recessive diseases and congenital malformations within Arab communities in Israel (Sharkia et al., 2010; Zoltogora et al., 2003). In addition, several studies among Arab societies show that there is a higher occurrence of consanguineous marriages among parents of offspring with congenital malformations than in the general population (Bener et al.,

2007; Tadmoure et al., 2009; Teebi, 2010, as cited in Teebi, 2010). A strong association between most of the examined disorders and consanguinity was demonstrated in the present study; approximately 56% of the children with one or more disorders were the offspring of consanguineous marriages, and in approximately 68% of these marriages the parents were first cousins or closer. This association between consanguinity and disorder rate as well as the familial effect of most disorders' types that were obtained by the current results indicate that genetic factors are involved with the underlying cause. In addition, we found that the frequency of the disorders' types were higher among males (60%) than females (40%) in our studied sample, possibly `reflecting the elevated levels of X-chromosome homozygosity inheritance. The relationship between consanguinity and genetic disorders is attributed to the fact that a high prevalence of consanguinity increases homozygosity and reduces the genetic variation which may protect against the expression of recessive genes that can lead to genetic disorders in a group. When a new mutation is inserted in such a population, it will rapidly spread, leading to an increased prevalence of carriers, and a high number of affected homozygous individuals. An analysis of data in the Catalogue for Transmission Genetics in Arabs (CTGA) carried out by Tadmouri et al., (2009), indicates that the overwhelming proportion of the disorders follow a recessive mode of inheritance of about 63% as compared to the smaller proportion of dominantly inherited traits (27%). A detailed analysis study of the molecular basis of autosomal recessive diseases among Palestinian Arabs in Israel found that most of the responsible mutations among the affected patients were homozygosity (Zlotogora, 2002). We believe that the genetic conditions of the disorders in the present studied sample probably relates to homozygosity autosomal recessive diseases.

The largest age distribution (70%) of affected children was in the 10 to 18-year range, in contrast to the 16% of affected children who were in the less than 5 year age group. Furthermore, most (97.6 %) of the disorders causes among the affected children were by illness and congenital, while only (2.4%) were caused by "during birth". These results demonstrated that implementing various health interventions and genetic counseling services in order to improve public health issues in the Israeli Arab community will have a positive effect, even if only partial. Therefore, such programs are needed, particularly, for identifying and diagnosing the molecular genetic basis of the most common disorders so that a preventive program can be launched, with the aim of minimizing the occurrence of different spectrum disorders in future generations.

5. Acknowledgements

This project was supported by the European Union, EU Partner for Peace. Dr. Sharkia was supported in partly by Beit-Berl College. We thank Eid Rohany for performing the statistical analysis and many thanks to the scientific director Dr. Ibrahim Yehya for his cooperation and extending various facilities of the Research and Development Center. We are grateful to the families who participated in this study.

6. References

Abu-Rabia, S. & Maroun, L. (2005). The effect of consanguineous marriage on reading disability in the Arab community. *Dyslexia*, Vol. 11, pp. 1-21

Al-Gazali, L.; Hamamy, H. & Al-Arrayad, Sh. (2009). Genetic disorders in Arab world. *British Medical Journa*, Vol. 333, pp. 831-843

Alwan, A. & Modell, B. (2003). Recommendations for introducing genetics services in developing countries. *Nat Rev Genet*, Vol.4, pp.61–68

Alper, OM.; Erengin, H.; Manguoglu, AE.; Bilgen, T.; Cetin, Z.; Dedeoglu, N. & Luleci, G. (2004). Consanguineous marriages in the province of Antalya, *Turkey*. *Ann Genet*, Vol. 47,pp 129-138

Ayesh, SK.; Al-Sharef, WA.; Nassar, SM.; Thawabteh, NA. & Abu-Libdeh, BY. (2005a). Prenatal diagnosis of beta-thalassemia in the West Bank and Gaza. *Saudi Med J*,Vol. 26,pp. 1771-1776

Ayesh, SK.; Al-Sharef, WA.; Nassar, SM.; Thawabteh, NA. & Abu-Libdeh, BY. (2005b). Genetic screening of familial Mediterranean fever mutations in the Palestinian population. *Saudi Med J*, Vol. 26, pp. 732-737

Bener, A.; Hussain, R. & Teebi, A.S.(2007). Consanguineous marriages and their effects on common adult diseases: studies from an endogamous population, *Med. Princ. Pract.* Vol. 16,pp. 262-267

Bittles ,AH. (2001). Consanguinity and its relevance to clinical genetics. *Clin Genet*.Vol.60, pp.89-98

Bittles, AH. & Hamamy, H. (2010). Endogamy and Consanguineous Marriage in Arab Populations, In: *Genetic disorders among Arab populations*, A. Teebi, (Ed.), 85-108, Springer , 978-3-642-05079-4 , Springer-Verlag Berlin Heidelberg

Bromiker, R.; Glam-Baruch, M.; Gofin, R.; Hammerman, C.& Amitai, Y. (2004). Association of parental consanguinity with congenital malformations among Arab newborns in Jerusalem. *Clin Genet*, Vol.66,pp.63-66

Central Bureau of Statistics.(2009). Israel, available in: www.cbs.gov.il. At: http://www.cbs.gov.il/shnaton61/st02_01.pdf

Fuster, V. & Colantonio, SE.(2004). Socioeconomic, demographic, and geographic variables affecting the diverse degrees of consanguineous marriages in Spain. *Hum Biol*, Vol. 76, pp.1-14

Hamamy, H.; Al-Darawsheh, J. & Ajlouni K. (2005). Consanguineous marriages in Jordan: why is the rate changing with time? *Clin Genet*,VOL. 67,pp.511-516

Jaber, L.;Bailey-Wilson, JE.; Haj-Yehia, M. Hernandez, J. & Shohat, M. (1994). Consanguineous matings in an Israeli-Arab community. *Arch Pediatr Adolesc Med*, Vol.148,pp.412-415

Jaber, L.; Halpern, GJ.& Shohat, M. (1998) . The impact of consanguinity worldwide. *Community Genet*,Vol. 1, pp.12-17

Jaber, L.; Halpern, GJ.; Shohat, T.(2000). Trends in the frequencies of consanguineous marriages in the Israeli Arab community. *Clin Genet*, Vol. 58, pp.106-110

Jaber, L.; Merlob, P.; Bu, X.; Rotter, JI. & Shobhat, M. (1992). Marked parental consanguinity as a cause for increased major malformations in an Arab community. *Am J Med Genet*,Vol. 44, pp.1-6

Jaber L, Shohat M, Halpern GJ. (1996). Demographic characteristics of the Israeli Arab community in connection with consanguinity. *Isr J Med Sci*, Vol. 32, pp.1286-1289

Khlat ,M. (1988) . Social correlates of consanguineous marriages in Beirut: a population-based study,*Hum Biol*,Vol.60, pp.541-548

Pedersen, J.(2002). The influence of consanguineous marriage on infant and child mortality among Palestinians in the West Bank and Gaza, Jordan, Lebanon and Syria, *Community Genet*, Vol. 5, pp. 178-181

Qidwai, W.; Sued, IA.& Khan, FM. (2003). Prevalence and perceptions about consanguineous marriages among patients presenting to family physicians, in 2001 at a teaching hospital in Karachi, Pakistan, *Asia Pacific Family Medicine*, Vol. 2,pp.27-31.

Sharkia, R.; Zaid, M.; Athamna, A.; Cohen, D.; Azem, A.& Zalan, A. (2008). The changing pattern of consanguinity in a selected region of the Israeli Arab community,*Am. J. Hum. Biol.*,Vol. 20,pp. 72-77

Sharkia, R.; Azem, A.; Kaiyal Q.; Zelink, N. & Mahajnah, M. (2010). Mental Retardation and Consanguinity in a selected Region of the Israeli Arab Community. *Cent. Eur. J. Med*,.Vol. 5(1), pp.91-96

Schull, WJ. (1958). Empirical risks in consanguineous marriage: sex ratio, malformation and viability, *Am J Hum Genet*,Vol. 10, pp.294-343

Tadmouri, G.; Nair, P.; Obeid, T.; Al Alim, M .; Alkhaja, N. & Hmamy, H.(2009). Consanguinity and reproductive health among Arabs, *Reproductive Health*. PP.1-9

Teebi, A. (2010). Genetic diversity among the Arabs, In: *Genetic disorders among Arab populations*, A. Teebi, (Ed.), 3-34, Springer , 978-3-642-05079-4 , Springer-Verlag Berlin Heidelberg

Teebi, A.S. & Teebi, S.A. (2005). Genetic diversity among the Arabs, *Community Genet*,Vol. 8, pp.21-26

Varela, TA. Ainsua, RL.& Farina, J.(2003). Consanguinity in the Bishopric of Ourense (Galicia, Spain) from 1900 to 1997. *Annals of Human Biology* Vol. 30, pp.419-433

Zlotogora, J. ; Habiballah, H.; Odatallah, A.& Barges, S. (2002). Changing family structure in a modernizing society: a study of marriage patterns in a single Muslim village in Israel, *American Journal of Human Biology*, Vol. 14, pp.680-682

Zlotogora, J.; Haklai, Z.; Rotem, N.; Georgi, M.; Berlovitz, I. ; Leventhal, A.& Amitai, Y. (2003). Relative prevalence of malformations at birth among different religious communities in Israel, *Am J Med Genet*, Vol. 15, pp.59-62

Zlotogora, J. (1997). Genetic disorders among Palestinian Arabs: effects of consanguinity. *Am J Med Genet*, Vol. 68, pp.472-475.

Zlotogora, J.(., 2002). Molecular basis of autosomal recessive diseases among the Palestinian Arabs, *Am. J. Med. Genet*,Vol. 109,pp. 176-182

16

Genethical Aspects of Research and Medical Services in Islamic Countries

Mohsen A.F. El-Hazmi
King Saud University, Riyadh
Kingdom of Saudi Arabia

1. Introduction

Islam has approximately 1.5 billion followers worldwide, the majority of whom live in Arabic/Islamic states with an appreciable number live in non-Islamic states.[1,2] In both environments the Muslims maintain a "Code of life", where they adhere to the instructions of Islam and respect its guidance in all aspects of their daily life. In this respect, Islam responds to person's need through the "Code of Conduct" drawn from Al-Sharea'h, the Islamic law.[3,4,5,6,7,8] . The Teaching of Islamic Law include all that is required to appropriately serve the needs of the individual, the family and the community at large [3]

To respond to various issues learned from Human Genome and associated studies, varieties of scientific activities, including conferences, symposia and workshops were held during the last 15 years in a number of Islamic countries to discuss the new issues arising from the scientific and technical developments and their applications in genetical practices. These include an international conference on Islamic medicine held, to discuss ethics of medicine in the light of Islamic views and a seminar on "Genetics, Genetic Engineering, the Human Genes, and Genetic Treatment - An Islamic Perspective".[9] Thereafter, World Health Organization (W.H.O) organized two relevant meetings. A meeting to discuss "Ethical aspects of scientific application in Genetics", followed by another meeting to discuss the "Ethical issues in application to genetics in developing countries", which include a large number of Islamic countries.[10,11] A complementary workshop entitled: "The 1st Regional workshop on Ethical issues in Genetic counseling" was held, thereafter.[12] The last three events benefited from the previously held conferences and from related "Fiqh" Council Fatwas, the guidelines of the Learned. Of significance also, is the United Nations Educational, Scientific and Cultural Organization (UNESCO) general guidelines on Bioethics and Human rights.[13]

2. Genetic investigations and community ethical beliefs

As Science has global identity, research was advanced by collaborative efforts between scientists from various countries. However, the genetic research outcome encroaches into the individuals and the family beliefs in all communities. Nevertheless, the basic ethical aspects remain universal, though with specific unique features that are relevant to the concerned community, its societal beliefs, customs and prevailing traditions.

In general, Medical Ethics combines a set of societal values and beliefs that are relevant to diagnosing illnesses, preventing and controlling diseases and provision of care for patients.

The health care teams are required to conduct research and acquire further knowledge and technology to help improving medical care. The balance between the medical services and research aimed to enrich knowledge, is necessary, but has to meet a battery of ethical elements, including:[6,14 -18]

- Autonomy
- Beneficence
- Non-maleficence
- Justice
- Confidentiality
- Medical professionalism

In Islam, the Holy Book of Moslems (The Qur'an) and the Prophet's instructions (The Hadeeth), Peace Be Upon Him (PBUH), the Consensus (Al Ijmaa') of the Learned (Al-Ulama) and Analogy (Al Qiyas) on the newly found matters of life, are the sources of religious practices and govern all aspects of life through Al-Sharea'h.[19-24] Consideration is also given to "Maslaha" (public interest) and urf (the local customary precedent).[21] These Islamic teachings are in line with the ethical elements observed in medical practices (Figure 1).

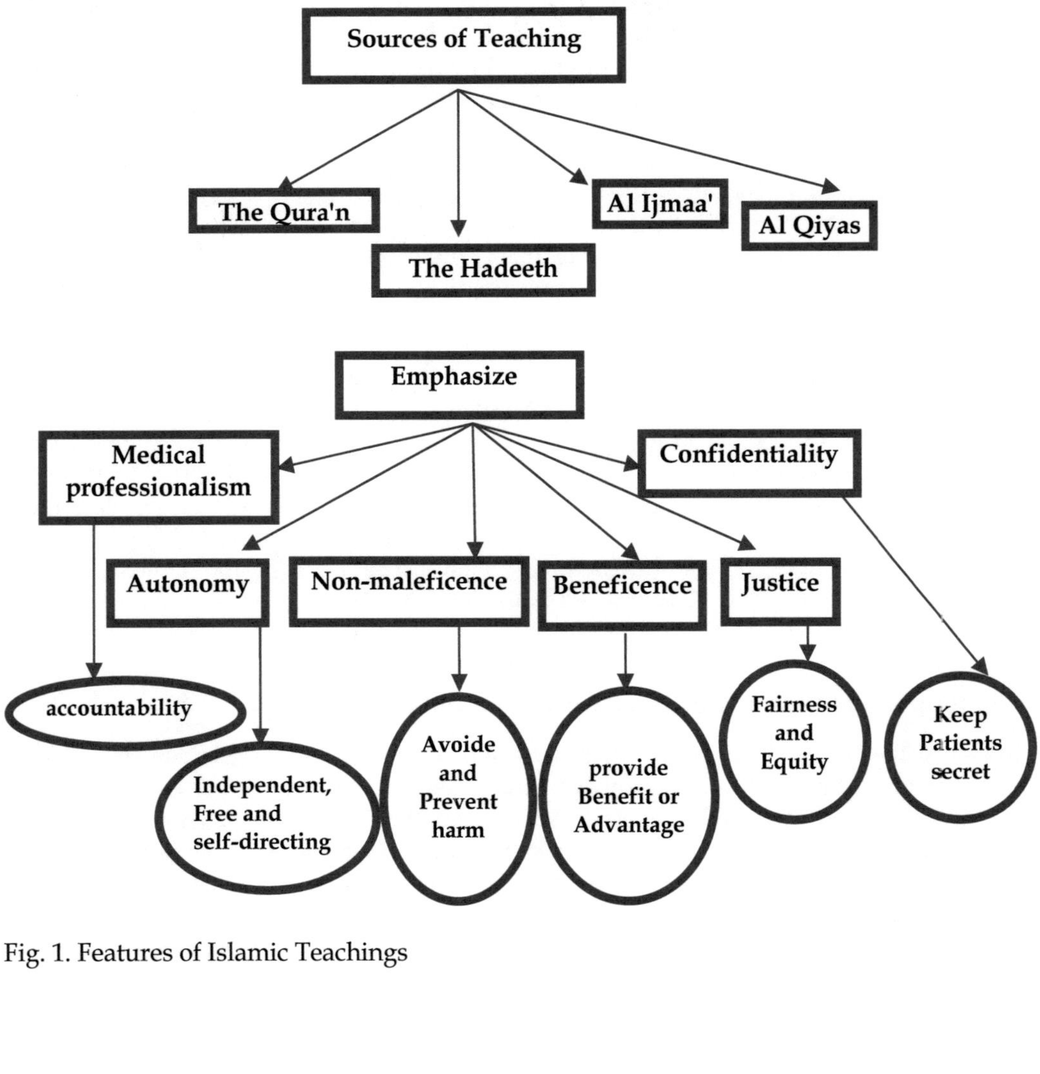

Fig. 1. Features of Islamic Teachings

The Arabian Peninsula is the cradle of Arabs and Islam, with the two Holy Mosques of Moslems in the cities of "Makkah Al Mokarramah" and "Al-Madinah Al-Monawarrah" in Saudi Arabia. Makkah Al-Mokarramah houses "The Islamic Jurisprudence (Figh) Council of Islamic World League of the Organization of Islamic Countries", with members representing Islamic States. In this article, this source of guidance, in addition to relevant verses of Qura' n and the Hadeeths are followed.

Cultural awareness and contextual knowledge are necessary prerequisites for health care in culturally sensitive communities with strong societal values and beliefs, as is the case in Islamic communities. An appreciation of the societal values and beliefs must be reflected in all aspects of life as well as in individual and family interactions. In Islamic countries, as well as among Islamic communities in non-Islamic countries, Islam continues to influence the societal conduct of life and customs of an estimated one fifth of the inhabitants of the globe [19] (Figure 2)

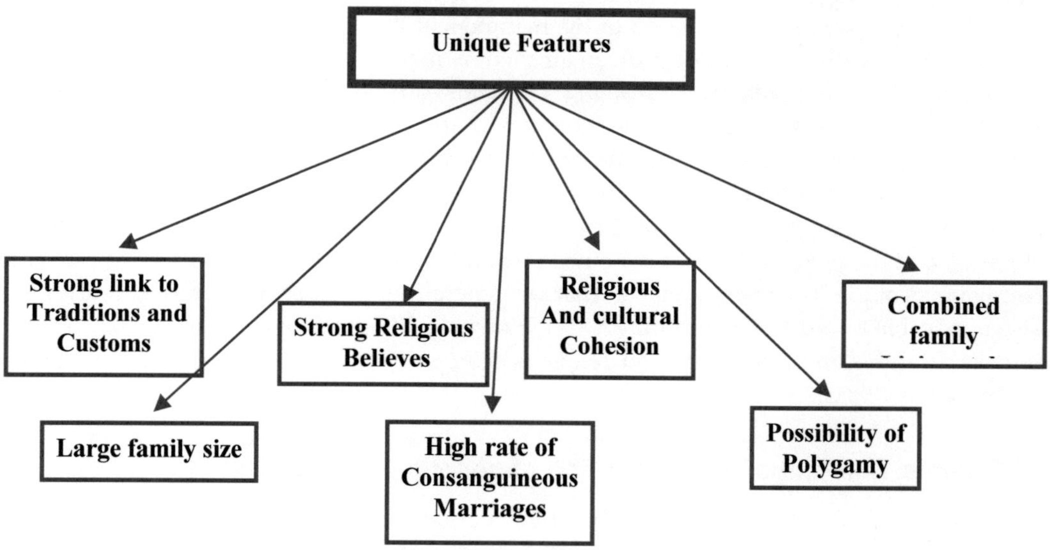

Fig. 2. Arabic/Islamic Communities - Pattern of life

In Islamic Teachings, preservation of the five necessities, "Magasid Al-Sharea'h" represents the respect for human being and human life[20]. The five necessities are:

1. Maintenance of religion (A-ddeen) ; including the five Pillars of Islam.
2. Maintenance of self (Al-nafs) ; including Human Dignity Prohibition of abortion and fetus rights to survive Prohibition of Killing and suicidal.
3. Maintenance of brain - intellect (Al-aql) ; including education freedom of intellect and research.
4. Preservation of Progeny (Al-nasl) ; including encourage of marriage and prohibition of adultery.
5. Preservation of wealth and honor (A-tharwal wa , Al-erdh) ; including freedom of commerce and offering of Alms "A-Zakat " to the needy.

In addition, varieties of costumes and traditions that, over the years, became part of the Islamic community practices and any instruction contrary to them looked at with suspicion.

3. Genetic screening and counseling as means of prevention of genetics diseases

The genetic disorders can give rise to chronic diseases that currently have no or limited definite cure. Preventive measures of genetic diseases, particularly at an earlier stage, proved to be of practical value. The main pillars of prevention are genetic screening and supportive counseling. Genetic screening or testing can be carried out at different stages, as follows[25 - 27]:

- Age of puberty
- School age
- Post-natal screening
- Screening during pregnancy
- Pre - implantation Genetic Screening - before implementation and after *in vitro fertilization* (IVF).

Genetic counseling is considered an important complementary approach to the screening procedure. As a service, it is offered to the members of the high risk groups, i.e. carriers of recessive genetic disease or those with an affected member of the family. [25 - 36]

As a profession, the genetic counseling demands certain ethical frameworks that are required by the very nature of the function of the counselor. Being considerate and compassionate should complement the counsellor and colour the communication with the client. The counseling process should be nondirective, where the decision-making should lie in the hands of the person concerned, but to be based on full understanding of the genetic situation and the pros and cons of the outcome of the probable condition. The principles and components of the "Informed Consent" that are generally acceptable in western countries are also applicable to Muslim community [28 - 44]. However, Muslims, in general, will often want to consult with family members and religious scholars, particularly in aspects of religious and social relevance.

4. "Islamic Teachings" on prevention of genetic disorders

Ethics in medical practices, within the framework of Islamic teaching, emphasizes the importance of educating the people and raising their awareness of the pattern of inheritance, its implications and the available means of prevention and care. On prevention side, pre-marital screening seems to be the preferable means of choice and appropriate counseling that takes into account the religious beliefs and prevailing traditions can be effective. These practices are carried out in a number of Islamic Countries and considered the method of choice in prevention of Single Gene Disorders. Similarly, neo-natal testing, avoiding of terratogenes and provision of folate and iodine in the diet is encouraged as supportive measures. On the care side, drug treatment, supportive care, Stem cell and gene therapy are welcomed.

Islam pays special attention to the reproduction of mankind and the maintenance of human race on earth. One of the necessaties in the Magasid Al Sharea'h is that progeny is to be protected throughout life, namely pre-marital, pre-conception, pre-natal, natal and post-natal stages. At pre-marital stage, selection of the parent (man/women) includes that the parent should be healthy, and perform a good deeds. At pre-conception stage, Islam prohibits any attempt to tamper with the productive process. At natal stage, Islam prohibits abortion after the fourth months of pregnancy, i.e. after the Spirit is blown into the foetus.

Thereafter, the parents should appropriately care for the newborn including advocacy for breastfeeding until two years of age. The parents looking after the children should include observing their rights of having a decent, peaceful and worthy life.

5. Directions regarding abortion of the genetically affected foetus

"The Fatwa" number 4 of "The Islamic Jurisprudence Council of Islamic World league of the Organization of Islamic Countries", at its 12th session,[47] allows for the option of abortion under certain specific conditions. The fatwa determined that the abortion may take place only if a committee of specialized, competent physicians has decided the foetus is grossly malformed, and that its life would be a calamity for both the family and itself. The malformation must be untreatable, unmanageable and very serious, and the abortion may only be carried out prior to the 120th day of conception (computed from the date of fertilization, not the last menstrual cycle). Beyond 120 days, i.e. after the sprit blown into the fetus, abortion only is allowed if there is a danger threatening the mothers' health.

6. The "Sharea'h" views toward human genetic research outcome and use

In Islamic communities, genomics research and the applications of its outcome into medical practices, are conducted within the context of culture and religion framework. In this respect, 'The Islamic jurisprudence Councils in Islamic Countries' paralleled the scientific advancements in looking into the usefulness of the genetic research outcome to human kind. "The Islamic Jurisprudence (Figh) Council of the Islamic World League of the Organization of Islamic Countries" in Makkah Al-Mukarama and The High Council of Al-Ulama" of Saudi Arabia, as well as similar bodies in other Islamic Countries, as the need rises, discuss and pass guidelines and "Fatwas" of the Learned, an authoritative ruling, on subjects of general concern to Islamic communities. The decision making leading to the Fatwas and the guidelines, are based on information provided by professionals and experts in the relevant field under discussion.

7. Guidelines on the use of genetic information and technologies in the management of genetic diseases

"The Islamic Jurisprudence Council of the Islamic World League of the Organization of Islamic Countries", in its 15th session gave the following guidance on the use of the genetic information and research technology [45]:

1. allow the use of genetic engineering for disease prevention, treatment, or amelioration on the condition that do not cause further damage;
2. forbid the use of engineering in evil and criminal use or what is forbidden religiously;
3. forbid using genetic engineering and its tool to change human personality and responsibility, or interfering with genes to improve the human race;
4. forbid any research or therapy of human genes except in extreme need, after critical evaluation of its benefits and dangers and after an official consent of the concerned, respecting the extreme confidentiality of the information and human rights and dignity as dictated by Islamic Sharea'h;
5. allow the use of bio-engineering in the field of agriculture and animals, on the condition that precautions are taken not to inflict harm (even in the long term) on humans, animals or vegetation;

6. call on biotechnology companies and food and medical factories to reveal the structure of these bioengineered products so they can be dealt with and used with caution in light of potential harm or if any are forbidden religiously;
7. recommend all doctors, factory and laboratory owners to fear Allah (GOD) and to watch out for Allah to avoid inflicting harm to humans, society or the environment

8. DNA fingerprinting and its use

On DNA fingerprinting, "The Islamic Jurisprudence Council of Islamic World league of the Organization of Islamic Countries", in its 16th session, issued the following guidance:[46]

1. It is religiously allowed to use DNA fingerprinting in forensic interrogations to prove crime which has no definite penalty in Islamic law (Share'ah) (Avoid punishment if there is any doubt, as doubt should always be used for the sake of the accused), this will lead to justice and to safety of the community, as the criminal will be punished and the innocent will be freed from guilt, which is one of the most important goals of Share'ah.
2. DNA fingerprinting may be used in lineage (genealogy) only with great caution and confidentiality as the Share'ah rules take precedence over DNA fingerprinting.
3. It is forbidden to use DNA fingerprinting in paternity (lineage) disputes, which should not precede the oath of condemnation (the sworn allegation of adultery committed by one's spouse).
4. It is forbidden to use DNA fingerprinting to confirm or refute legally proven lineage; the state should forbid this and inflict punishment, in order to protect people's honor and to preserve their lineage.
5. It is allowed to use DNA fingerprinting in proving lineage on the following conditions;
   - in case of a dispute about unknown lineage, as mentioned by the Islamic scholars because the evidence is either absent or equivocal, and to overcome (inundate) the vagueness (suspicion).
   - in case of a dispute over babies in hospitals and nurseries or test tube babies;
   - in case of children lost because of war, accidents or natural disasters, where there family could not be found;
   - to identify babies or prisoners of war.
6. The human genome of an individual, nation or race should not be sold for any reason; neither should it be given because of the harm it can cause. The counsel recommends that:
   i. the state to forbid DNA fingerprinting testing except on judge's orders and performed in the state laboratories; the private sector should be forbidden from doing such tests because of the great danger and harm.
   ii. each state should have a committee on DNA fingerprinting tests which should include legal scholars, physicians and administrators to supervise and approve the result of such tests.
   iii. there should be a precise mechanism to prevent deceit, cheating, contamination or human error in such laboratories, so the results are compatible with reality. The accuracy of these laboratories needs to be confirmed.
   iv. the number of genes used for a test should be sufficient, in the opinion of specialists, to overcome any doubts about the accuracy of the results.

9. Cloning and stem cell research

"The Islamic Jurisprudence Council of Islamic World League of the Organization of Islamic Countries", in its 10th session,[48] explored all the research papers and recommendations of the 9th Medical and Fiqh Seminar held by the Islamic Medical Organization during 14-17 June 1987 and agreed on the Decree no. 2/100D 10, which states that:

1. Human Cloning is forbidden in these two (or any other) methods that lead to human reproduction.
2. If the first legal rule is overstepped, the consequences should follow the legal rulings.
3. It is forbidden in all cases to introduce a third party into marriage, i.e an egg donor, a surrogate womb, a sperm donor, or a cloned cell.
4. It is permissible to use genetic engineering and cloning in the fields of germs, microorganisms, plants, and animals following legitimate rules which lead to benefits and prevent harm.
5. All Muslim countries are called upon to formulate the necessary legislation to prevent foreign research institutes, organizations and experts from directly or indirectly using Muslim countries for experimentations on human cloning or promoting it.
6. The Islamic Organization for Medical Sciences and other similar bodies are called upon to monitor all scientific developments in the field of cloning and define its terminology and organize seminars and meetings, as required, to determine and articulate the Islamic rulings and principles pertaining thereto.
7. Specialized committees should be set up to look into the ethics of biological research and adopt protocols for study and research in Muslim countries.
8. Biological and bioengineering research institutions (other than cloning research) should be supported and established, according to the Islamic rulings, so that Muslim world will not be dependent on others in this field.

"The communication media are called upon to deal with recent scientific advances from an Islamic perspective in a faithful way and avoid employing their services against Islam, aiming to educate the public to be confident before any decision. According to God saying (When there comes to them some matter touching (Public) safety or fear, they divulge it. If they had only referred it to the Messenger, or to those charged with authority among them, the proper investigations would have tested it from them (direct). Were it not for the Grace and Mercy of Allah unto you, all but a few of you would have fallen into the clutches of Satan (The Holy Qura'n, Sorat Al Nesae, Ayat 83)".

After listening to the research papers and the opinion of the Council members and the experts with relevant knowledge, the Council made the following decree:

FIRST: It is permissible to obtain stem cells, to be grown and used for therapy or for permissible scientific research, if its course is legitimate, as for example:

1. adults if they give permission, without inflicting harm on them.
2. children provided that their guardians allow it, for a legal benefit and without inflicting harm on the children.
3. the placenta or umbilical cord, with the permission of parents.
4. a fetus is spontaneously aborted or when aborted for a therapeutic reason permitted by Shareah, with parents' permission. (Be reminded of decree No. 7 of the counsel in its 12th session about abortion).
5. left over zygotes remaining from in vitro fertilization, if donated by the parents, when it is ascertained that they will not be used in an illegal pregnancy.

SECOND: It is forbidden to use stem cells, if their source is illegal. As for example:
1. intentionally aborted fetuses (that is, abortion without a legal medical reason).
2. intentional fertilization between a donated ovum and sperm.
3. therapeutic human cloning".

10. Conclusions

Islamic teachings in all aspects of life are drown from the Holy Book of all Muslims (The Qura'n), the Prophet (PBUH) speech (The Hadeeths), then Consensus *(Al ijma)* and Analogy *(Al Qiyas)*, resulting in "Islamic Jurisprudence". Where appropriate, consideration is also given to public interest " *Maslaha*" through the decision of the Learned, i.e. the "Fatwa", and local customary precedent, i.e. "The *urf* " [49].
Bio- and medical ethics are extension of Sharea'h, where decision-making observe Magasid Al-Isalm, that emphasizes the need for preservation of the components of human being and the patterns of human life. In these principles, Islam shares many foundational values with the other Abrahamic" religions, Judaism and Christianity, where similar teachings are given [50-54]. Of relevance are these religions teachings regarding the restriction on abortion and the wrights of the foetus. Like other religions, Islam has diverse sects and, therefore, diversity of views in bioethical matters does exist. However, there is little that is controversial, concerning pre-natal diagnosis and abortion of the malformed or genetically disordered foetus. The Islamic Teachings in medical practices, particularly those related to genetic services as outlined in this article, are not meant to be exclusive, where there may be different opinions based on other "Fatwas", or sources related to other Islamic sects. It is hoped that the insights gained from this presentation will aid clinicians and other health care workers providing genetics services to better serve their Moslem patients, their families and the whole community and deliver care that pays due respect to their beliefs, customs and prevailing traditions.

11. References

[1] Bill J. Muslims everywhere yet still in chains. *Mahajuba* 1994; 13:5-6

[2] Hedayat K, Pirzadeh R. Issues in Islamic Biomedical ethics: A Primer for Pediatrician. *Pediatrics* 2001;108:965-71

[3] El-Hazmi MAF. Ethics of genetic counseling in Islamic Communities (in Arabic) Al-Obeikan Bookstore, Riyadh, 2002

[4] Rehman F. Legacy and prospects. Islam. 2nd ed. Chicago: University of Chicago Press; 1979:235-54.

[5] Rispler-Chaim. V Islamic medical ethics in 20th century: *J Med Ethics* 1989;15:203-208

[6] Von Bommel. A Medical ethics from the Muslim perspective: *Acta Neurochir* 1999;17-27

[7] Paladin A.V Ethics and neurology in the Islamic World: Ital *J Neurol Sci* 1998;19:255-258.

[8] El-Hashemite N. The Islamic view in genetic preventing procedures: *The Lancet* 1997;350:223

[9] http://www.islamset.com/bioethics/genetics/index.html

[10] World Health Organization. Proposed International Guidelines in Ethical Issues in Medical Genetics and Genetic Services: *WHO/HGN/GL/ETH*/98;1:1997.

[11] World Health Organization. Services for the prevention and management of genetic disorders and birth defects in developing countries:

WHO/HGN/GL/WAOPBD/99;1:1999
[12] The first Regional Workshop on Ethical issues in genetic counseling. College of Medicine, King Saud University; Riyadh. Saudi Arabia 1999.
[13] Unesco Universal Declaration on Bioethics and Human Rights, 19 Oct.,2005
[14] Genomics and World Health. Report of the Advisory Committee on health research. Geneva, Switzerland: World Health Organization; 2002
[15] Weijer C, Dickens D, Meslin Eric. Bioethics for clinicians: 10. Research ethics. *Can Med Assoc J* 1997;156:1153-7.
[16] Daar AS, Al Khitamy AB. Bioethics for clinicians: 21. Islamic Bioethics. *Can Med Assoc J* 2001;164:60-63
[17] Michael M. Burgess, Claude M. Laberge, Bartha Maria Knoppers. Bioethics for clinicians: 14. Ethics and genetics in medicine *CMAJ* 1998;158:1309-13.
[18] Etchells E, Sharpe G, Burgees MM, Singer PA. Bioethics clinicians: Disclosure. *CMAJ* 1996;155:387-91.
[19] G.I. Seroura,b, B.M. Dickens. Ethical and legal issues in reproductive health. Assisted reproduction developments in the Islamic World: *International Journal of Gynecology & Obstetrics* 2001; 74: 187-193.
[20] Grated AR, Sheikh A. Medical ethics and Islam: principles and practice. *Arch Dis Child* 2001; 84:72-75.
[21] Kamali MH. Urf (custom). In: Principles of Islamic Jurisprudence. Cambridge: *Islamic Text Society*; 1991;283-96
[22] AlAjlooni IM: Kashef Al Khafa'a wa Muzeel Al Ilbas, *Mu'ssast Al Risala* H, Beirut, 1983, 2:491, Hadith No 3075 (Available only in Arabic).
[23] Albar M.A. Ethical considerations in prevention of management of genetic disorders with special emphasis on religious considerations: *Saudi Medical Journal* 2002;23:627-32.
[24] Bacaille M. Human reproduction. In: The Bible, the Qur'an and science. Indianapolis: *North American Trust Publications*; 1979:198-210.
[25] Model B, Darr A. Genetic counseling and customary consanguineous marriage. *Nature Review/Genetics* 2002; 3:225-29.
[26] Scriver CR. Genetic screening, testing and treatment: how far can we go? *J Inher Metab Pis* 1996; 19:401-11.
[27] Sermon K, Andre Van Steirteghem, Inge Liebaers. Preimplantation genetic diagnosis (Review).*The Lancet* 2004; 363:1633-41.
[28] Donnai D. Genetic Services. *Clinical genetics*.2002; 61:1-6
[29] El-Hazmi MAF. Genetic counseling theory and practice. In: Proceedings of the Symposium on Medical Genetics in the setting of the Middle Eastern Population. KACST Press, Riyadh; 1995 , 243-248
[30] El-Hazmi, M.A.F.Ethics of Medical Practice and Genetic counselling in Islamic Communities. *Saudi Medical Journal* 2002; 23: 233-47.
[31] M.A. Albar. Counselling about genetic diseases: an Islamic perspective. *Easter Med Health J* 1999; 5:1129-33
[32] El-Hazmi, M.A.F.Ethics of genetic counselling – basic concepts and relevance to Islamic communities, *Annals of Saudi Med. Journal* 2004.
[33] El-Hazmi,M.A.F. Pre-marital screening for prevention from genetic diseases – scientific background and objectives (in Arabic), Dar Al-Oloum Bookstore ,Riyadh, 2005

[34] El-Hazmi,M.A.F. Genetic diseases in Arab populations. East Mediterr. Health J.,1999;5(6): 1102-13
[35] Hussain FA. Reproductive issues from the Islamic Prespective. *Hum Fertil (Camb)*.2003;3:124-28
[36] Salih HM. Genetic counseling among Muslims: questions remain unanswered. *The Lancet* 2004;364:209-14.
[37] Jackie Leach Scully, Christine Rippberger and Christoph Rehmann-Sutter. Non-professionals' evaluations of gene therapy ethics .*Social Science & medicine* 2004; 58:1415-25.
[38] Marshal E. Clinical promise, ethical quandary. *Science* 1996; 271: 586-88.
[39] Carol A Tauer. International policy failures: cloning and stem-cell research. *The Lancet* 2004; 364:209-14.
[40] Wakayama T, On the road to therapeutic cloning. *Nat Biotechnol*2004; 22: 399--400.
[41] Strong C. Fetal anomalies: ethical and legal considerations in screening, detection, and management. *Clin Perinatol*. 2003 ; 30: 113-26.
[42] T.Smith. *Ethics in medical research. A handbook of good practice,* Cambridge University Press, Cambridge 1999.
[43] Robertson J. Extending pre implantation genetic diagnosis: the ethical debate-ethical issues in new uses of preimplantation genetic diagnosis. *Hum Reprod* 2003; 18: 465-71.
[44] Pennings G, Schots R, Liebaers. Ethical considerations on preimplantation genetic diagnosis for HLA typing to match a future child as a donor of hematopoietic stem cells to a sibling. *Hum Reprod* 2002; 17: 534-38.
[45] The Islamic Jurisprudence Council of the Islamic World League of the Organization of Islamic Countries, in its 15th session, 1998
[46] The Islamic Jurisprudence Council of the Islamic World League of the Organization of Islamic Countries, 16th session 2002.
[47] The Islamic Jurisprudence Council of the Islamic World League of the Organization of Islamic Countries, 12th session 1990.
[48] The Islamic Jurisprudence Counsel of the Islamic World League of the Organization of Islamic Countries), 10th session 1987.
[49] Kamali MH. Urf (custom). In: *Principles of Islamic jurisprudence*. Cambridge: Islamic Texts Society; 1991. p. 283-96.
[50] Daar AS. Xenotransplantation and the major monotheistic religions. *Xeno* 1994;2(4):61-4.
[51] Daar AS: A survey of religious attitudes towards donation and transplantation. In: Collins GM, Dubernard JM, Land W, Persijn GG, editors. *Procurement and preservation and allocation of vascularized organs*. Dordecht: Kluwer Academic Publishers; 1997. p. 333-8.
[52] Hathout H. Why an Islamic perspective? In: El-Gindy AR, editor. *Health policy, ethics and human values: Islamic perspective*. Kuwait: Islamic Organization of Medical Sciences; 1995. p. 81-5.
[53] *Qur'an*. Sorat Al-Toor, Ayat 21
[54] *Qur'an*. Sorat Al-Nisae, Ayat 85 and 86.